TESTICULAR TUMORS

Second Edition

Edited by

Douglas E. Johnson, M.D.

Professor (Urology) and

Chief, Section of Urology

The University of Texas System Cancer Center,

M.D. Anderson Hospital

and Tumor Institute,

Houston, Texas

MEDICAL EXAMINATION PUBLISHING COMPANY, INC.

65-36 Fresh Meadow Lane

Flushing, N.Y. 11365

Library of Congress Card Number
75-8134

ISBN 0-87488-743-7

November, 1976

Printed in the United States of America

SIMULTANEOUSLY PUBLISHED:

IN GREAT BRITAIN: LONDON
H. K. LEWIS & Co. Ltd.
1976

IN BRAZIL: GUANABARA KOOGAN
1976

IN SINGAPORE: TOPPAN COMPANY (S) Pte. Ltd.
NO.38, LIU FANG ROAD, JURONG TOWN
SINGAPORE-22, SINGAPORE
1976
TOPPAN PUBLISHING

IN INDIA: SCIENTIFIC BOOK AGENCY
22 Raja Woodmunt Street
Calcutta, India
1976

PREFACE

Testicular tumors rank second only to reticulo-endothelial neoplasms as a cause of death from cancer in young men. The tragic loss of these lives during early adulthood is all too frequently the result of a delay in diagnosis. Fear, as well as ignorance on the part of the patient contribute to his procrastination in seeking medical attention. The physician in evaluating the patient is often misled by the symptomatology and clinical findings with an initial error in diagnosis made in one-fourth to one-half of the cases. Once a correct diagnosis is established, the physician is confronted with the dilemma of recommending the most appropriate therapy for the individual patient.

Proper selection of therapy requires free communication and close co-operation among multiple disciplines — pathology, radiology, radiotherapy and chemotherapy. Without the combined skills, experience and knowledge of the various specialists, the patient is deprived of the benefits of modern medicine.

This monograph is an attempt to collect, review and discuss the diagnosis and treatment of patients with testicular tumors. It represents not the work of any single individual, but is the product of innumerable contributions made by investigators in the past and those pursuing the studies in the present. It is intended for the urologists, general surgeons, radiologists and radiotherapists, who frequently deal with the disease, as well as the general practitioners, internists and pediatricians to whom the responsibility for the diagnosis is often entrusted. If this monograph, in some small way, provides help to a physician in the management of a patient with testicular malignant disease, it will have served its purpose.

ACKNOWLEDGMENTS

I would like to express my deep appreciation to the publishers who are responsible for the conception of this monograph and to my contributors who assured its completion. Considerable credit must be given to Mr. Gero Van Le Fort of the Art Unit and Mr. Donald Kelly of the Photographic Service of the Medical Communications Department for the illustrative material. I am indebted to Mrs. Betty Shields and Mrs. Mary Lou Rogge for their generous secretarial help. Lastly, I am forever grateful to my wife and sons who have given so much of their time in order that I might complete this small endeavor.

CONTRIBUTING AUTHORS

The University of Texas System Cancer Center
M.D. Anderson Hospital and Tumor Institute
of Houston

AYALA, ALBERTO G., B.A., M.D.
Associate Pathologist, Section of Anatomical Pathology,
Department of Pathology and *Associate Professor of Pathology.*

BUTLER, JAMES J., M.D.
Pathologist, Section of Anatomical Pathology,
Department of Pathology and *Associate Professor of Pathology.*

DAVIS, WILLIAM D., M.D.
Faculty Associate (Urology), Section of Urology,
Department of Surgery.

DOORNBOS, JOHN F., M.D.
Fellow, Department of Radiotherapy.

GALLAGER, H. STEPHEN, A.B., M.D.
Pathologist, Section of Anatomical Pathology,
Department of Pathology and *Professor of Pathology.*

GUINN, GENE A., M.D.
Assistant Professor of Surgery at Baylor Medical School,
Assistant Chief of the Surgical Service at the Veterans Administration
Hospital, and *Chief,* Thoracic and Cardiovascular Surgery,
Veterans Administration Hospital, Houston, Texas.

HOGAN, JOHN M., M.D.
Resident in Urology, Section of Urology, Department of Surgery.

HUSSEY, DAVID H., M.D.
Associate Radiotherapist, Department of Radiotherapy and
Associate Professor of Radiotherapy.

JING, BAO-SHAN, M.D.
Radiologist, Section of Clinical Diagnostic Radiology,
Department of Diagnostic Radiology and *Professor of Radiology.*

JOHNSON, DOUGLAS E., B.A., M.D.
Surgeon (Urology), Chief, Section of Urology,
Department of Surgery and *Professor of Urology.*

LUNA, MARIO A., M.D.
Associate Pathologist, Section of Anatomical Pathology, Department of Pathology and *Associate Professor of Pathology.*

SAMUELS, MELVIN L., M.D.
Internist, Chief, Section of General Medicine and Clinical Oncology and *Professor of Medicine.*

WALLACE, SIDNEY, B.A., M.D.
Radiologist, Chief, Section of Clinical Diagnostic Radiology, Department of Diagnostic Radiology and *Professor of Radiology.*

TESTICULAR TUMORS
Second Edition

TABLE OF CONTENTS

CHAPTER 1

PATHOLOGY OF TESTICULAR AND PARATESTICULAR NEOPLASMS

by

H. Stephen Gallager

In the medical literature of recent years, testicular neoplasms are accorded an amount of scientific attention quite disproportionate to their low incidence. There is some justification for this. Tumors of the testis represent only about one per cent of all malignant disease in men, but their peak incidence falls in the third, fourth and fifth decades, man's most productive years. In this age range, they constitute a leading neoplastic cause of death, second in frequency only to the neoplasms of the reticuloendothelial system.

For pathologists, the extreme variability of the testicular germinomas pose both a challenge and a problem. The publications of Friedman and Moore (1946) and Dixon and Moore (1952), based upon their monumental study of material accumulated from Armed Forces personnel during World War II, have done much to clarify the biology of these tumors and to establish a basis for logical understanding and sound diagnosis. Individual neoplasms, however, continue to present conceptual problems. The surgical pathologist's anxiety is accentuated by the knowledge that accurate histologic interpretation is a major determinant of treatment and prognosis. With few notable exceptions, recent publications have tended to de-emphasize practical considerations of histologic diagnosis in favor of more esoteric matters. Lengthy speculation on questions of histogenesis is, while fascinating, less than helpful to the pathologist whose primary concern is the care of the patient.

It has often been pointed out (Teilum 1959) that there is a homology between the neoplasms of testis and those of ovary. This is true for the germinal neoplasms, duplicates of which occur in both male and female gonads, although applicable terminology differs. Tumors of Müllerian derivation, however, which make up some 75 per cent of the primary neoplasms of the ovary, are all but unknown in the testis. While it is correct to say histologically similar tumors occur in both ovary and testis, it must be added that the distribution of various types of neoplasms is widely dissimilar in the two organs.

It will be the intent of this presentation to provide a clinically oriented overview of the pathology of primary neoplasms of the testicle. Pathologic criteria for diagnosis will be described and related to pertinent clinical features and biologic behavior. Histogenetic considerations will be avoided not because they are uninteresting, but because they contribute little to solving the problems of diagnosis and management which are our primary concern.

CLASSIFICATION

The classification of intrascrotal neoplasms in use at The University of Texas System Cancer Center, M. D. Anderson Hospital and Tumor Institute (Table I) is based upon that of Dixon and Moore and is quite similar to the classification employed at the Armed Forces Institute of Pathology (Sulak 1970). Tumors of the testis fall readily into two large groups: those which are derived from germinal epithelium, and those which are of gonadal stromal origin. As a rule of thumb, tumors of the first group are almost universally malignant, while the stromal tumors are usually benign. In accord with the clinical approach adopted for this chapter, a category of intrascrotal neoplasms not testicular in origin has been included. These require, at least during clinical examination, differentiation from testicular neoplasms.

The British scheme of classification for germinal tumors, proposed by Collins and Pugh in 1964 (Table II) indicates a slightly different set of concepts of histogenesis and narrows somewhat the histologic definitions of several entities. This categorization has not received widespread acceptance in the United States. It is presented here for comparison and for clarification of the terminology used in the two tabulations.

GERMINAL TUMORS

Tumors of germinal origin comprise about 90 per cent of all neoplasms of the testis. They occur slightly more frequently on the right than on the left and are bilateral in only one to two per cent of patients (Johnson and Morneau 1974). The incidence of these neoplasms in Negroes is significantly lower than in Caucasians; germinal tumors in Negroes are distinct rarities. The incidence in Asiatics and North Africans is about one-third of that reported in Europeans. Tumors of this group occur over a wide range of ages and have been reported from infancy to senility. The peak incidence is between 20 and 40 years of age.

Cryptorchidism is a significant factor in the etiology of germinal neoplasms. Twenty per cent of such tumors occur in patients with cryptorchidism and some twenty per cent of these arise in the descended testicle. These facts suggest that there is a basic defect in gonadogenesis which is responsible for both lack of descent and for a predilection to tumor development. The frequency of tumor development in undescended testes is not affected by orchiopexy done after early childhood. In adolescents and older patients presenting with cryptorchidism, orchiectomy should be considered in preference to orchiopexy (Johnson et al. 1968).

The occurrence of extratesticular germinomas without evident testicular primaries has given rise to the impression that spontaneous regression is a common phenomenon in these tumors. Experience fails to support this contention. There are three possible explanations for the occurrence of germinal tumors in non-gonadal tissues. First of all, and perhaps most common, is the situation in which there are massive metastases from a small, nonpalpable intratesticular tumor (Meares and Briggs 1972). Not infrequently, the presenting symptom of a germinal neoplasm is the presence of an abdominal mass due to retroperitoneal lymph node metastases. Second, it is reasonably well established that embryologically displaced germ cells may occur in a variety of extragonadal locations, particularly the mediastinum, and serve as sources for the development of germinal tumors. The third possible explanation is the only one which involves the phenomenon of spontaneous regression of a testicular primary. Occasional reports have called attention to the presence of fibrous scars in testes in the presence of extragonadal

TABLE I: CLASSIFICATION

NEOPLASMS OF THE TESTIS AND RELATED STRUCTURES

(The University of Texas System Cancer Center,
M. D. Anderson Hospital, 1975)

- I. Neoplasms of testis proper
  - A. Germinal tumors
    - 1. Seminoma, pure
      - a. Classic type
      - b. Anaplastic type
      - c. Spermatocytic type
    - 2. Embryonal carcinoma, pure, or with seminoma
      - a. Juvenile variant
    - 3. Teratoma, pure, or with seminoma
      - a. Mature
      - b. Immature
    - 4. Teratoma with embryonal carcinoma or choriocarcinoma or both, with or without seminoma
    - 5. Choriocarcinoma, pure, or with embryonal carcinoma or seminoma or both
  - B. Gonadal stromal tumors
    - 1. Interstitial cell tumor
    - 2. Tumor of specialized gonadal stroma
      - a. Androblastoma
      - b. Sertoli cell tumor
      - c. Granulosa cell tumor
  - C. Secondary neoplasms
    - 1. Reticuloendothelial neoplasms
      - a. Malignant lymphoma, various types
    - 2. Metastatic neoplasms
      - a. Adenocarcinoma of prostate
      - b. Malignant melanoma
      - c. Bronchogenic carcinoma
      - d. Other

- II. Neoplasms of related structures
  - A. Connective tissue neoplasms
    - 1. Paratesticular rhabdomyosarcoma
    - 2. Nonspecific connective tissue neoplasms
  - B. Other neoplasms
    - 1. Adenomatoid tumor of epididymis
    - 2. Papillary cystadenoma of epididymis
    - 3. Mesothelioma of tunica vaginalis testis

TABLE II

CLASSIFICATION OF TUMOURS OF TESTIS, EPIDIDYMIS AND RELATED STRUCTURES

(Collins and Pugh 1964)

Tumours of testis

- Seminoma
- Teratoma
  - Teratoma differentiated (T. D.)
  - Malignant teratoma intermediate (M. T. I.)
    - with differentiated or organoid components (M. T. I. A.)
    - without differentiated or organoid components (M. T. I. B.)
  - Malignant teratoma anaplastic (M. T. A.)
  - Malignant teratoma trophoblastic (M. T. T.)
- Combined tumour
- Sertoli cell tumour
- Interstitial cell tumour
- Orchioblastoma
- Malignant lymphoma
- Miscellaneous tumours
- Metastases
- Tumours of uncertain diagnosis

Tumours of epididymis and cord

- Adenomatoid tumour
- Tumours of connective tissue and muscle
  - Benign: Fibroma, leiomyoma, lipoma, etc.
  - Malignant: Embryonic sarcoma, rhabdomyosarcoma, fibrosarcoma, leiomyosarcoma, etc.
- Miscellaneous tumours
- Metastases
- Tumours of uncertain diagnosis

germinal neoplasms.

Such cases, however, are rarities and the regression phenomenon must be regarded as being distinctly uncommon (Johnson et al. 1973).

Macroscopic Appearances

There are no pathognomonic gross appearances among the germinal tumors. They range in size from a few millimeters in diameter to tumors weighing 1,000 grams and more. Seminomas tend to produce large masses while choriocarcinomas are often quite small at the time they are removed. For obvious reasons, those tumors which arise from intra-abdominal testes are among the largest to have been reported. Tumors which do not enlarge the testis are usually sharply circumscribed, but not encapsulted, and have smoothly rounded or bosselated margins. Larger tumors compress the surrounding testicular parenchyma and produce nodular bulges beneath the capsule, which may be focally thickened and present opaque white areas over the nodules. Blood vessels in the capsule may be increased in prominence. Seminomas are usually homogenous and vary from moderately firm to soft in consistency and from light gray to pale yellow-brown in color. Areas of necroses are common in the larger examples, and tend to be centrally located, bright yellow, amorphous and to have irregularly scalloped borders surrounded by narrow hemorrhagic bands. Spermatocytic seminomas characteristically have a slimy, mucoid cut surface appearance. Embryonal carcinomas tend to be firm and somewhat granular in their cut surface appearance. In both these and choriocarcinomas, hemorrhage is common in small masses. Teratomas, particularly those containing differentiated elements, are often multiply cystic and may have a sponge-like appearance in section. The cysts are filled either with pasty yellow-gray grumous material or with thick white mucoid fluid. Rarely in these tumors is it possible to see or palpate tiny spicules of bone or islands of cartilaginous material.

Tumors whose microscopic composition is significantly mixed, of course, partake of all of these characteristics. Large masses give the appearance of being composed of multiple nodules, sometimes confluent, sometimes entirely separate from one another. Associated nodules may be similar in appearance or may show widely differing structure. Frequently, hemorrhage and degeneration is much more pronounced in one mass than in another.

Processing the Orchiectomy Specimen

The accurate diagnosis of germinal tumors depends upon the preparation of histologic sections of high quality. For this reason it seems appropriate to discuss briefly some procedures which have been found to be effective in achieving satisfactory histologic results.

Since the cells of many germinal tumors are exceedingly fragile, it is important that specimens be processed promptly after surgical removal. The tunica albuginea is relatively impervious to aqueous fixatives, and an intact testis allowed to repose for many hours in formalin (particularly in an inadequate volume of formalin) is likely to undergo a degree of autolysis which may seriously impede histologic diagnosis. The pathologist should insist that the specimen be sent immediately to the laboratory without having been erratically incised by an over-anxious surgeon, and should begin the processing promptly.

The following procedure is routine at the University of Texas System Cancer Center, M. D. Anderson Hospital. The external aspect of the specimen is first examined and photographed. If a hydrocele is present, the reflected or scrotal portion of the

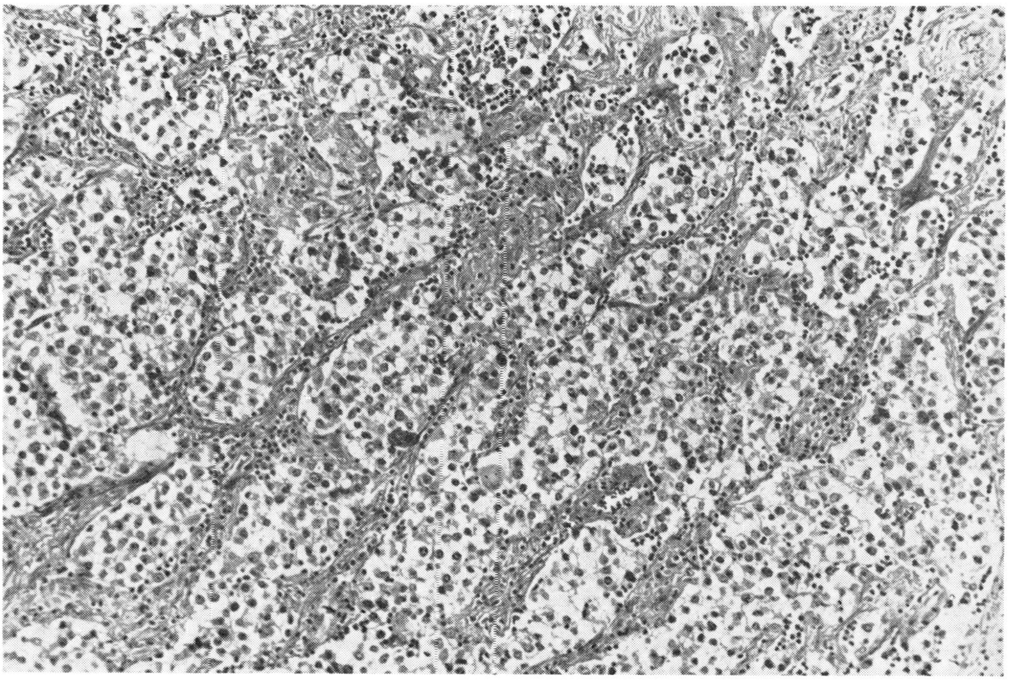

Fig. 1-1. Classical seminoma. The polyhedral cells with clear or granular cytoplasm, the clustered arrangement and the delicate, lymphocytic infiltrated stroma are typical. X 100.

sac is cut free leaving a narrow rim attached to the testis. The testis is sliced longitudinally through the entire structure, the plane of sectioning being placed in such a way as to pass through the mediastinum of the testis and the head of the epididymis. Parallel cuts are spaced not more than 3 mm apart. The slices are arrayed upon an appropriate transilluminated background and again photographed. The making of thin slices is facilitated by the use of a straight-bladed, very sharp knife such as the knife of a Stadie-Riggs slicer, or a large razor blade. If time permits, it is sometimes helpful to allow the specimen, wrapped in saline-moistened gauze, to chill at refrigerator temperature for a brief period.

Small tumors are serially embedded. An attempt is made to select blocks which will show the relationship of the tumor to the residual normal testicular tissue and to the epididymis. If the tumor is so large as to make serial blocking impractical, numerous blocks are taken in such a way as to represent all of the grossly differing kinds of tissue present. The spermatic cord is transversely sectioned at intervals of 3-5 mm. If no gross changes are present, a number of representative blocks are submitted. There should be not less than one block for every centimeter of the cord included with the specimen.

Formalin fixation, dehydration, infiltration and paraffin embedding follow in the usual way. Sections are cut at a thickness of 5 microns or less and stained with Harris hematoxylin and eosin. Special stains are only of occasional value and these being for the specific identification of differentiated elements in teratomas.

Microscopic Appearances

The tumorigenic versatility of germinal epithelium is reflected by the variety of histologic appearances which may occur in a neoplastic single mass, a prime source of confusion in microscopic interpretation. Much of the perplexity can be eliminated by recognizing that among germinal tumors there are four fairly discrete histologic patterns--seminoma, embryonal carcinoma, teratoma and choriocarcinoma. Any can occur in pure form or two or more types can be intermixed in any conceivable combination. Each basic pattern has a number of variants. It is convenient to describe the several histologic patterns individually.

Classical Seminoma: The cells of seminoma are fragile and exceedingly subject to artefactual distortion. When well preserved, they are polyhedral, have fine, definite cytoplasmic membranes, copious, finely granular or clear cytoplasm, centrally placed rounded nuclei with well dispersed chromatin and one or two nucleoli. They may be arranged in small clusters surrounded by delicate fibrillary connective tissue somewhat suggesting seminiferous tubules, or they may be arranged in broad sheets without detectable organization (Fig. 1-1). When the tissue is less than optimally preserved, there is a tendency for the cells to shrink and to assume a stellate outline. The cells tend to arrange themselves in rosette-like clusters and there is pyknosis and wrinkling of the nuclei.

The stroma associated with seminomas is variable in both quality and quantity. It may consist of only the slender fibers which separate cell clusters, or may form a dense, sclerotic, collagenous matrix, within which clusters of epithelial cells are embedded. Lymphocytic infiltration, a characteristic feature of seminoma, is also exceedingly variable, both from tumor to tumor and from place to place within the same tumor. In some tumors, lymphocytosis is so intense that a reticuloendothelial neoplasm is suggested, while in others only a sparse sprinkling of lymphocytes is present. Adequate sampling usually reveals at least some foci with moderate lymphocytic infiltration.

Secondary changes in seminomas are so common as to be almost diagnostic. One of these is the phenomenon of eosinophilic necrobiosis (Fig. 1-2). Large areas of the tumor become necrotic but the cells, while losing their internal structure, maintain their individual outlines. Necrobiotic areas are usually sharply circumscribed and are separated from viable tumor only by a narrow band of reactive connective tissue, often infiltrated with lymphocytes. A second phenomenon is the formation of granulomas. Small nodules of epithelioid cells with variable admixtures of lymphocytes, plasma cells and occasional Langhans' giant cells may be present and may, upon occasion, be exceedingly numerous (Fig. 1-3).

Anaplastic Seminoma: In this variant, the cells of the seminoma retain their regular arrangement and cytoplasmic characteristics but the nuclei are considerably more variable. They may be ballooned, with irregularly clumped chromatin and prominent nucleoli, or they may be small and hyperchromatic. Mitotic figures are frequent. Tumor giant cells which resemble trophoblastic giant cells are often found but other trophoblastic elements are never present. In other respects the structure is similar to that of classical seminoma (Fig. 1-5).

It is somewhat misleading to imply that anaplastic seminoma is a distinctive neoplasm, since it represents simply one extreme of the range of anaplasia which seminoma may exhibit. The grading of seminomas, however, is difficult and has not been shown to have prognostic significance. The anaplastic pattern may make up the entire mass of an individual tumor, or may be irregularly intermingled with areas showing the classical pattern.

Spermatocytic Seminoma: This rare tumor, which comprises four to eight per cent of all seminomas, is sufficiently different from classical seminoma, both in its histology and its clinical setting, that it may indeed represent, as Scully (1961) has suggested, a different tumor. While having a general similarity in microscopic appearance to classical seminoma, the cells of spermatocytic seminoma are more variable in size and their cytoplasm is more homogenous and stains a deeper color (Fig. 1-6). The nuclei are round with coarsely granular condensed chromatin resembling the nuclei of spermatogonia and spermatocytes. Mitotic figures are usually present, as are giant cells, and both may be numerous. The cells are almost always arranged in broad sheets without the intervening stromal characteristics of the classical pattern. Lymphocytic infiltration and granulomatous reaction are absent. Reported cases of spermatocytic seminoma have invariably been pure and this pattern has not been associated with either other patterns of seminoma or with other forms of germinal neoplasia. Over half of the reported patients have been over 50 years of age. Too little experience has accumulated thus far to justify any statement as to prognosis.

Embryonal Carcinoma: The range of variability within this pattern is very wide (Marin-Padilla 1968). It is characterized by having both epithelial and stromal components. The epithelium varies from low cuboidal to columnar and may be arranged in irregular glands, about small spaces, or in large sheets (Fig. 1-7). In the least differentiated areas, blood vessels are scanty and necrosis and hemorrhage are common. When glands are present they vary in shape and are lined by cuboidal or columnar cells with clear cytoplasm and hyperchromatic nuclei. Frequently, irregular papillary projections extend into the glands sometimes with the formation of the so-called extraembryonic yolk sac body (Pierce et al. 1970). Invari-

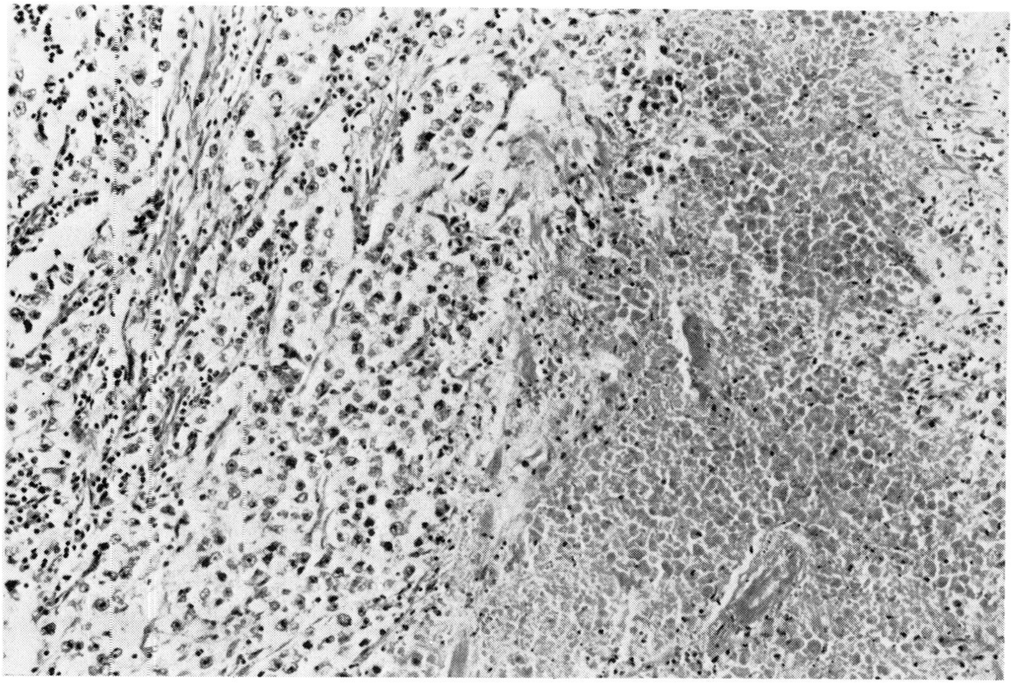

Fig. 1-2. Eosinophilic necrobiosis in seminoma. At the left half of this field, the neoplasm is well preserved. On the right, however, is a typical area of necrobiosis showing only cell outline but no nuclei or other internal cellular structures. X 120.

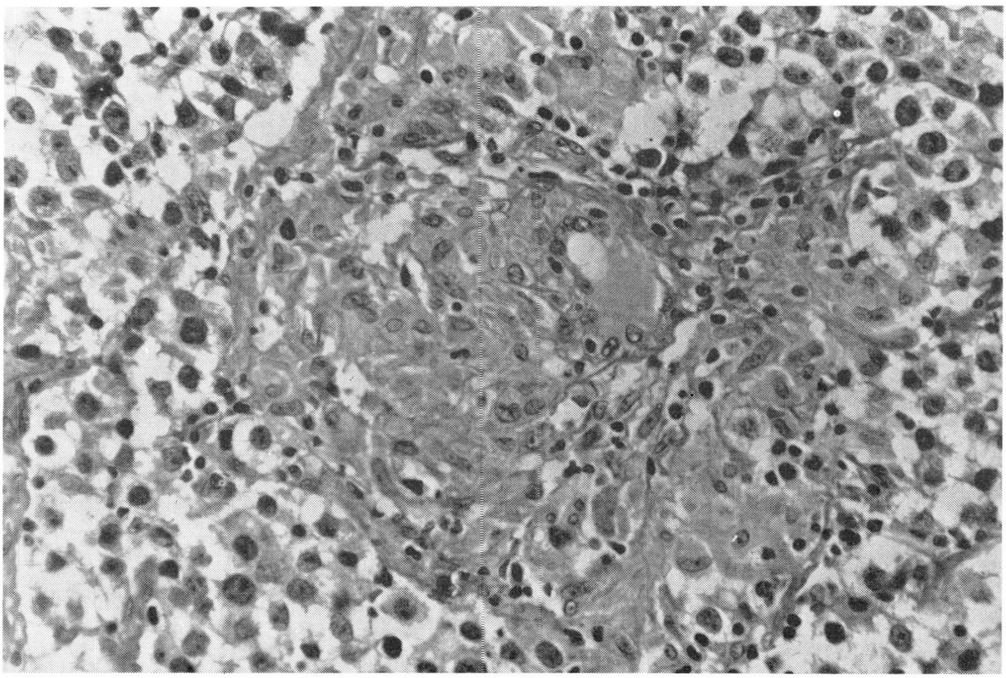

Fig. 1-3. A granulomatous nodule in seminoma. At the right of the nodule is a formative giant cell with cytoplasmic vacuolation. X 275.

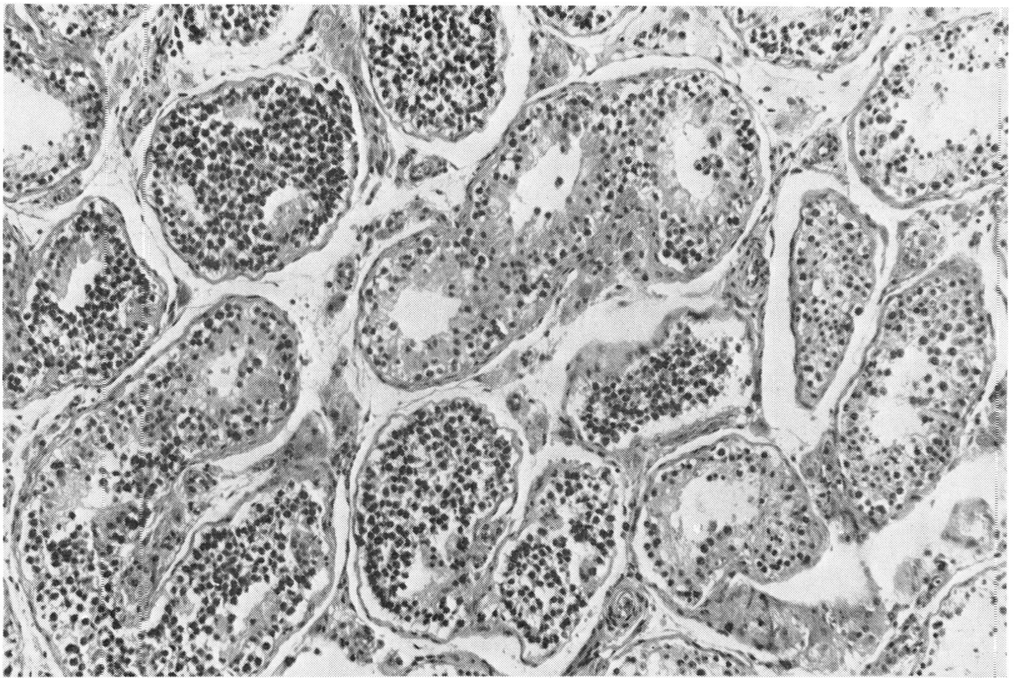

Fig. 1-4. Seminoma growing within seminiferous tubules at the margin of a mass. The presence of this phenomenon has been considered by some to indicate an unfavorable prognosis. X 90.

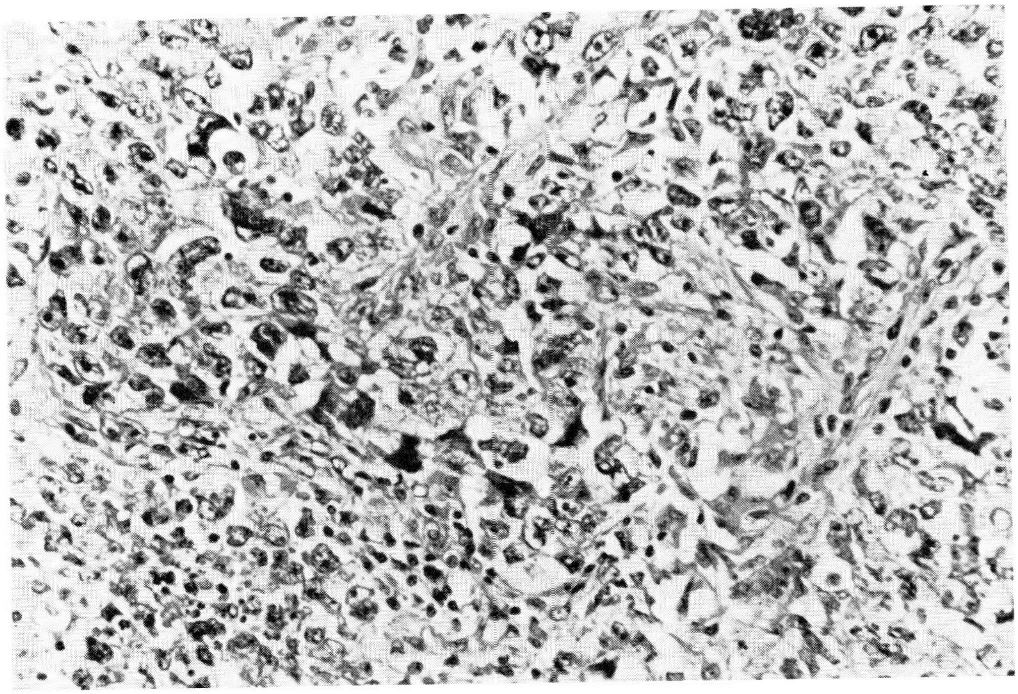

Fig. 1-5. Anaplastic seminoma. The nuclei are variable, often vesicular, and some mitoses are present. Several giant cells resembling syncytiotrophoblast are also present. X 250.

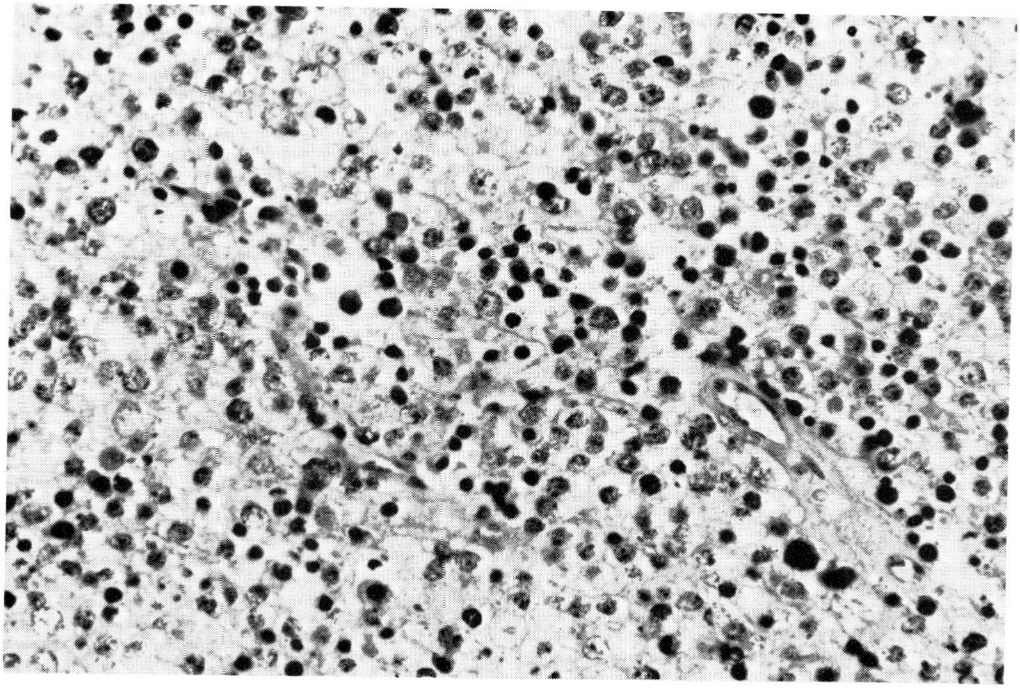

Fig. 1-6. Spermatocytic seminoma. The nuclei resemble those of spermatogonia and spermatocytes. X 250.

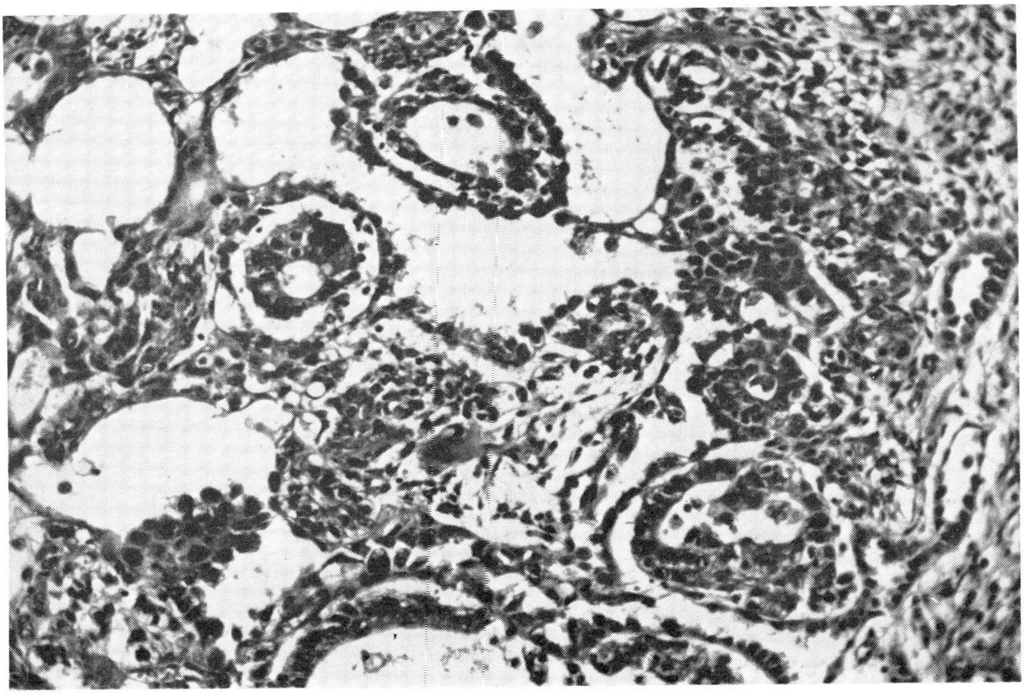

Fig. 1-7. Embryonal carcinoma.

ably associated with the protean epithelium is an equally primitive stroma. This is composed of small spindle cells with dark ovoid or irregular nuclei and scanty cytoplasm. The stroma may be compact or loosely arranged, or it may be reticulated, the small cells connected to one another by delicate cytoplasmic processes. Mitoses, many of them abnormal, are frequent in both the epithelium and stroma. While the well differentiated areas of epithelium are often set off from the stroma by definite basement membranes, one can usually find areas which suggest a transition from stroma to epithelium, or in which it is difficult to ascertain whether a specific group of cells represent stroma or a solid epithelial formation.

So-called embryoid bodies may occasionally be found. These are structures suggesting an early stage of embryogenesis and consist of two adjacent cystic structures within one of which the separating wall is covered by a cluster of epithelial cells resembling an embryonic plate.

Embryonal Carcinoma, Juvenile Variant: This rare tumor is regarded by many as a distinctive neoplasm having a histogenesis different from that of other germinal tumors (Brown 1964). Accordingly, it has been called by a variety of names, including adenocarcinoma of infantile testis, testicular adenocarcinoma with clear cells (Magner et al. 1962), endodermal sinus tumor, extraembryonic yolk sac tumor and orchioblastoma. It occurs exclusively in young children, almost all of the reported cases being under age two. Some have imputed to it a degree of aggressiveness less than that of other embryonal carcinomas, but other workers have failed to confirm this (Abell and Holtz 1963).

Histologically, the juvenile embryonal carcinoma is a poorly differentiated papillary adenocarcinoma, differing in only a few respects from its adult counterpart (Fig. 1-8). The cells contain intracellular mucin and PAS positive material, and small mucin-filled pools may be found in solid clusters of epithelial cells. The structure is usually uniform throughout the entire mass, lacking the pleomorphism typical of adult embryonal carcinoma. Teratoma, choriocarcinoma and seminoma are rarely found in association with this tumor when it occurs in children (Young et al. 1970), but mixtures are common in adults.

Teratoma: This pattern of germinal tumor is recognizable by the presence of differentiated or partially differentiated somatic tissues. The most frequently recognizable elements are glial tissue, gastrointestinal or respiratory epithelium, cartilage, bone and smooth muscle (Fig. 1-9). Occasionally there is organoid development. The heterologous tissues may be fully differentiated or may show neoplastic transformation such as might be found in the tissue in its normal location. In well differentiated teratomas the heterologous tissues are embedded in a fibrous stroma of varying cellularity. Immature teratomas often have areas of primitive mesenchyme composing a part or all of the background stroma.

Teratomas containing only fully differentiated tissues occur rarely in testes, and are relatively more frequent in infants and very young children. It is unjustifiable, either in a child or an adult, to assume that all fully differentiated teratomas are benign. Frequently more extensive sampling of the original mass will reveal undifferentiated foci. Even when this is not the case, subsequent metastases may demonstrate that fully malignant components were present but undetected in the primary. Some reports have implied that differentiated teratomas in infants are always benign (Abell and Holtz 1963). More extensive experience, however, indicates that this is not the case (Pugh and Smith 1964).

Choriocarcinoma: Testicular choriocarcinoma closely resembles choriocarcinoma arising in the uterus. Two cell types are invariably present.

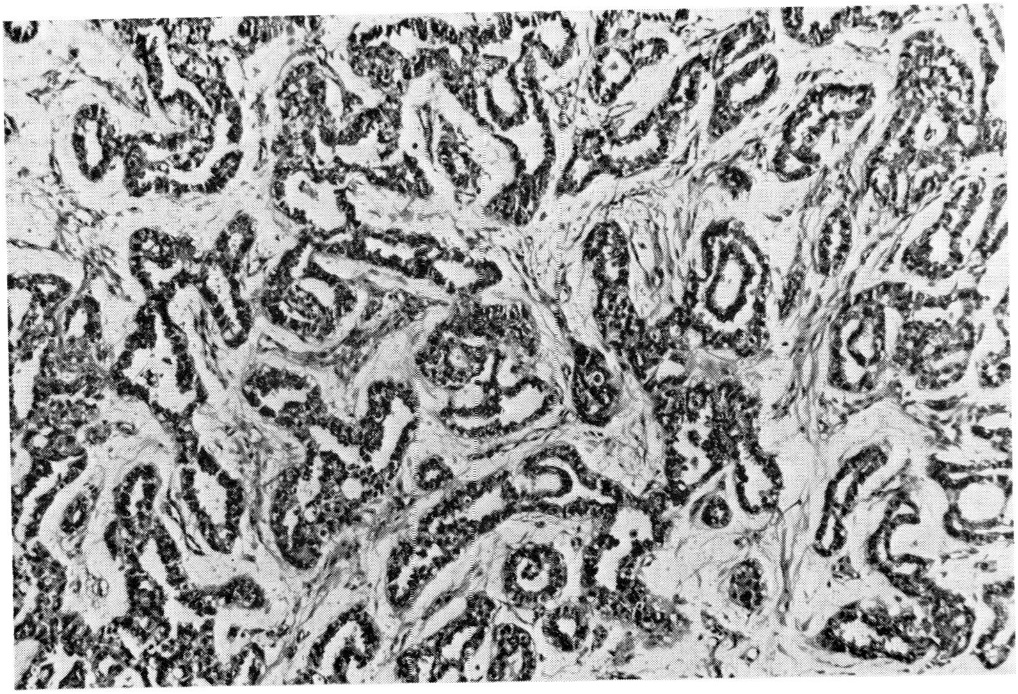

Fig. 1-8. Embryonal carcinoma, juvenile variant. This particular tumor occurred in a boy 14 months old. X 80.

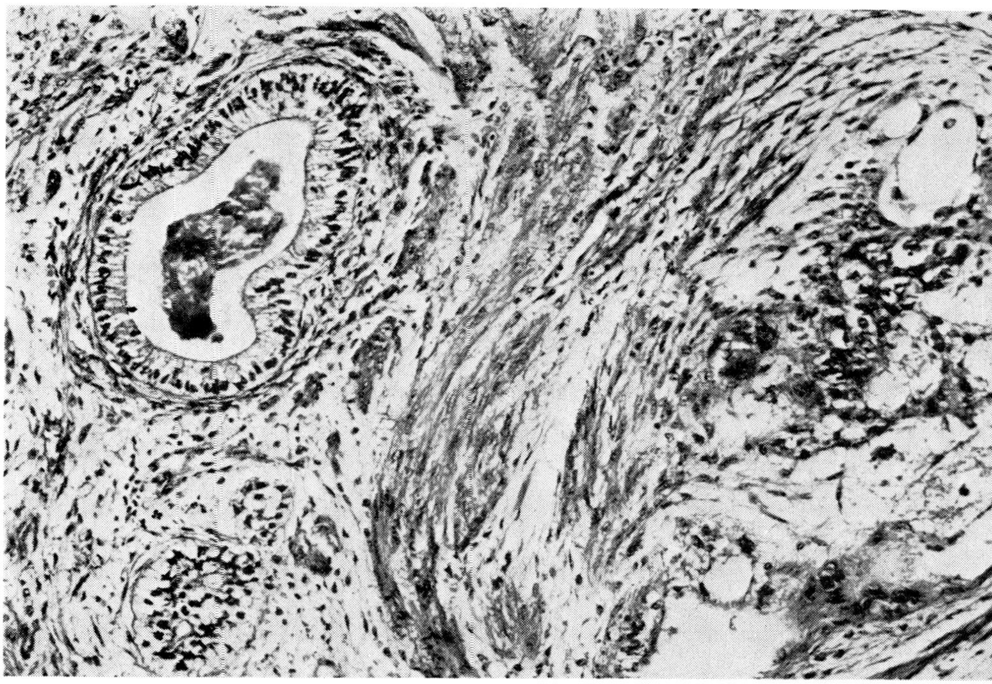

Fig. 1-9. Teratoma, immature type. Both differentiated and undifferentiated epithelial elements are embedded in a stroma containing recognizable smooth muscle and embryonic mesenchyme. X 120.

One of these, the cytotrophoblastic cell, is small and polyhedral, with a definite cell membrane and clear cytoplasm. Nuclei are small, regular, centrally placed and usually contain small nucleoli. The second cell type, the syncytiotrophoblastic cell, is a bizarre giant cell composed of abundant brightly eosinophilic cytoplasm which is poorly delineated peripherally. Nuclei usually number three to ten and are variable in size, shape and appearance even within a single cell. Chromatin is clumped in an irregular fashion and may be concentrated about the nuclear membrane. These two types of cells are arranged in irregular sheets with many spaces into which broad tongue-like villi protrude (Fig. 1-10). Frequently, the villi are composed of cytotrophoblasts, about which the syncytial giant cells form a cap. Necrosis and hemorrhage are common (Fig. 1-11).

Germinal Tumors: Combined Forms: In most large studies, pure seminomas make up about 40 per cent of all testicular germinal neoplasms (Sulak 1970). Autopsy findings, however, show that in 20 to 35 per cent of patients with tumors classified as pure seminomas which ultimately metastasize, the metastases are another form of germinal tumor, usually embryonal carcinoma or choriocarcinoma. This implies that the primary mass contained undetected foci of the more aggressive pattern and that the true incidence of pure seminoma is somewhat lower than usually reported.

Mixtures of embryonal carcinoma and teratoma are often difficult to substantiate, and the evaluation of such tumors depends on the criteria adopted for the diagnosis of each specific pattern. To distinguish, for example, between a poorly differentiated adenocarcinoma arising in teratoma and the tubular component of embryonal carcinoma is difficult and may, indeed, be an exercise without prognostic importance. In our experience, the occurrence of a teratoma in an adult male without some admixture of elements interpretable as embryonal carcinoma is most unusual.

Choriocarcinoma in a mixed germinal tumor is usually easy to recognize. Occasionally, however, a seminoma which produces numerous giant cells may be confusing, since these cells are indistinguishable from syncytiotrophoblast. A diagnosis of choriocarcinoma in a mixed germinal tumor should not be entertained unless both villi and recognizable cytotrophoblastic cells are present.

Within any mass showing mixed patterns, embryonal carcinoma, teratoma and choriocarcinoma tend to be intimately intermingled, and areas of transition are difficult to characterize specifically. The seminomatous component of combined tumors, on the other hand, is usually separate, arranged in fairly discrete nodules which vary from a few millimeters to a significant proportion of the tumor. Transitions between seminoma and the other elements are never observed. Halley (1963), in a whole organ section study of germinal tumors, pointed out that in mixtures of seminoma, embryonal carcinoma and teratoma, the nodules of seminoma often surround the other components and suggested that such an arrangement may provide a measure of protection when the quantity of the seminomatous component exceeds that of other elements.

It is our policy to base treatment upon the most ominous element present in a testicular tumor, even if this element is present in only one or two foci.

NON-GERMINAL TUMORS

Interstitial-Cell Tumors

These rare tumors, believed to arise from the interstitial or Leydig cells of the testis, constitute one to two per cent of all testicular tumors (Collins

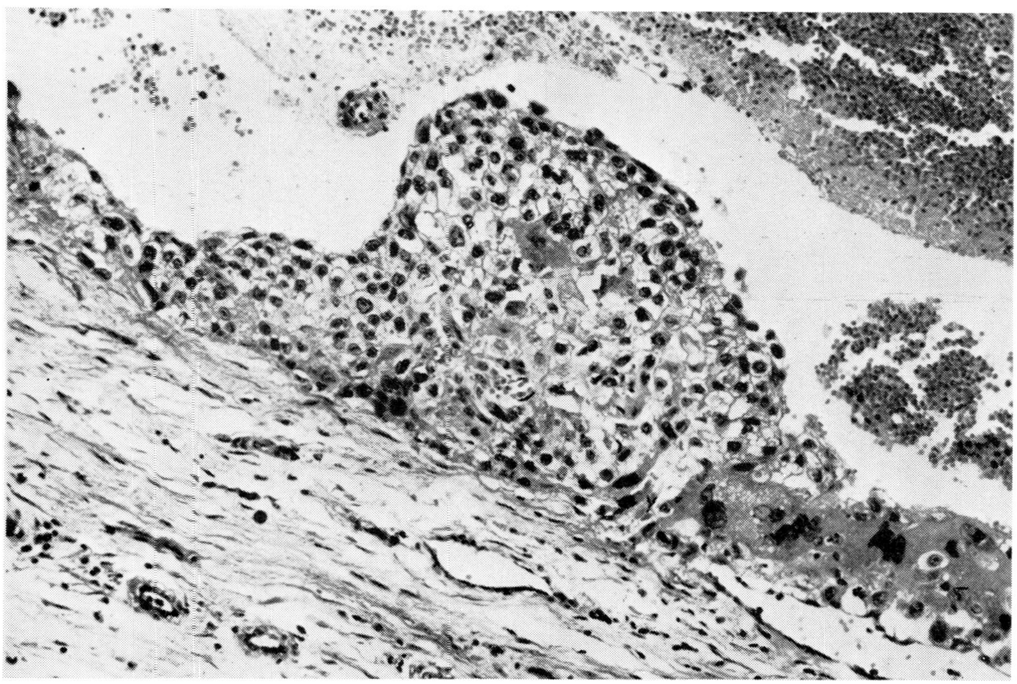

Fig. 1-10. A villus in choriocarcinoma. Most of the broad projection is composed of cytotrophoblast. Some syncytial giant cells are visible at the lower right. X 130.

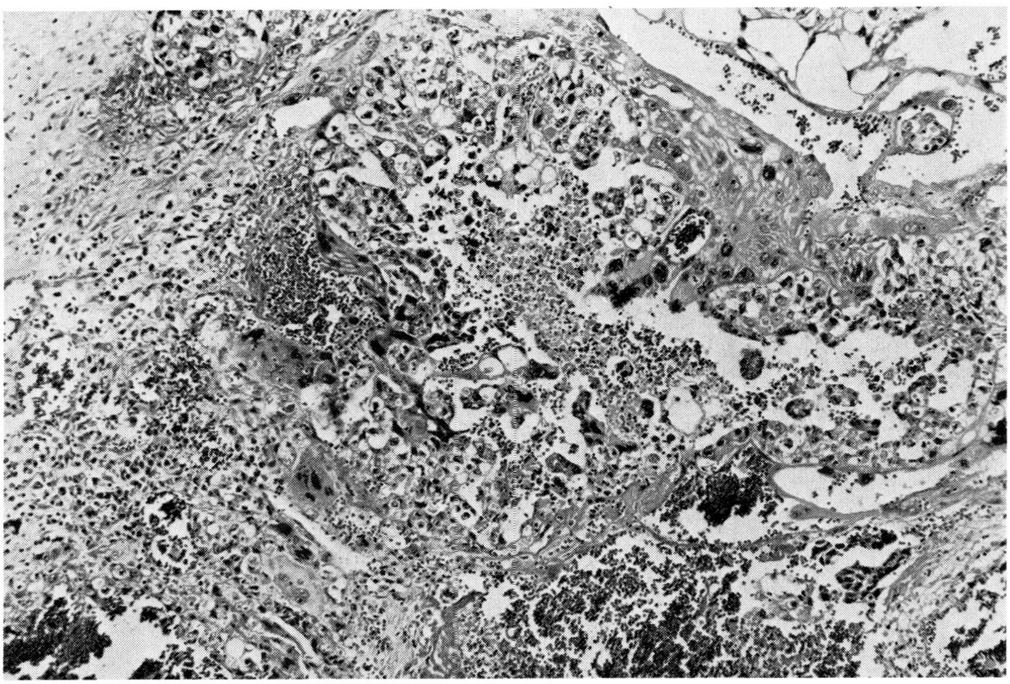

Fig. 1-11. Necrosis and hemorrhage in a choriocarcinoma. X 100.

and Cameron 1964). They occur at all ages but are most frequent between 30 and 50. Size varies from a few millimeters in diameter to several hundred grams. Usually benign, an occasional tumor of this type has metastasized (Livesay et al. 1972). No special predilection has been found for occurrence in cryptorchidism, but these tumors have been found in undescended gonads (Bader and Proctor 1964).

Grossly, tumors of interstitial cells are spherical, sharply circumscribed but not encapsulated and compress the surrounding testicular tissue. They are usually bright yellow to yellow-brown and firmer than the surrounding tissue. As a rule there is no invasion of the testicular capsule or involvement of the epididymis.

The cells of the tumor are irregularly angular and fit together in mosaic fashion. Their cytoplasm is uniformly and brightly eosinophilic, finely granular and sometimes contains vacuoles in which lipoid materials may be demonstrated by appropriate stains. The nuclei in most examples are bland, rounded, have finely dispersed chromatin and small central nucleoli (Fig. 1-12). Occasional examples show some degree of nuclear pleomorphism and anaplasia but these changes are not indicative of malignant behavior. In many examples of interstitial-cell tumor it is possible to demonstrate crystalloids of Reinke (Fig. 1-13) which are diagnostic of testicular interstitial-cells. These bodies are homogenous, cylindrical, have round or pointed ends, and stain faintly with eosin. One or two may be found in a single cell. They usually distort the shape of the cell, extending beyond the contour of the cytoplasmic membrane.

Tumors of Specialized Gonadal Stroma

This term was first proposed by Mostofi in 1952 to designate the rare tumors of testicle which reciprocate the development of specialized gonadal stromal cells and are homologues of the arrhenoblastoma of the ovary. Such tumors occur over a wide range of age, from infancy to senility, and are often associated with evidence of estrogen production in the form of gynecomastia. They occur with increased frequency in undescended testes and have been reported to occur in association with germinal testicular tumors. We have recently observed two instances of specialized gonadal stromal tumors in the intra-abdominal testes of phenotypic females with testicular feminization syndrome.

Grossly, tumors of specialized gonadal stroma are sharply circumscribed, encapsulated or non-encapsulated, spherical, single or multiple, and range from a few millimeters to about ten centimeters in diameter. They are firm and light yellow-brown. Degeneration, hemorrhage and cyst formation are uncommon. Microscopically, these neoplasms contain an epithelial and a stromal component, each of which may vary in its pattern of differentiation, its arrangement and the proportion of the tumor which it makes up. The epithelial cells when well differentiated are columnar and tend to be arranged in tubular fashion around small central lumens, producing an appearance reminiscent of a fetal testis (Fig. 1-14). Nodules composed almost entirely of such cells with scanty stroma have, in the past, been designated "androblastoma" or "tubular adenoma" and are identical with the Sertoli cell tumors common in dogs. Differentiation ranges downward to poorly formed tubules, usually with a greater amount of stroma, to irregular sheets and clusters of vacuolated polyhedral cells (Fig. 1-15). Occasionally, areas suggesting the pattern of granulosa cell tumor may be also found. Such an appearance has been described by Norris and Scully (1958) as occurring also in arrhenoblastoma of ovary. Clusters of irregularly ovoid cells with homogeneous eosinophilic cytoplasm

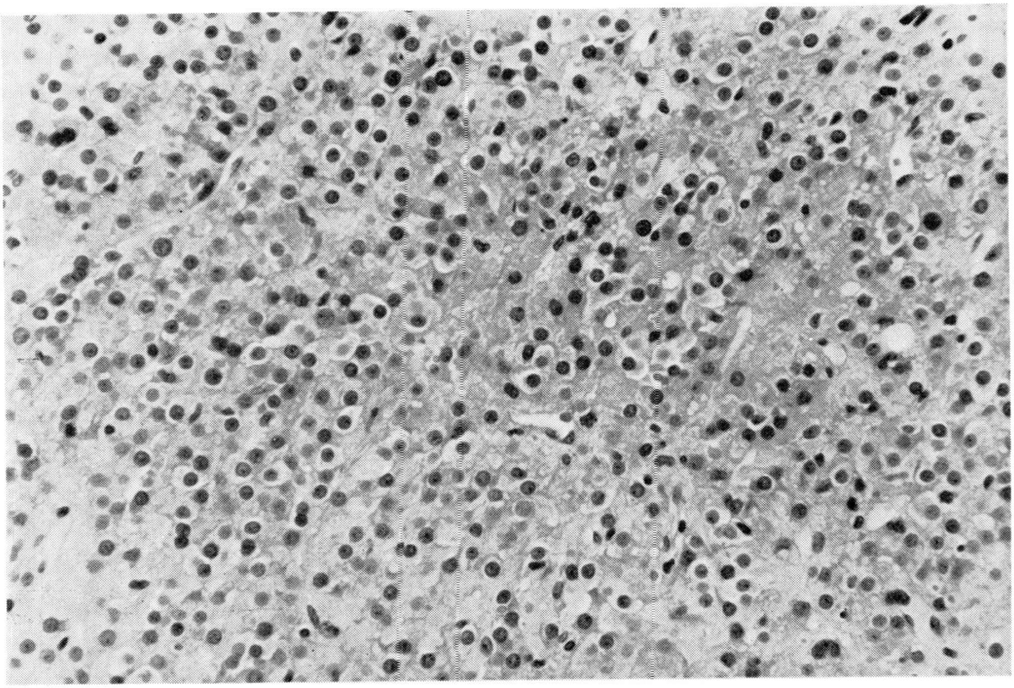

Fig. 1-12. Interstitial cell tumor. X 300.

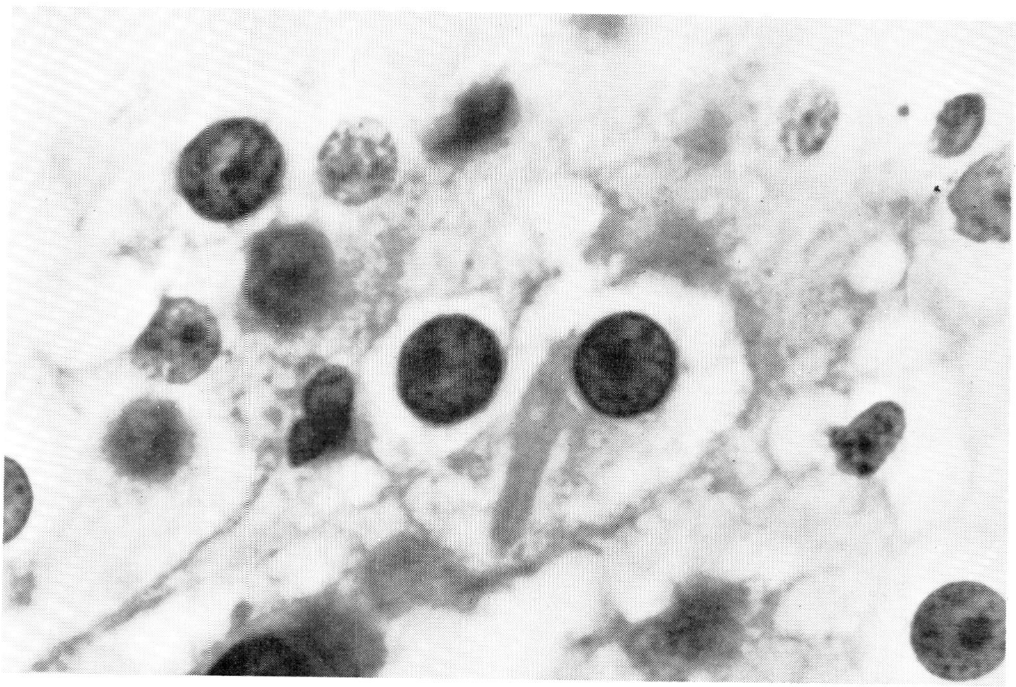

Fig. 1-13. Interstitial cell tumor. The large cell near the center contains a typical rod-shaped, round-ended Reinke crystalloid. X 1800.

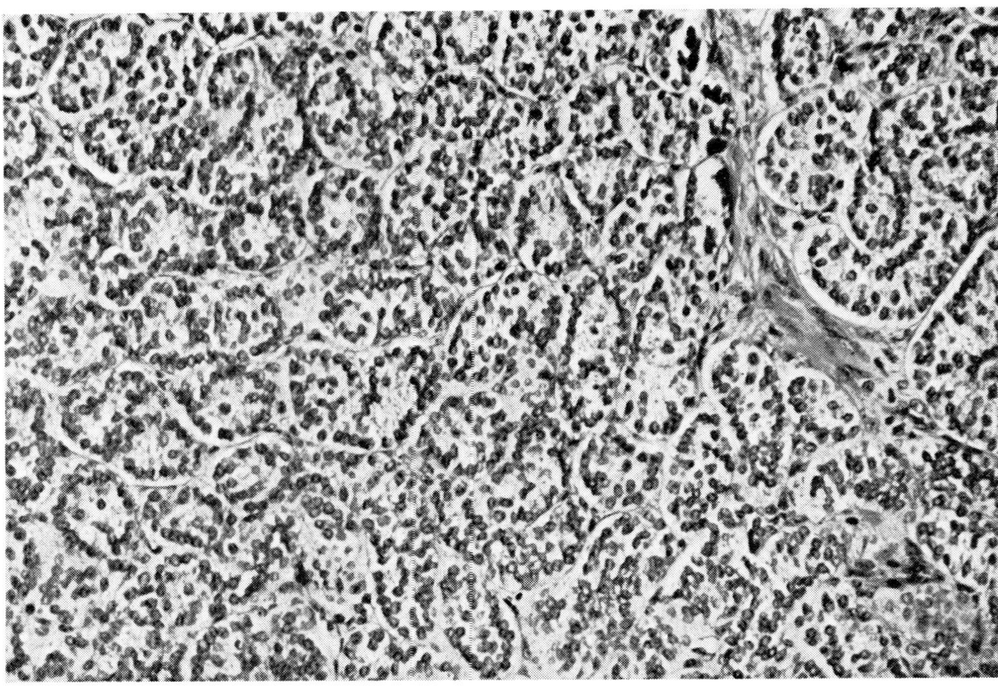

Fig. 1-14. Tumor of specialized gonadal stroma of the differentiated type, a lesion often called androblastoma. X 120.

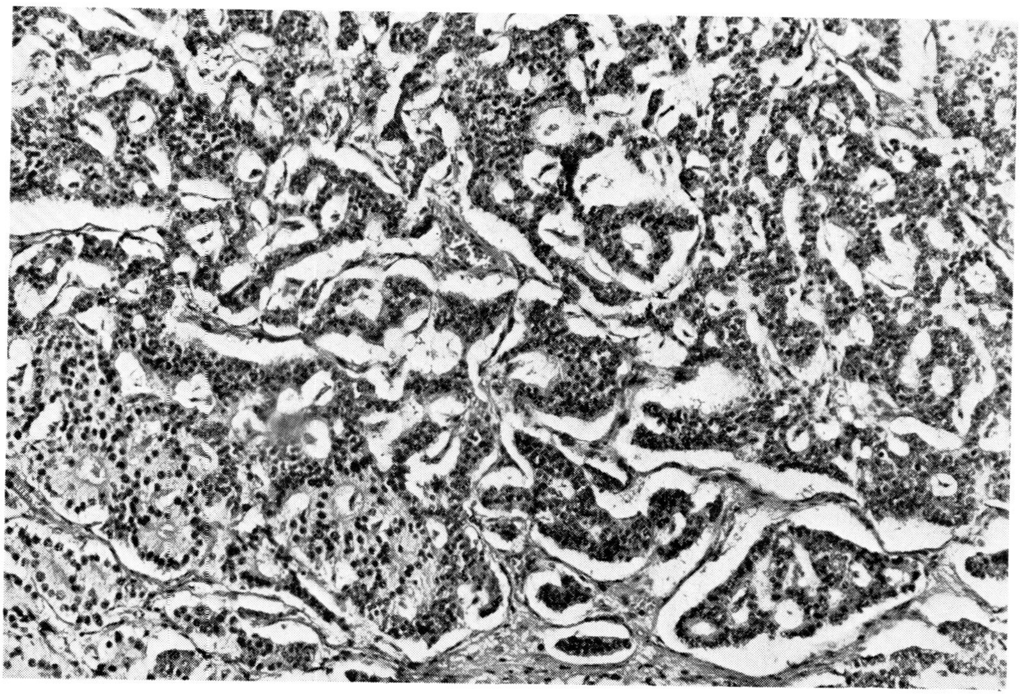

Fig. 1-15. Tumor of specialized gonadal stroma of intermediate type. It contains a mixture of Sertoli cells and smaller cells of indeterminate type. X 120.

resembling interstitial cells may also be found. Reinke crystalloids in such cells are rare or absent. The stromal component, when copious, may be arranged in a variety of ways. The cells may be elongated, spindle-shaped, compact and fibromatous. Occasionally, their nuclei exhibit considerable pleomorphism, suggesting a connective tissue neoplasm. In other examples the stromal cells are short, plump, stellate and arranged in a reticular fashion. Specialized gonadal stromal tumors are almost invariably benign, but rare examples of malignant behavior have been reported. There is no correlation between clinical behavior and the degree of pleomorphism in the tumor. Gynecomastia is usually reported to regress after the removal of these tumors but the regression is often incomplete.

SECONDARY TESTICULAR NEOPLASMS

Metastases to the testes from solid primary tumors are by no means common. They occur with just sufficient frequency that the possibility must be borne in mind in differential diagnosis. In our autopsy material, the neoplasms which have most frequently produced testicular metastases have been malignant melanoma, bronchogenic carcinoma (usually the small cell undifferentiated type) and adenocarcinoma of the prostate (Johnson et al. 1971). In only one case was testicular enlargement the initial manifestation of disease. The histologic appearance in each case was comparable to that of the primary neoplasm.

Reticuloendothelial neoplasms are, by far, the most common secondary tumors of the testis and present special problems (Gowing 1964). They occur predominantly during the age span in which malignant lymphomas are prevalent. More than 60 per cent are found after age 50. These tumors have a high rate of bilaterality, either simultaneously or sequentially. They may involve the testis diffusely or form single or multiple nodules. Grossly, the masses have a glassy cut surface which is light yellow-brown and homogeneous. Microscopically, the malignant reticuloendothelial cells infiltrate between testicular tubules, separating them but sparing both the tubules and the small intratesticular arteries (Fig. 1-16). Most commonly, the cells are of the reticulum cell sarcoma type or of the poorly differentiated lymphocytic lymphosarcoma type. A few cases of plasmacytoma have been reported. No cases of testicular involvement by Hodgkin's disease are reported in the available literature.

The bulk of patients either have systemic reticuloendothelial neoplasia at the time of testicular enlargement or they develop it within a few months thereafter (Johnson et al. 1972). There are, however, a few patients who have survived for periods of years after removal of lymphomatous testicular masses without further evidence of disease. This is true also of localized lymphomas arising in other non-lymphoid tissues such as stomach or breast. It is probable that many such lesions represent pseudolymphomas or peculiar inflammatory reactions, which in the case of the testicle are possibly related to granulomatous orchitis. No specific histologic criteria for their distinction exist.

PARATESTICULAR NEOPLASMS

Paratesticular Rhabdomyosarcoma: Malignant connective tissue neoplasms occur occasionally in the paratesticular region. Such tumors as leiomyosarcoma, fibrosarcoma and liposarcoma apparently arise fortuitously from the epididymis, spermatic cord or scrotal sac and are not grossly or histologically different from similar tumors occurring in other soft tissue areas (Spark 1972; Ray et al. 1972; Remzi 1973). One group of tu-

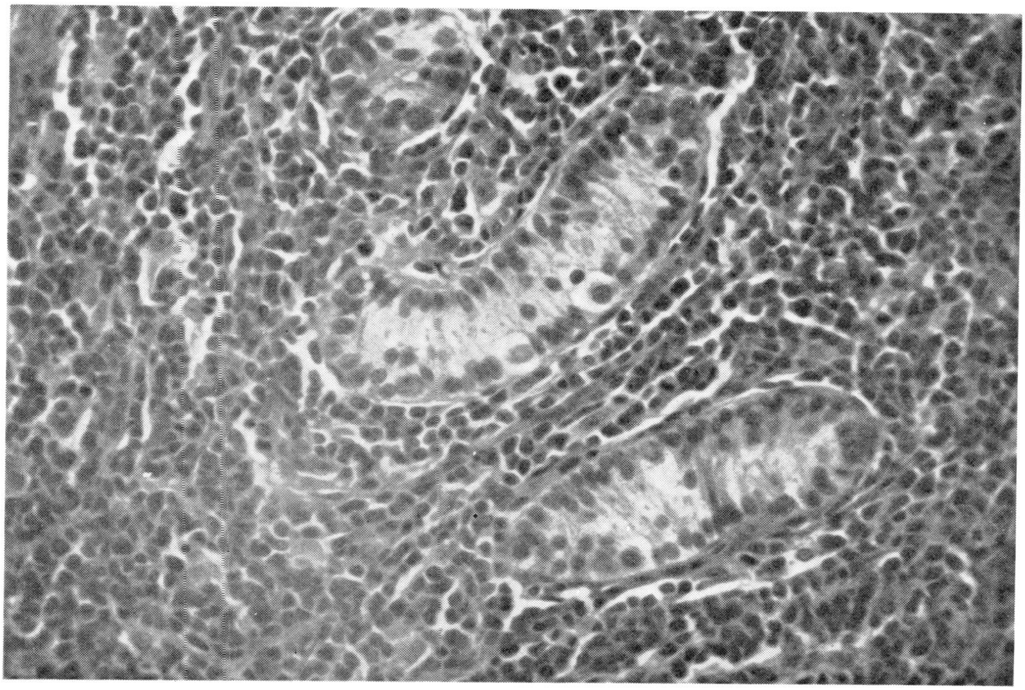

Fig. 1-16. Reticulum cell sarcoma in testis. The lymphomatous cells infiltrate between seminiferous tubules which show no striking alteration. The patient had widely disseminated reticulum cell sarcoma.

mors, however, is sufficiently numerous and consistent in its behavior as to be recognized as a clinicopathologic entity. This is the rhabdomyosarcoma of paratesticular tissue.

Paratesticular rhabdomyosarcomas occur almost exclusively in patients under age 20 (Arean and Kreager 1965; Gowing and Morgan 1964; Rosas-Uribe et al. 1970). Usually they are rapidly growing, but an occasional tumor has been reported to have been present for several years before removal. They arise from the tunica vaginalis or other paratesticular structures and usually displace the testis without invading it.

A typical rhabdomyosarcoma appears grossly as a single or multilobulated, rubbery-firm, gray-tan mass, separate and distinct from the testicle. Histologically there is great variability in appearance, both from tumor to tumor and within a single mass. Most common is the embryonal rhabdomyosarcoma (Fig. 1-17) pattern (Horn and Enterline 1958) which is composed of slender spindle cells, closely arranged and often arrayed radially about small arteries. These cells have single nuclei, sharply marginated eosinophilic cytoplasma and are intermingled with small racket-shaped or comma-shaped cells of similar structure. Areas of myxoid degeneration are common. Foci corresponding to the pleomorphic pattern of Horn and Enterline may also be encountered. Here the cells are large and variable in shape with eosinophilic cytoplasm, multiple nuclei arranged in tandem and cross striations. Other characteristic cells are large and ovoid with sharply defined eosinophilic cytoplasm and eccentrically placed large nuclei with bizarre chromatin arrangement. Smaller ovoid cells of similar structure may also be present. All of these cell types contain abundant cytoplasmic glycogen. The alveolar pattern of rhabdomyosarcoma has rarely been reported to occur in paratesticular tumors.

Adenomatoid tumors:

Adenomatoid tumors are slow growing, encapsulated, usually symptomless, small, firm nodules which occur in the body and tail of the epididymis or within the testis, usually toward the lower pole. They are spherical, white or cream colored, and have a distinct peripheral cleavage plane. Histologically they may be composed of solid cords of cells or may contain spaces resembling tubules or small vessels (Fig. 1-18). The typical cell is round or polyhedral and has a centrally-placed, small, bland nucleus. Within the eosinophilic cytoplasm, vacuoles are frequent. The cells contain hyaluronic acid and have ultrastructural features suggesting mesothelial origin (Mackay et al. 1971). Larger spaces apparently form as the result of the coalescence of enlarging vacuoles of adjacent cells in a single cell cord, the cells being compressed about the space and assuming either epithelial or endothelial characteristics. These tumors are completely benign and are often disposed in such a way that they can be removed without damage to the testis, epididymis or other structures.

Papillary cystadenoma of the epididymis:

This rare benign lesion, apparently a hamartoma, is believed to be the epididymal component of Lindau's disease (Price 1971). The circumscribed nodules may range up to 5 cm in diameter, occur usually in the head of the epididymis and are bilateral in about a third of cases. Histologically, the lesion consists of complex papillary processes covered by epithelial cells having clear or vacuolated cytoplasm and duct-like spaces lined by similar cells. Patients who present with bilateral nodules of this type are especially prone to subsequent development of central nervous system manifestations of Lindau's disease.

Mesothelioma of the tunica vaginalis:

Only four well-documented examples of this neoplasm have been reported (Johnson et al. 1973). In a personally studied case, the presenting symptoms were those of hydrocele, rapidly recurrent after repeated aspiration. Scrotal hydrocelectomy yielded a thick-walled sac, on the inner surface of which was a verrucoid plaque 4 cm in diameter. Histologically, this was composed of coarse, fibrous papillae covered by one to three layers of low columnar cells. Irregular calcifications were found in the stroma. Such lesions may be mimicked by metastatic adenocarcinomas in this location.

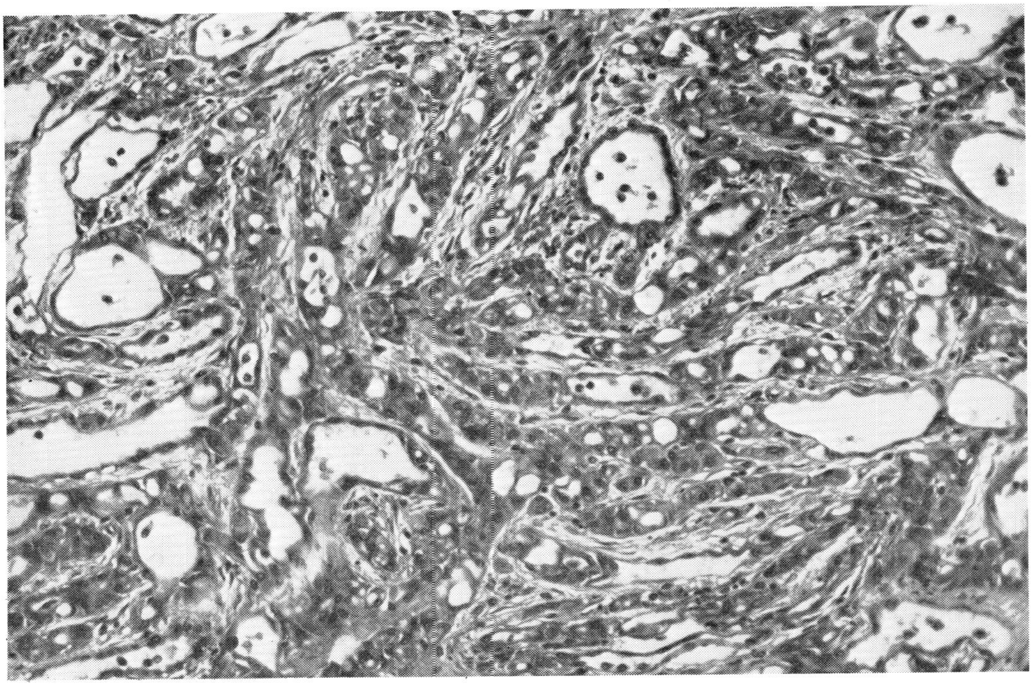

Fig. 1-18. Adenomatoid tumor of the epididymis.

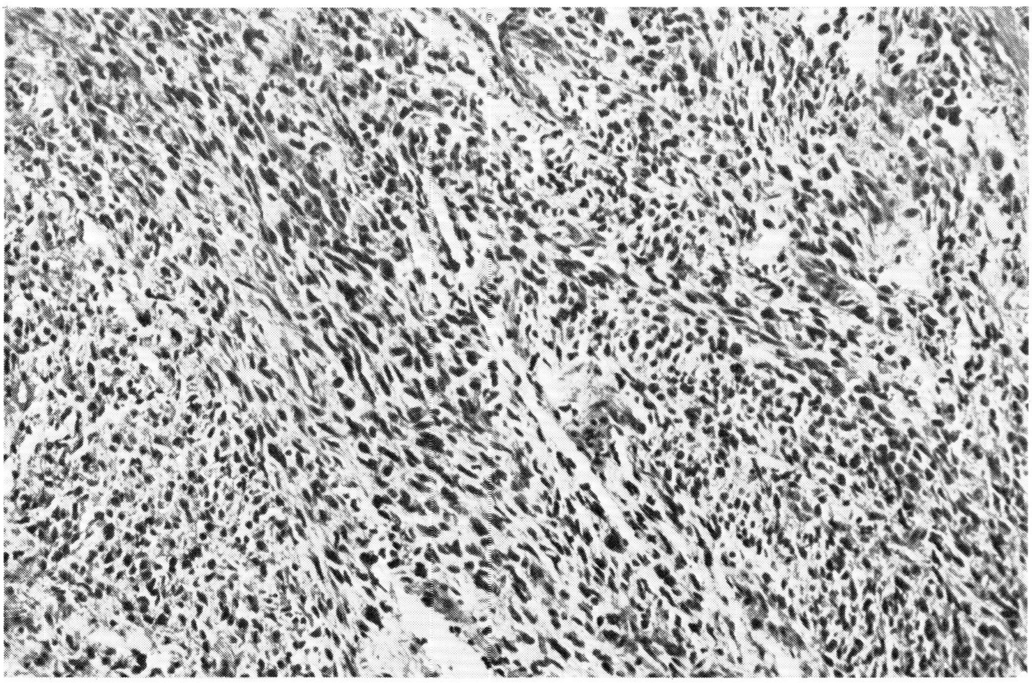

Fig. 1-17. Paratesticular rhabdomyosarcoma. In this case, the tumor is entirely of the embryonal pattern.

CHAPTER 2

ETIOLOGY OF TESTICULAR TUMORS

by

John M. Hogan and Douglas E. Johnson

HISTOGENESIS

The cellular origin of testicular neoplasms has remained in dispute since 1696 when Saint Donat recorded the first case of a testis tumor with teratomatous elements. Over the ensuing centuries, various theories attempting to explain the histogenesis of these tumors have been suggested, but none have met with universal acceptance. The current classification and nomenclature of testicular tumors which is used extensively in this country is based on the work of Freidman and Moore (1946), Dixon and Moore (1952) and Melicow (1956).

Testicular tumors are divided into two general groups: 1) germinal tumors composed of seminomatous, embryonal carcinomatous, teratomatous and choriocarcinomatous elements, which are thought to arise from cells of the sex or germ series and 2) non-germinal tumors (interstitial-cell tumors, tumors of specialized gonadal stroma, sarcoma, etc.) which arise from the non-germinal elements of the testes. There are few arguments as to the histogenesis of non-germinal tumors since they resemble, for the most part, their parent cells (Dixon and Moore 1953). The major controversy, however, surrounds the origin of germinal tumors.

An intratubular site of origin for seminoma was suggested initially on the basis of the close resemblance of seminoma cells to spermatogonia and the frequent finding of seminoma cells within the seminiferous tubules (Dixon and Moore 1952). Most investigators now agree that the origin of seminoma is from germinal epithelium of the seminiferous tubules, but the exact type of cell (undifferentiated germ cell, spermatogonia or spermatocyte) has remained speculative. Collins and Pugh (1964) trace the histogenesis of seminoma no further back than the spermatic epithelium of the differentiated seminiferous tubules. Pierce (1966), in studying the ultrastructure of seminomas, found a close resemblance among undifferentiated seminoma cells and primordial germ cells, spermatogonia and spermatocytes. His work suggests that seminomas arise from any or all of the spermatocytic elements, depending upon the availability and responsiveness of these cells to the carcinogenic stimulus.

It has not been as firmly established that the other morphological types of germinal testicular tumors (embryonal, teratoma or choriocarcinoma) are derived from primordial germ cells (Collins and Pugh 1964). However, there is increasing circumstantial and direct evidence to substantiate the hypothesis that these tumors develop from totipotential primordial germ cells (Melicow 1965; Stevens 1967). It is postulated that when an oncological factor or factors stimulate the primordial germ cells to divide, development proceeds in either somatic, trophoblastic or combined directions (Fig. 2-1). An embryonal carcinoma is the result of early differentiation before definite teratoid or choriocarcinomatous structures have formed. Its morphological features lie in the gray zone between the totipotential primordial germ cell and well differentiated somatic and trophoblastic tissue. Complete trophoblastic differentiation results in choriocarcinoma, whereas, somatic differentiation results in the formation of teratomatous elements (ectoderm, endoderm and mesoderm). Occasionally, malignant transformation of the teratomatous tissue may occur.

The following evidence has been offered in support of the hypothesis that these tumors arise from primordial germ cells: 1) The majority of germinal (teratoid) tumors occur in the gonads which suggest a germ cell origin (Dixon and Moore 1952); 2) All early testicular teratomas in the mouse are completely enclosed by the seminiferous epithelium, which indicate that they are derived from cells within the seminiferous tubules; 3) Human teratomas (Melicow 1940; Evans 1957), as well as transplanted teratomas of the mouse (Pierce and Dixon 1959; Stevens 1959), will, under certain conditions, form structures (embryoid bodies) which resemble normal early embryos; 4) Testicular teratomas of strain 129 mice have been manipulated experimentally to show that their somatic and trophoblastic tissues developed from embryonal carcinoma cells. They both possess similar embryonic potentialities (Kleinsmith and Pierce 1964; Pierce 1961; Pierce and Dixon 1959; Pierce et al. 1960; Stevens 1960, 1962, 1964); 5) The ultrastructure of human embryonal carcinoma, either alone or as a component of a teratocarcinoma, closely resembles its counterpart in the rodent which has been shown to be the multipotential stem cell of murine teratocarcinoma (Pierce 1966); and 6) Gonads with few germ cells have fewer teratomas than gonads with normal numbers of germ cells, as would be expected if teratoma were derived from primordial germ cells (Stevens 1967).

TUMORIGENESIS

There are few established oncological factors responsible for testicular tumorigenesis. Although environmental, occupational, genetic, traumatic, vascular and viral influences, occurring separately or in various combinations, have been implicated as possible inciting causes leading to the formation of testicular tumors, their carcinogenicity has been difficult to demonstrate in the research laboratory. To date, the mechanisms responsible for the development of testicular tumors remain largely unknown. It does appear significant, however, that the majority of germinal testicular tumors occur during the age of greatest sexual activity.

Trauma

A relationship between trauma and the subsequent discovery of a testicular tumor has been recognized for centuries and through the years attempts have been made to demonstrated that injury plays a part in the initiation of tumor development. In fowls the intratesticular injection of zinc chloride (Michalowsky 1928; Guthrie 1964), zinc sulphate (Falin 1940), cooper sulphate (Falin and Anissimowa 1940) and cadmium chloride (Guthrie 1964) results in severe coagulation necrosis with subsequent development of teratomas. Falin (1940) has suggested that in these instances tumorigenesis is the result of embryonic inductor substances liberated from the areas of necrosis which incite the germ cells. Ganina

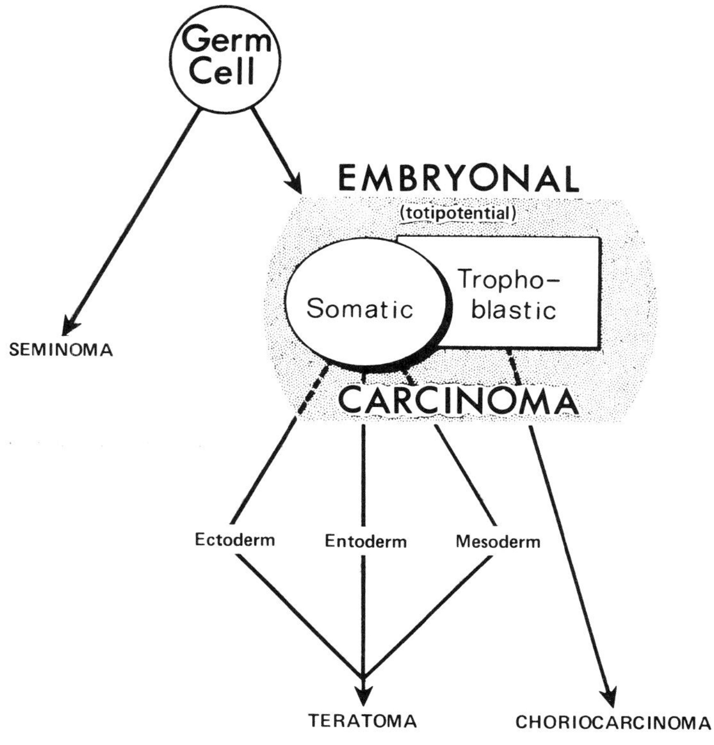

Fig. 2-1. Diagram of histogenesis of germ cell testicular tumors.

(1964) produced seminomas in albino rats by repeated mechanical trauma to the testis. He concluded that trauma produces conditions for the development of precancerous lesions which in turn lead to tumor formation. Other investigators (Willis 1934; Elwin and El-Katib 1960 and Hunt et al. 1962) have been unable to produce teratomatous growths by employing a wide variety of chemical and traumatic testicular injuries. Clinical studies suggest, likewise, that trauma plays no direct role in the etiology of testicular neoplasms (Field 1963).

Atrophy

The occasional development of testicular malignant disease in an atrophic testis has suggested to some observers a potential etiological relationship between testicular malignancy and testicular atrophy (Haines and Grabstald 1950; Hausfeld and Schrandt 1965). In a collective review from the literature of 5,500 cases of testicular tumors, Gilbert (1944) found 80 cases which had developed in a nonspecific atrophic testis (1.5 per cent) and an additional 24 cases with a history of previous mumps orchitis leading to atrophy of the testis (0.5 per cent). Giertsen (1958), in reviewing 120 cases of malignant testicular tumors, found five cases with previous mumps orchitis, an incidence of four per cent. Other authors (Lewis 1950) believe that the incidence of testicular tumors is as great in the descended atrophic testis as in the cryptorchid testis.

The role which atrophy plays in testicular tumorigenesis is not understood. It is possible that during the initial atrophic process an inductor substance is liberated by the necrotic tissue which incites other cells to undergo malignant transformation (Falin 1940). Testicular atrophy may result in hormonal imbalance which under certain conditions can be a tumor-inciting factor. A hormonal influence has been shown necessary for the experimental production of testicular tumors in fowls (Guthrie 1964). Hinman and Smith (1960) in producing Leydig cell neoplasia in dogs by temporarily occluding the spermatic vessels, concluded that increased pituitary gonadotropin activity was responsible for tumor development. However, further investigation is needed to clarify the association between atrophy and the subsequent development of a testicular tumor. In the meantime, it is suggested that whenever an asymptomatic atrophic testis is discovered in a young male patient, the testis should be closely observed for malignant degeneration (Haines and Grabstald 1950; Hausfeld and Schrandt 1965). If during periodic examinations suspicion is aroused, immediate orchiectomy is warranted.

Cryptorchidism

The role that cryptorchidism plays in testicular tumorigenesis has been of concern to physicians since Le Comte (1851) first focused attention on the tumor potentiality of an undescended testicle. Today, there is no doubt that the incidence of tumors in patients with cryptorchidism is higher than in those with normally descended testes.

Various series (Grove 1954; Campbell 1959; Collins and Pugh 1964; Johnson et al. 1968) have demonstrated that 3.6 to 11.6 per cent of testicular tumors arise in cryptorchid testis. Cryptorchidism occurs in only about 1 out of 500 men (Campbell 1942; Gilbert and Hamilton 1940) with the probability of malignant degeneration occurring in an undescended testis estimated to be 20 to 40 times greater than in a normally located scrotal testis (Hinman and Benteen 1936; Gilbert and Hamilton 1940; Campbell 1959; Thurzo and Pinter 1961).

Fear of malignant degeneration prompted Szymsnowski, in 1868, to advocate prophylactic excision of all non-scrotal testes. However, in the absence of adequate statistics demonstrating the actual incidence rate of malignant degeneration of cryptorchidism, physicians have felt obligated to perform orchidopexy. The development of subsequent malignant disease is not necessarily prevented by orchidopexy.

Cunningham (1921) described the first case of a testicular tumor developing after orchidopexy and numerous cases have subsequently appeared in the literature. Recent cumulative reports (Sumner 1959; Dow and Mostofi 1967; Johnson et al. 1968) have raised serious doubts as to the effectiveness of this operation, if performed after puberty, in preventing cancer of the testis. Testicular tumors have been reported in only three patients, however, who have undergone orchidopexy prior to the age of 10 years. In addition, an increased incidence of neoplasia in the normal descended testis in patients with unilateral cryptorchidism has been demonstrated (Johnson et al. 1968). Approximately one out of five testicular tumors developing in patients with a history of cryptorchidism, arise in the contralateral normal scrotal testis (Table III). An inherent developmental defect within the germinal cells may prove to be responsible for both maldescent and testicular tumorigenesis.

Studies by Sohval (1956) have suggested that testicular dysgenesis may be responsible for the development of testicular neoplasms. The increased incidence of dysgenetic tissue reported in cryptorchid testes Sohval 1954) may account for the relative susceptibility to malignant degeneration. If dysgenesis is a factor in testicular tumorigenesis, dysgenetic tissue in the contralateral scrotal testis should be present in a significant number of patients with unilateral cryptorchidism.

If testicular function is to be preserved and the risk of later malignant transformation is to be reduced, orchidopexy should be performed prior to six years of age (Hinman 1955; Lesson 1966; Giarolo 1967). No demonstrable histologic differences have been observed between the undescended and the normally descended testis of the infant from birth to five years of age. At five years of age a normally descended testis undergoes progressive maturation, but an undescended testis undergoes gradual involution and degeneration (Hinman 1955; De La Bolze et al. 1960). It is recommended, therefore, that: 1) orchidopexy be performed prior to the age of six years and not after the age of 10 years; 2) strong consideration be given to performing an orchiectomy in patients with unilateral cryptorchidism diagnosed after the age of 10 years; and 3) careful periodic examinations of both scrotal compartments be performed after orchidopexy or orchiectomy.

TABLE III

TESTICULAR TUMORS ASSOCIATED WITH CRYPTORCHISM

Series	No. of cases	No. of patients with cryptorchism	No. of cryptorchid patients with malignancy in contralateral scrotal testis
Collins and Pugh 1964	995	58	9
Field 1962	135	9	2
Hope-Stone et al. 1963	282	17	2
Schwartz and Reed 1956	167	15	3
Thurzo and Pinter 1961	139	9	3
Johnson et al. 1968	147	12	3
Gehring et al. 1973	529	37	7
Total Cases	2,394	157 (6.6%)	29 (18.5%)

CHAPTER 3

EPIDEMIOLOGY

by

Douglas E. Johnson

INCIDENCE

Testicular tumors comprise one to two per cent of all malignant neoplasms in the male (Gilbert and Hamilton 1940; Leadbetter 1958; Host and Stokke 1959; Perttala 1964; Blandy et al. 1970), and account for 4 to 10 per cent of all malignant disease occurring within the male genitourinary system (Pack and LeFevre 1930; Pessin 1957; Wershub 1962; MacKay and Sellers 1966). Similar findings have been observed at the University of Texas System Cancer Center, M. D. Anderson Hospital and Tumor Institute at Houston (Fig. 3-1). More importantly, testicular tumors are the most common malignant disease, excluding leukemia, developing in men between 20 and 34 years of age (Ackerman and del Regato 1954; Patton et al. 1959; MacKay and Sellers 1966).

Estimates of the annual incidence rate for all testicular tumors range from two to three per 100,000 men. Dixon and Moore (1952) reported an incidence of testicular tumors occurring in the male Army population from 1940-47 of 2.88 per 100,000. Griswold et al. (1955) found an annual incidence rate of 2.1 per 100,000 males in Connecticut during the period 1935-51. Ferber et al. (1962) reports a similar figure for New York State during 1941-60. Collins and Pugh (1964) placed new registrations in England for all types of testicular tumors at 2.3 per 100,000 males and estimated that between 550 and 600 new cases occur annually. Krain (1973) reports an incidence rate for California of 2. 6 per 100, 000.

Recent computations by Clemmesen (1968) have suggested a marked increase in the incidence of testicular cancers in Denmark, noticeably within the larger metropolitan areas. The age-adjusted incidence rate for Copenhagen during the period 1943-62 rose from 3.2 to 6.3 new cases per 100,000 population per year; in provincial towns, an increase was reported from 3.8 to 5.3 per 100,000. A much smaller rise was noted in rural areas (Editorial, Lancet 1968). On the other hand, Lipworth and Dayan (1969) in studying the incidence of seminoma of the testis in England and Wales during the years 1961 through 1967, found a significantly higher incidence in rural areas when compared with urban communities. Sharma et al. (1972) in reviewing the experience at Roswell Park Memorial Institute for the years 1959 through 1969, likewise reported a significantly higher rural preponderance in seminoma patients as compared with other testicular tumors. Talerman et al. (1974) also report a significantly higher incidence of testicular neoplasms in a rural district as compared to urban communities. Although Krain (1973) reports a 67 per cent increase in the prevalence of testicular cancer in California between 1945 through 1954 and

Frequency of Testicular Tumors at M. D. Anderson Hospital
March 1944 – August 1973

Patients with Genito – Urinary Malignancy	4,753
Patients with Testicular Tumors	652
	13.7 %
Patients with Malignant Disease	34,375
Patients with Testicular Tumors	652
	1.9 %

Fig. 3-1

1955 through 1969, he could find no significant difference in the urban versus rural distribution of testicular cancer or seminomas as separate groupings. In view of these conflicting reports further epidemiological studies would appear warranted.

FREQUENCY OF HISTOLOGIC TYPES

Prior to the classic work of Friedman and Moore (1946), the multiple variations in histologic criteria and nomenclature did not allow a comparison of series from different institutions. With the publication of the Armed Forces Institute of Pathology Atlas (Dixon and Moore 1952) standardization in terminology was firmly established.

Germinal tumors constitute approximately 97 per cent of all primary testicular tumors with the remaining three per cent comprised of non-germinal neoplasms (O'Connell and Geschickter 1950; Dixon and Moore 1952; Melicow 1956; Patton et al. 1960). The relative incidence of the various histologic types of germinal tumors is summarized in Table IV. Although there is a considerable range in the incidence of various morphological types, most investigators (Grabstald et al. 1957; Collins and Pugh 1964; Reddy and Ranganayakamma 1966; Blandy et al. 1970) agree that seminoma is the most frequently encountered testicular tumor. Occasionally, seminoma has comprised an overwhelming majority of germinal tumors reported in individual series (Hope-Stone et al. 1963; Navarro and Martinez 1964; Van Welkenhuyzen and Henry 1965; Correa and Tallman 1965). The incidence of embryonal carcinoma among most reported series has varied from 30 to 35 per cent, but occasionally it has been recorded as low as 14 to 20 per cent (Rusche 1952; Melicow 1955). Friedman and Moore (1946) reported an incidence of 35 per cent for teratocarcinomas, but again statistics vary to a low of nine per cent (Culp 1953). Although fully developed adult teratomas have been absent in many series (Merren et al. 1951; Thomas and Bischoff 1954; Schwartz and Mallis 1954; Parker and Holyoke 1960), their incidence is usually given as seven per cent or less (Grabstald et al. 1957). Pure choriocarcinoma is rare, accounting for one or less per cent of the reported germinal tumors. However, choriocarcinomatous tissue is not infrequently found admixed with other histologic types.

AGE

Neoplasms of the testis may present at any age. Reports in the literature describe occurrences in the newborn (Julien 1925) to as late as the eighty-ninth year (Jackson and Magner 1965). The majority of germinal testicular tumors, however, arise in men 15 to 44 years of age. Seminomas tend to develop later than other histologic types with an average age incidence reported to be from 30.7 to 41.9 years (Patton and Mallis 1959; Parker and Holyoke 1960; Thackray 1964). Embryonal carcinomas and teratocarcinomas as compared with seminomas arise four to five years earlier, with the average age incidence ranging from 26.1 to 33.0 years (Kaplan et al. 1951; Patton and Mallis 1959). Choriocarcinomas, on the other hand, occur in men about 10 years younger than those affected by seminoma, with an average age for this group fluctuating between 24.0 and 26.3 years (Kaplan et al. 1951). An analysis of the age incidence for germinal testicular tumors evaluated at Anderson Hospital is given in Fig. 3-2. The pattern of the age distribution for each histologic type is shown in Fig. 3-3.

RACE

Testicular tumors occur infrequently in Negroes, especially under 45 years of age (Schrek 1944; Grumet and MacMahon 1958; Tulinius et al.

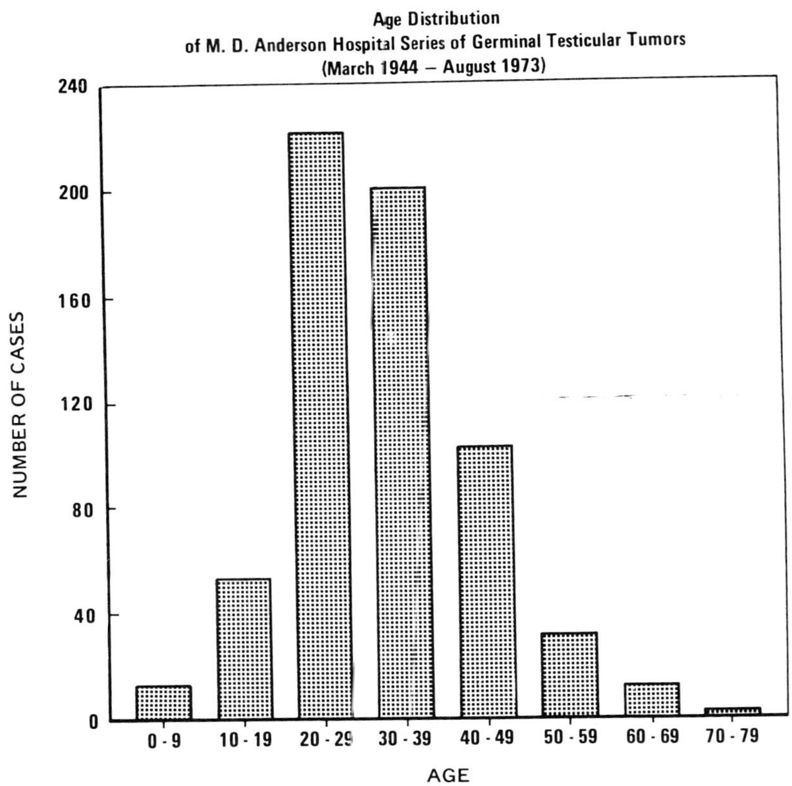
Age Distribution
of M. D. Anderson Hospital Series of Germinal Testicular Tumors
(March 1944 – August 1973)
NUMBER OF CASES
240
200
160
120
80
40
0
0 - 9
10 - 19
20 - 29
30 - 39
40 - 49
50 - 59
60 - 69
70 - 79
AGE

Fig. 3-2

1973). Dixon and Moore (1952) found that 1. 5 per cent of testis tumors occurred in non-whites, although the Army population of non-whites varied from 6. 0 to 8. 5 per cent. In the Anderson Hospital Series of 652 testicular tumors, 17 cases occurred in Negroes, an incidence of three per cent. Koehler et al. (1962) in compiling the racial incidence from questionnaires sent to 12 medical institutions where high Negro patient densities were to be expected, found 17 instances (1. 5 per cent) in 1127 cases of testicular tumors. A similar incidence of testicular tumors among Negroes has been reported by other authors (Table V).

Higginson and Oettlé (1960), Davies et al. (1964), Oettlé (1964) and Templeton (1972) have called attention to the rarity of these tumors in Africans. The rarity of testicular tumors in Africans appears related to a deficiency of seminoma and teratoma since other tumors of the testis are seen approximately as frequently as in other races (Templeton 1972). Walter et al. (1964) have likewise found testicular tumors uncommon in Jamaicans. Whether these findings represent a true difference between races or reflect the effect of latitude or mean annual temperature requires further epidemiological evaluation (Blandy et al. 1970).

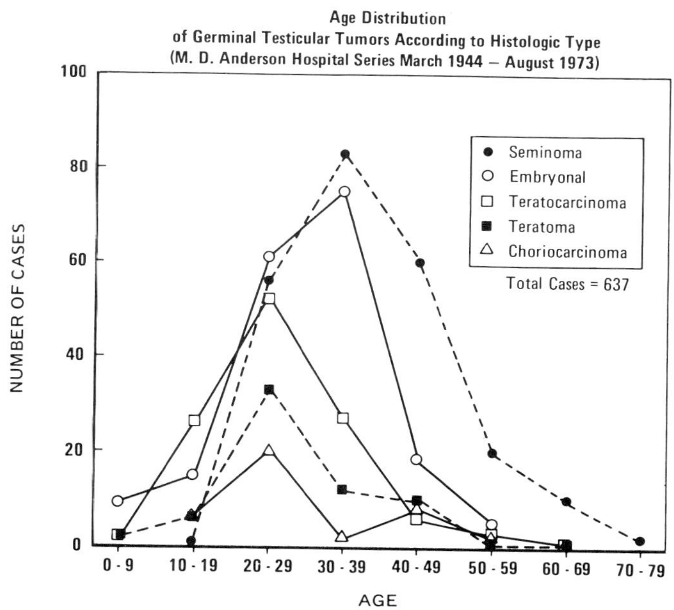

Fig. 3-3

SIDE

There appears to be a slight but definite predilection for testicular tumors to involve the right side (Gray et al. 1950; Thompson 1953; Schwartz and Mallis 1954; Grabstald et al. 1957; Collins and Pugh 1964; Kurohara et al. 1968; Keller 1974). To date, this finding remains a curiosity. Similarly, cryptorchidism has a predilection for affecting the right testicle. Since cryptorchidism favors malignant degeneration, some investigators have speculated that the factor operative in testicular maldescent may be to a lesser extent responsible for the slightly increased tendency to malignancy of the normal right testicle (Leadbetter 1958; Hickinbotham 1950; Blandy et al. 1970).

BILATERAL TESTICULAR TUMORS

The documentation of malignant disease in both testes, either simultaneously or at successive intervals of time, has been reported with such frequency as to remove the condition from the realm of medical curiosity. Livingstone (1805) is credited with describing the first case of bilateral testicular cancer. Hamilton and Gilbert (1942), in a review of 7,000 cases of testicular tumors found in the literature from 1805 to 1939, located 144 cases, an incidence of two per cent. A similar frequency has subsequently been confirmed in other series (Abeshouse et al. 1955; Whittle 1957; Stephen 1958; Collins and Pugh 1964; Shepherd 1966; Johnson and Morneau 1974) with the incidence ranging from two to three per cent.

The most common bilateral testicular tumor is malignant lymphoma (See Chapter 12), accounting for approximately 50 per cent of the cases. Next in frequency of occurrence has been seminoma (Ulm and Draper 1961; Collins and Pugh 1964; MacKay and Sellers 1966; Blandy et al. 1970) with occasional cases of simultaneous development being reported (Arduino and Sola 1957; Dodson and Hooper 1954; Smart and Escamilla 1961; McLean et al. 1973). The concomitant finding of bilateral embryonal carcinoma has also been documented (Hotchkiss and Laury 1950; Abeshouse et al. 1955; Dunlap and Ochsner 1967). Occasionally, histologically different tumors have occurred (Coleman and McKeown 1954; Harper et al. 1954; Brady et al. 1963; Ellner et al. 1966). Bilateral tumors have been associated with bilaterally cryptorchid testes (Friedman and Purkayashtha 1960; Vallega and Magrassi 1966) and have followed either unilateral (Blandy et al. 1970) or bilateral orchidopexy (Kaplan and Roswit 1950).

It has been estimated that after the removal of one testicle due to malignancy, the possibility of the development of a neoplasm in the remaining testicle is 700 times greater than in the general population (Gonick and Lancaster 1959). All patients, therefore, should be observed indefinitely following orchiectomy for malignancy. Prognosis is not necessarily poor should a second tumor develop. Treatment should be instituted on the basis of its histologic characteristics and the stage of the disease.

FAMILIAL INCIDENCE

A familial tendency to the formation of testicular tumors has been recorded on rare occasions (Silber et al. 1972; Arcadi 1973). Cases occurring in brothers have been described by Ravin (1934), Lownes and Leberman (1939), Gordon-Taylor and Wyndham (1947), Collins and Pugh (1964), Hutter et al. (1967); Door et al. (1971), Myers and MacPherson (1972) and Young and Bohne (1972). Howden (1968) reports a patient with seminoma of the testicle who had previously lost two older brothers, each from a seminoma of the testis. The development of testicular malignant disease in twins has been

TABLE IV

FREQUENCY OF HISTOLOGIC TYPES
(2561 Cases)

Series		Total No. Cases	Histologic Types (Per Cent) Seminoma	Embryonal	Teratocarcinoma	Teratoma	Choriocarcinoma
Dixon & Moore	1953	955	38	20	32	9	1
Melicow	1955	100	55	23	17	5	
Staubitz et al.	1958	59	37	31	29	-	3
Parker & Holyoke	1960	91	54	32	21	-	2
Patton et al.	1960	556	37	32	27	2	2
Fons et al.	1964	93	53	28	17	1	1
Vechinski et al.	1965	104	45	34	9	8	4
Kurohara et al.	1967	190	35	33	28	3	1
Kurohara et al.	1968	414	50	27	20	1	2
	Range		34-55%	23-34%	9-32%	1-9%	1-4%

TABLE V

INCIDENCE OF TESTICULAR TUMORS IN NEGROES

Author		Total Cases	Caucasian	Negro	
			%	%	Cases
Kaplan[1]	1951	158	100%	0%	(0)
Merren	1951	41	97	3	(1)
Schwartz	1954	100	99	1	(1)
Thomas	1954	80	99	1	(1)
Raines	1955	50	92	8	(4)
Grabstald	1957	115	97	3	(3)
Cohen	1961	56	91	9	(5)
Thompson	1961	178	99	1	(2)
Krantz	1965	102	98	2	(2)
Kurohara	1967	196	100	0	(0)
Kurohara	1968	425	99	1	(4)
Maier[2]	1968	277	98	2	
Keller	1974	910	96	4	(33)
Total cases		2,688		2.0	(56)

1-Hospital Negro population was 12%
2-Seminomas only

found to occur less often. Champlin (1930), Dormich (1940), Gordon-Taylor and Wyndham (1947), Salm and Adlington (1962), Stewart and Bagshaw (1965), and Villani (1967) cite cases of testicular tumors developing in pairs of twins. There have been reports (Villani 1967) of concordant tumors occurring at about the same age and with the same histologic features in only four pairs of twins. At present, there is no evidence to suggest that the actual incidence of testicular tumors is increased in twins. Harvald and Hauge (1963), having traced nearly 7, 000 sets of unselected twins from the Danish Twin Registry, found the incidence of cancer in twins to be no higher than the expected rate.

TRAUMA

The role of trauma in the etiology, detection and dissemination of testicular tumors has been the subject of considerable conjecture and little experimental or clinical investigation. A history of prior testicular injury is a frequent recording in most series, with the incidence ranging from 8 to 25 per cent (Kimbrough and Denslow 1951; Thomas and Bischoff 1954; Parker and Holyoke 1960; Thompson et al. 1961; Notter and Ranudd 1964; Collins and Pugh 1964; Robson et al. 1965; Kurohara et al. 1968). Only one author has reported the absence of a history of trauma in all his cases (Reddy and Ranganayakamma 1966).

The work of Michalowsky (1928) as well as others (Ljvraga 1934; Bagg 1936; Falin 1940; Carleton et al. 1953) in producing testicular teratomas in fowls suggested an etiological association between trauma and testicular neoplasms. However, Willis (1934) was unable to produce testicular tumors in rats using a variety of chemical and traumatic injuries. He considered the history of previous injuries in patients displaying testicular tumors to be nothing more than a coincidental finding. Most investigators currently agree that trauma bears no relationship to testicular malignancy except as a circumstance leading to the discovery of the lesion (Parker and Holyoke 1960; Field 1963). Attempts at correlating injury with survival has failed to show a relationship (Jones 1955; Kurohara et al. 1968).

METASTASES ON ADMISSION

Metastases from testicular tumors may occur by any of the three classic routes: direct extension; the blood stream; or through the lymphatic system. Direct extension to the scrotum or spermatic tunics is rare and carries a grave prognosis (Patton et al. 1960). The vast majority of tumors metastasize by way of the lymphatics, except for choriocarcinoma which is notorious for its hematogenic spread. The frequency with which metastases may be found on admission is largely dependent upon the thoroughness of the physical examination, the morphological composition of the tumor and the completeness of the radiographic assessment of the stage of the disease.

When the presence of metastases at the time of admission is based solely upon clinical and radiological means the overall incidence varies from 14 to 39 per cent (Higgins and Arber 1953; Schwartz and Mallis 1954; Reinhard and Climie 1960; Patton et al. 1963; Prossor 1964; Sandeman 1964; MacKay and Sellers 1966). An additional 10 to 30 per cent of the cases reveal metastases when lymphadenectomy is performed (Staubitz et al. 1958; Patton and Mallis 1958). The incidence of metastases present at the time of admission according to the various histologic types is given in Table VI. The frequency is significantly lower for seminoma than for the other histologic types.

TABLE VI

FREQUENCY OF METASTASES ON ADMISSION
ACCORDING TO HISTOLOGIC TYPE

Author	Total No. Cases	Cases with Metastases on Admission	Seminoma	Embryonal Carcinoma	Terato-Carcinoma	Teratoma	Choriocarcinoma
		%	PER CENT				
Merren et al. (1951)	44	27.3	25 (3/12)	45 (7/15)	(0/2)	(0/1)	100 (2/2)
Kimbrough & Denslow* (1951)	30	43	20 (2/10)	57 (4/7)	38 (3/8)	(0/0)	80 (4/5)
Rusche (1952)	131	----	15 (6/41)	26 (11/26)	42 (8/18)	35 (7/20)	100 (3/3)
Dixon & Moore (1953)	955	----	11 (----)	32 (----)	19 (----)	24 (----)	--------
Schwartz & Mallis (1954)	100	39	35 (8/23)	35 (17/18)	48 (11/23)	50 (1/2)	67 (2/3)
Reinhard & Climie (1960)	29	19	16 (3/19)	25 (1/4)	0 (0/2)	0 (0/2)	100 (2/2)
Thompson et al. (1964)	175	19	15 (11/75)	17 (7/42)	17 (9/58)		--------
Shepherd (1966)	254	----	44 (80/184)	27 (4/15)	50 (1/2)	51 (20/39)	--------
MacKay & Sellers (1966)	827	25	24 (----)	34 (----)	33 (----)	--------	--------

* All patients had lymphadenectomy
--Not stated by author

CHAPTER 4

CLINICAL DIAGNOSIS

by

Douglas E. Johnson

The early diagnosis of a malignant testicular lesion requires a high index of suspicion on the part of the patient, as well as the physician. A delay in seeking medical treatment is an all too frequent and tragic experience, with the average time lag between the onset of the patient's symptoms and his first examination by a physician exceeding five months (Kimbrough and Cook 1953; Thomas and Bischoff 1954; Patton et al. 1960; Thompson et al. 1961; Kurohara et al. 1968). A campaign to encourage self examination of the testes in men, similar to the self examination stressed in the detection of breast cancer in women, has been recommended (Santos 1963; Markland 1968) and could stimulate an increased awareness of this problem.

Although it is axiomatic that every scrotal mass should be considered malignant until proven otherwise, in at least one-fourth of the cases an erroneous initial diagnosis is made by the examining physician (Kimbrough and Denslow 1951; Patton et al. 1963). The tumor is most frequently mistaken for epididymitis or hydrocele, but on occasion has been confused with hematocele, varicocele, spermatocele and torsion. As with any disease, a correct diagnosis is dependent upon a careful history, a thorough physical examination, and the obtainment of proper laboratory and radiographic studies.

HISTORY

There are no pathognomonic symptoms of a testicular tumor. Patients presenting with testicular neoplasms offer a wide spectrum of unusual symptoms which are frequently misleading, even to the most astute clinician. Many of the difficulties which may be encountered have been aptly discussed by Gordon-Taylor and Wyndham (1947), Rose (1960) and Stephen (1962). These presentations range from the "obvious to the bizarre."

In an attempt to systematize the various clinical expressions of testicular tumors, Kimbrough and Denslow (1951) described four clinical types which are usually seen: 1) tumors with slow, insidious, painless, but progressive onset; 2) a "hurricane" type with an acute onset and rapid progression; 3) the chronic type with a slow onset and a variable latent period followed by a sudden increase in size; and 4) the unobtrusive type first recognized by metastases. Although it helps to keep these various types in mind during an examination for a suspected testicular tumor, the rarity of the lesion prevents such an orderly categorization in clinical practice. The alarming frequency of mistaken diagnoses suggests that the more common symptoms need emphasis (Table VII).

Testicular neoplasms most

TABLE VII

PRESENTING SYMPTOMS
(2926 PATIENTS)

Author	No. Cases	Testicular Mass/Swelling	Testicular Pain	Symptoms of Metastatic Disease	No. Symptoms	History of Trauma
Patton et al. (1960)	491	74%	23%	10%	5%	7%
Thompson et al. (1961)	178	76%	33%	---	--	21%
Collins & Pugh (1964)	858	91%	32%	14%	2%	10%
Robson et al. (1965)	360	80%	26%	5%	4%	19%
Vechinski et al. (1965)	112	88%	13%	11%	4%	---
MacKay & Sellers (1966)	731	78%	15%	4%	1%	6%
Kurohara et al. (1967)	196	85%	49%	10%	8%	7%

commonly present as a painless enlargement of the testis, which may be accompanied by a feeling of heaviness of the scrotum. The enlargement is usually discovered accidently, often during bathing or after minor trauma. Although a history of trauma to the affected testis has been reported in 6 to 21 per cent of the patients with testicular tumors, trauma by itself has never been documented as a factor in the oncogenesis of these tumors. It may, however, play a significant role in the dissemination of the disease.

The relative mildness of the typical early symptomatology combined with ignorance or fear on the part of the patient results frequently in his procrastination to seek medical attention. It is only with progressive enlargement that he becomes concerned. At the time of the examination, a history of associated testicular pain or tenderness can be elicited in 30 to 50 per cent of the patients. Acute testicular pain, on the other hand, is an uncommon presenting symptom providing the lesion has developed within a scrotal testis (Milner and Gilbert 1950; Arvola and Lilius 1972). Acute testicular pain can, however, result from hemorrhage, necrosis or infarction within the tumor or a combination of these factors. Rarely, the clinical picture may simulate a strangulated inguinal hernia (Williams 1955; Hira 1965). It, therefore, behooves the clinician to recognize the possibility of an underlying testicular tumor in any patient presenting with an acute onset of scrotal pain.

Acute abdominal pain developing in a patient with abdominal cryptorchidism should alert the physician to the possibility of torsion of an intra-abdominal testicular tumor. Gerster in 1898 reported the first such instance with an additional 22 cases having subsequently appeared in the literature (Crowe 1951; Packham 1965; Garber and Kauffer 1968; Passanante et al. 1968). These patients have characteristically presented with sudden, lower abdominal pain accompanied by nausea, vomiting and low grade fever. Physical examination usually demonstrates tenderness and guarding in the lower abdomen. When rupture of the testis occurs, there is evidence of intra-abdominal hemorrhage, abdominal wall rigidity, rebound tenderness, increased pulse rate, shoulder pain, etc. Although rectal tenderness is usually present, a mass is rarely palpable. A correct preoperative diagnosis has been made infrequently (Chitty 1933). The condition is most frequently diagnosed as acute appendicitis.

Gynecomastia may be the first sign or symptom of a testicular tumor. Treves (1958) reported the occurrence of breast enlargement in 54 of 525 patients with testicular tumors; in three patients it was the first sign or symptom of the testicular lesion. Cairns (1926), Copeman (1959) and Wright (1964) cite additional examples of breast hypertrophy preceding recognition of a palpable testicular tumor. In most large series (Rusche 1952; Collins and Pugh 1964; Vechinski et al. 1965; MacKay and Sellers 1966; Kurohara et al. 1967) gynecomastia has been initially present in two to four per cent of the patients presenting with a germinal testicular tumor. When gynecomastia is associated with malignant testicular disease, it is usually bilateral and fails to regress following orchiectomy. It is most frequently associated with embryonal carcinoma followed in descending order by seminoma, choriocarcinoma and teratoma.

Infertility has been the presenting complaint on occasion and was noted by Collins and Pugh (1964) in 10 of 400 cases with seminoma (2.5 per cent). Borski and Kimbrough (1954) reported a case of cystic adult testicular teratoma associated with an absence of the ductus deferens discovered during an examination for sterility in a 24 year-old male. Bunge and Bradbury (1965) described a case of an early seminoma which was originally missed on microscopic examination of a testicular biopsy specimen performed as part of a fertility potential evaluation in a 27 year-old man. Similar observations have been reported recently by Skakkebaek (1972) and Neilsen et al. (1974).

In 5 to 10 per cent of patients with malignant testicular disease the first manifestations are those resulting from metastatic deposits. Back pain, usually lumbar in position, is a relatively common complaint noted in 7 to 10 per cent of most large series. Its presence usually indicates retroperitoneal lymph node metastases. Less commonly, back pain may be due to the extension of the malignant disease through the vertebral foramina with direct involvement of the spinal cord. Occasionally, backache may result from reflex pain due to an unusually enlarged primary tumor.

Specific gastrointestinal complaints are uncommon as presenting symptoms. Vague abdominal pain, nausea, vomiting, anorexia and weight loss are frequently noted, however, as late systemic manifestations of generalized metastatic disease. With secondary enlargement of the epigastric lymph nodes, a patient may suffer from pyloric outlet obstruction (Dean 1951). The patient has a good appetite, eats heartily, but vomits shortly after each meal. Rarely, metastases to the gastrointestinal tract, especially from choriocarcinoma, may present initially with gastrointestinal hemorrhage.

Skeletal pain resulting from metastatic disease is rare, even late in the course of malignant testicular disease. Although cancer of the testis seldom metastasizes to the bone (Ackerman and Del Regato 1954), skeletal pain may indicate the presence of metastatic osseous deposits even when they are not demonstrable on radiographic examination. Reports of metastatic osseous involvement of the skull, maxilla, vertebrae, ribs, ilium, femora, humerus and scapula have been recorded in the literature (Lafferty and Pendergrass 1950; Sum et al. 1960; Kranz 1966). Roentgenograms have more commonly demonstrated osteolytic lesions, but osteoblastic foci may occur.

On rare occasions, swelling, adenopathy or a mass in the inguinal area are caused from metastatic disease and may be the presenting complaint in patients with undiagnosed testicular malignancy (Witus et al. 1959; Murugasu 1961; Bowles 1962; Altman and Malament 1967). Most frequently this is a result of disruption of the normal lymphatic drainage with establishment of alternate lymph channels through the inguinal nodes resulting from previous scrotal and inguinal surgical procedures. Less commonly, lymphatic spread to the inguinal lymphatics may be caused by invasion of the overlying scrotal skin or to retrograde lymphatic spread from massive retroperitoneal lymph node involvement.

Visual impairment has been reported as a presenting complaint due to the metastatic involvement of the orbital contents from testicular malignant disease. MacDonald (1936) was the first to report a case of choroidal metastasis from a chorioepithelioma of the testis and at least five similar cases have subsequently appeared in the literature (Kulvin 1951; Chitwood 1953). Mann (1967) reported a case of bilateral exophthalmos in a patient complaining of diplopia, as well as, swelling of the eyes. The patient had regression of his symptoms following orchiectomy for a testicular tumor composed of both seminoma and trophoblastic elements.

Other unusual presenting symptoms include a case reported by Betts (1954) of Horner's syndrome with ulnar nerve palsy resulting from massive left supraclavicular lymphadenopathy. Although the patient had noted testicular enlargement for two years, he did not seek medical attention until he had lost sensation in the fourth and fifth fingers of his left hand and developed pain down his left arm. Evans and Kaufman (1971) report a case of testicular seminoma presenting as peripheral sensorimotor neuropathy, which resolved after orchiectomy and radiation therapy. Resnick et al. (1973) describe a patient with embryonal carcinoma of the testicle whose initial complaint was pain and swelling of the lower extremity which was secondary to inferior vena caval thrombosis resulting from metastatic tumor compression. Heuson (1966) reports a case of typical Addison's disease resulting from an occult metastatic seminoma. The etiology of adrenal failure in this case was unsuspected for more than a year and became apparent only with the discovery of the testicular tumor. Schiff (1955) described a case wherein metastatic tumors of the scalp were the first clue to the presence of a primary testicular tumor. Nelson and Ruffolo (1966) report a case of seminoma previously undiagnosed which initially presented as a rapidly developing paraplegia.

Unfortunately, in a small group of patients, symptoms are either absent or they are of such minor significance as not to call the patient's attention to the testicular lesion. In approximately four per cent of patients, the tumor is discovered incidentally during the course of a routine physical examination (Patton et al. 1959; Vechinski et al. 1965). It becomes, therefore, mandatory that careful scrutiny of the scrotal contents be an integral part of all complete physical examinations.

PHYSICAL EXAMINATION

Examination of the patient should be undertaken only after he has been instructed to remove all of his clothing. The examination requires careful inspection and palpation of the patient in both an erect and supine position. Inspection will frequently show a variation in the size of the scrotal contents (Fig. 4-1). The presence or absence of varicocele should be noted. The overlying skin is usually normal, but in cases of large tumors the scrotal skin may appear tense and glazed (Fig. 4-2). Ecchymotic areas, suggesting trauma are rare. Hydroceles and testicular tumors can often be differentiated by inspection alone. Hydroceles of any significant size extend along the spermatic cord and cause a swelling at the base of the penis which makes the penis appear shortened, while a tumor is usually confined to the testis without apparent shortening of the penis (Dean 1951).

Palpation should be gentle so as to prevent the dissemination of the malignant cells into the vascular and lymphatic channels and thorough so as not to overlook a small, poorly defined tumor. Palpation of the testis should always be performed bimanually. The testicle should be held between the fingers and thumb of one hand and the spermatic cord and epididymis palpated with the other hand (Campbell 1950). In order to carry out a thorough examination of the testis, it is wise to palpate its constituent parts in a definitive order (Bailey 1960), beginning initially with the unaffected testis, which can serve as a baseline for comparison. Such an examination is best begun by first palpating the body of the testis, keeping in mind its relationship to the tunica vaginalis; then examining the head, body and tail of the epididymis, and lastly palpating the spermatic cord up to the level of the external inguinal ring.

The normal testicular parenchyma is usually uniform in consistency and any area of induration, nodularity or irregularity should be considered a tumor until proven otherwise. Occasionally, the entire testis may be replaced by neoplasm and in this situation the consistency will be firm to hard. In cases of teratoma, cystic depressions as well as hard nodules repre-

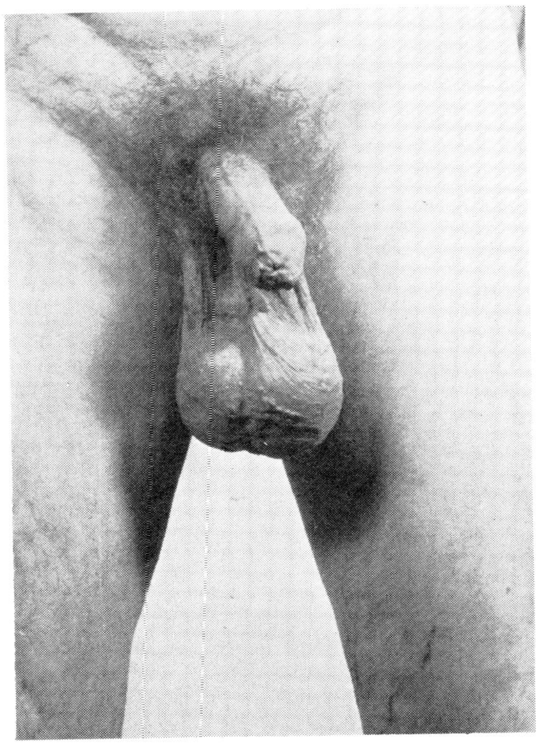

Fig. 4-1. Left testicular tumor. Note the asymmetrical enlargement of the left scrotum.

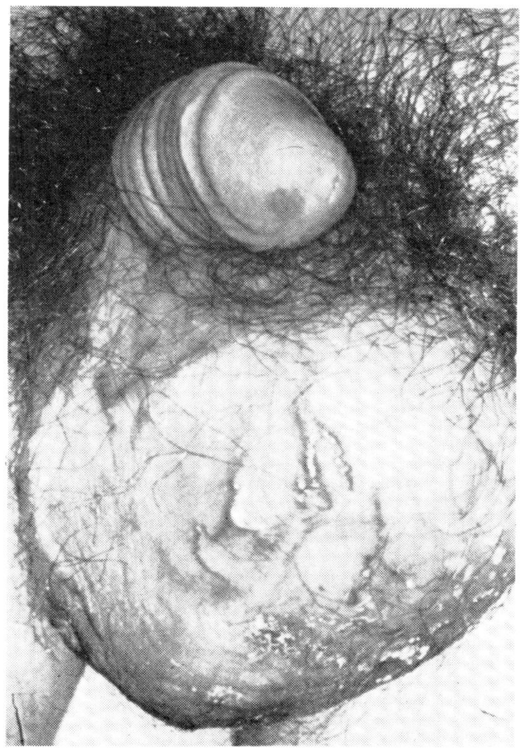

Fig. 4-2. Large testicular tumor with the overlying skin appearing tense and glazed.

senting cartilage or bone may be palpated.

In addition to increased firmness, the affected testis is usually relatively heavy. Testicular "weighing" should be performed by balancing each testicle in the palm of each hand and comparing their weights. Testicular sensation is usually diminished or absent, but in the presence of acute infarction, tenderness may be severe. Gentle squeezing of the testis in an attempt to elicit the presence or absence of normal testicular sensation should be omitted in patients with suspected neoplasia. Manipulation can force tumor cells into either the venous or lymphatic circulation, thereby risking dissemination of the disease.

The presence of a hydrocele has been demonstrated in 5 to 10 per cent of patients with testicular malignant disease. The finding of a hydrocele in a young male patient should arouse suspicion as to possible associated neoplasia. If thorough examination of the testis is prevented by the surrounding fluid within the tunica vaginalis, aspiration should be done and re-examination of the testis performed immediately. Care should be exercised to avoid perforating the tunica albuginea. The hydrocele fluid is usually clear and amber, and when bloody suggests either invasion of the tunica albuginea or infiltration of the epididymis.

The epididymis is usually easily identified separately from the testicular mass. The dense tunica albuginea provides a strong barrier to penetration by the testicular malignant disease and the tumor, therefore, retains the shape of the normal organ. Occasionally, direct extension of the tumor or a superimposed inflammatory reaction may result in the failure to differentiate these structures separately.

The Sign of the Vas (Bailey 1960) can aid in differentiating a testicular neoplasm from an inflammatory lesion of the testis. Inflammatory lesions involving the vas deferens causes it to become thickened; with testicular neoplasms the vas remains normal. These findings refer only to the vas deferens and not to the spermatic cord. The spermatic cord is usually uninvolved unless there is venous or lymphatic extension of the malignant disease. In rare cases, isolated metastatic deposits may be palpable along the spermatic cord. When a testicular tumor becomes larger, the spermatic cord may become bulky due to cremasteric muscle hypertrophy and engorgement of the veins of the pampiniform plexus. Rarely, increased vascularity of the tumor results in an easily palpable spermatic artery.

After the genitalia have been thoroughly examined, a complete physical examination is mandatory. In 14 to 44 per cent of the cases, metastases will have occurred by the time the diagnosis of malignant testicular disease has been established. In examining the patient, careful attention should be given toward detecting the presence or absence of enlarged lymph nodes, especially in the supraclavicular and cervical regions. Although it is more common for the subdiaphragmatic lymph channels to drain into the left supraclavicular lymph nodes, anomalous lymphatic drainage into either the right or both supraclavicular areas can occur. The supraclavicular lymph nodes are best examined with the patient in an upright position.

Inspection and palpation of the breasts for gynecomastia should be performed (Fig. 4-3). Its presence is usually indicative of trophoblastic elements within the tumor with secretion of chorionic gonadotropins. It frequently has a grave prognostic significance. Auscultation and percussion of the chest may reveal evidence of pulmonary metastases which can later be confirmed by chest roentgenograms.

The abdomen should be palpated for abnormal masses, as well as for evidence of visceromegaly. Early lymphatic metastases are usually retro-

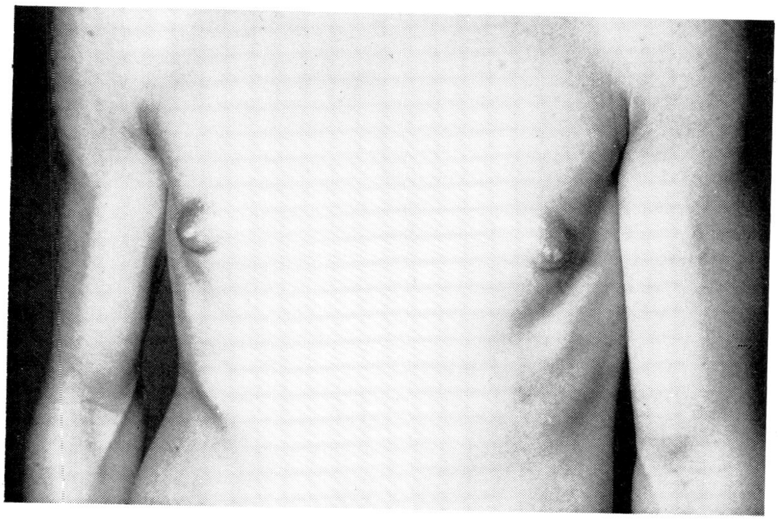

Fig. 4-3. Gynecomastia in a 16 year-old boy with teratocarcinoma of the testis.

peritoneal in position and located on the same side as the affected testis, slightly cephelad to the umbilicus in the angle formed by the renal artery and aorta. The mass is frequently non-tender, round, firm and fixed. Late in the course of the disease, either or both ureters may become obstructed by enlarged lymph nodes. With progressing hydroureteronephrosis, a palpable renal mass may be present. Inspection and palpation of the inguinal areas may reveal nodal metastases. Inguinal lymph node metastases signal local invasion of the overlying scrotal investments by the testicular neoplasm or altered lymphatic drainage, usually the result of previous inguinal or surgical procedures. The presence of such metastases is of prime importance if lymphadenectomy is to be considered as a part of the definitive treatment.

No physical examination is complete without digital examination of the prostate. On occasion, metastases to the testis from an unsuspected prostatic malignancy have been mistaken for a primary testicular tumor. In addition, the findings of either an acute or chronic prostatitis may aid in establishing a diagnosis of epididymitis and help in distinguishing an inflammatory scrotal lesion from a testicular tumor.

DIFFERENTIAL DIAGNOSIS

The accessibility of the scrotum and its contents to the examining fingers should facilitate the physician in establishing a correct diagnosis of testicular malignant disease. However, the fact remains that in over one-fourth of the cases an erroneous diagnosis is made by a physician (Table VIII), resulting in either a delay in treatment or an inappropriate surgical procedure.

Epididymitis or epididymo-orchitis is the most frequent diagnostic error in the cases subsequently proven to be neoplastic. Gordon-Taylor and Wyndham (1947) described a "pseudo-inflammatory" presentation as one of the more common clinical patterns in patients with underlying testicular tumors. Patton et al. (1959) in reviewing 510 cases of testicular tumors treated at Walter Reed Army Hospital found 16.3 per cent had an initial diagnosis of epididymitis. Thompson et al. (1961) in a survey of 178 cases found 19 patients which were mistakenly diagnosed as having epididymo-orchitis. Cohen and Tomskey (1961) found a history of unsuccessful treatment of epididymitis to be the most common presentation of teratocarcinoma and embryonal carcinoma. In Fergusson's (1962) survey of 527 cases of testicular tumors, six per cent were initially diagnosed as epididymo-orchitis. Other authors (Jensen 1952; Seddon 1962; Field 1964; Hosney 1965) have reported similar difficulties in differentiating inflammatory lesions of the epididymis from testicular tumors. The diagnosis of epididymitis is ordinarily not difficult, but it should be made with extreme caution in young men who do not have confirmatory signs and symptoms of urinary tract infection. If the testis cannot be distinguished from the epididymis and pyuria is absent, the diagnosis of epididymitis must remain in doubt. It is better to err on the side of surgical exploration than to allow a tumor to go undetected.

Hydrocele is the second most common mistaken diagnosis for a testicular tumor, being incorrectly made in two to five per cent of patients with testicular malignant disease (Higgins and Arber 1953; Patton et al. 1959; Field 1964). The error often results from failure to aspirate an associated hydrocele and to re-examine the testis immediately after removal of the fluid. Less commonly, a tumor may be of soft consistency and look and feel like a common idiopathic vaginal hydrocele. However, tumors are not translucent and transillumination remains the <u>sine que non</u> for a diagnosis of hydrocele. Occasionally, the parietal layer of a

TABLE VIII

ERRORS IN DIAGNOSIS

Epididymitis	Hematoma
Epididymo-orchitis	Torsion
Hydrocele	Spermatocele
Inguinal Hernia	Varicocele
Hematocele	Gumma

hydrocele sac may become thick, fibrous or partly calcified and may present a perplexing problem in differential diagnosis (Schmitz 1953). In these cases transillumination of the swelling can be difficult, but a past history of repeated aspirations can be helpful. In all suspicious cases, exploration should be carried out forthwith.

Thompson and associates (1961) reported an erroneous diagnosis of inguinal hernia in 10 of 155 patients (6.4 per cent) in whom the testicular lesion was the instigation for medical attention. Other authors have reported similar errors in diagnosis (Williams 1955; Field 1964; Hira 1965). However, this mistaken diagnosis is unlikely to be made when the physician performs a careful and thorough examination of the scrotal and inguinal areas.

Infrequently, a testicular tumor may either be mistaken for testicular torsion or is found in association with torsion at the time of exploration. Smith and Riese (1958) after reviewing the literature concluded that differentiation between torsion and tumor in infants could not be made on the basis of physical examination. Adolescents and adults with torsion of a completely descended testis classically present with an acute onset of severe testicular pain without associated urinary tract signs or symptoms. The pain may be indistinguishable from the pain resulting from hemorrhage or infarction of a tumor. Inspection will frequently reveal the affected testis to lie higher in the scrotum than its contralateral mate. The acute swelling frequently prevents the testis and epididymis to be palpated separately. However, treatment for each disease requires immediate surgical intervention.

Rarely, a hematocele or hematoma may mimic a testicular tumor. These lesions are frequently associated with trauma and necessitate excluding rupture of the tunica albuginea (Pohl et al. 1968). Early surgical intervention is usually the preferred treatment, especially if the differential diagnosis includes an underlying testicular tumor.

On occasion, a tumor has been mistaken for a spermatocele. A spermatocele is characteristically an extravaginal cystic mass communicating with the rete testis and is located behind and above the testis. It, like a hydrocele, is translucent and should not be confused with a tumor.

Varicocele ordinarily should present no problem in diagnosis. It results from dilatation of the pampiniform plexus of the spermatic cord and may be found in 10 per cent of the male population (Johnson et al. 1970). Palpation in the upright position reveals engorgement of the veins which collapse in the Trendelenburg position.

Gumma of the testis is now very rare. There is no way of distinguishing it from a tumor and a positive serology should not be relied upon to aid in the diagnosis. In any event, a gummatous testicle is best removed (Walton 1954).

CHAPTER 5

LABORATORY AND RADIOLOGICAL INVESTIGATION

by

Douglas E. Johnson

The diagnosis of a testicular tumor may be suspected on clinical findings, but it can only be proven by careful histologic examination of the excised tissue. Laboratory and radiographic investigations serve chiefly as ancillary studies for determining the extent of the disease and provide additional means for more accurately assigning a clinical stage. The importance of clinical staging, however, cannot be overemphasized, since it is this knowledge which allows the planning of appropriate treatment and serves as a guide for prognosis.

LABORATORY STUDIES

The usual routine laboratory screening procedures should be performed in all patients suspected of having a testicular tumor. These studies should include a complete blood count, urinalysis and a Simultaneous Multiple Analysis - 12/60 (Technicon Corporation, Tarrytown, New York). Anemia is seldom present until late in the course of the disease when widespread metastases have occurred. Urinalysis is of no aid in diagnosis, but the presence of pyuria may help to confirm the diagnosis of an inflammatory scrotal swelling (Kaufman 1967). The Simultaneous Multiple Analysis may detect early or occult lesions in the viscera or bones and provides necessary information about the patient's general medical condition.

Urinary Gonadotropins

The usefulness of urinary gonadotropin assays for diagnostic and prognostic purposes in patients with testicular tumors has been clouded by controversy and confusion since Zondek (1937) reported finding gonadotropins in the urine of a patient with testicular cancer. The failure to distinguish between pituitary and chorionic gonadotropins, as well as the lack of uniformity and standardization among assay procedures and an overinterpretation of results, has contributed to the many conflicting reports in the literature (Moore 1950; Ghormley and Jacek 1954; Hurley 1962; Symington and Wallace 1964).

Elevated pituitary gonadotropin excretion (follicle-stimulating hormone, FSH and interstitial-cell stimulating hormone, ICSH) has been observed frequently in patients with malignant testicular disease (Hamburger et al. 1936; Hamburger 1941; Wyndham 1948; Moore 1951; Umiker 1954; Hurley 1962; Notter and Ranudd 1964). This finding has never been adequately explained, but may result from a reduced production of androgens secondary to tumor growth in the testicle (Hamburger 1958), a reduction of functional tissue after orchiectomy (Melicow 1955; Notter and Ranudd 1964) or radiation damage to the remaining testis (Garvin 1962). Production of pituitary-like hormones within testicular tumors has not been demonstrated. An elevation of urinary pituitary gonadotropins has no prognostic significance (Notter and Ranudd 1964; Nielsen 1953).

Chorionic gonadotropin is produced only in chorionic epithelial cells occurring in trophoblastic and placental tissue (pregnancy), placental neoplasms and testicular tumors. The site of origin for chorionic gonadotropin in testicular tumors is thought to be the syncytiotrophoblastic and the cytotrophoblastic cells which have a highly developed endoplasmic reticulum (Pierce and Midgley 1963). The presence of chorionic gonadotropin in the urine may be taken as positive proof of the existence of chorionic elements within the testicular tumor, regardless of the ability to demonstrate them histologically (Nishimura et al. 1964; Hobson 1965; Gangai 1965).

An elevated chorionic gonadotropin titer on admission is usually an ominous sign (Kurohara et al. 1968; Boctor et al. 1969). A persistent elevation following orchiectomy or the subsequent demonstration of a rising titer on serial examinations suggests active metastatic disease and is also a poor prognostic sign (Shively 1950; Dixon and Moore 1953; Johnson 1957; Krantz et al. 1965; Wilson and Woodhead 1972).

In a review of 140 patients with testicular carcinoma studied by Wilson and Woodhead (1972) elevated urinary gonadotropins were demonstrated in 30 per cent of the patients at some point during their clinical course. Of these, 63 per cent subsequently died or were proven to have metastatic disease. However, only 18 per cent of those patients without elevation of urinary gonadotropin levels died or subsequently developed metastasis, emphasizing the prognostic and therapeutic significance of this examination.

A urine or serum specimen should be collected for a chorionic gonadotropin assay prior to exploration and orchiectomy in every patient suspected of harboring a testicular tumor. It is mandatory that the assay reflect only the presence of chorionic gonadotropins. In the past, examinations have frequently failed to distinguish between pituitary and chorionic gonadotropins, accounting for the conflicting conclusions.

An immunoassay or bioassay determination may be performed, but in either case the specimen should be sent to a laboratory that has the capabilities to perform an accurate, quantitative examination.* For either determination, a 100 milliliter aliquot of a 24-hour urine specimen or four milliliters of serum is sufficient. The urine specimen should have an adjusted pH in the range of 2-3. Serial determinations should similarly be performed at three month intervals in all patients with testicular tumors. The persistence of chorionic gonadotropin titers after completion of conventional therapy or the documentation of a rising titer on serial examinations dictates the institution of appropriate chemotherapeutic agents even though metastatic disease may not be apparent.

Alpha-Fetoprotein

Alpha-1 fetoprotein, a specific fetal globulin which is absent from the sera of adults and children, has been found in 21 to 43 per cent of patients with testicular tumors (Al-Sarraf et al. 1972; Merrin et al. 1973). Its importance as a biological marker lies in (1) assessing the results of therapy, (2) detecting the development of recurrences and (3) monitoring the progress

*Bio-Science Laboratories, 7600 Tyrone Avenue, Van Nuys, California, 91405

of the disease (Smith 1971; Kithier et al. 1972; Merrin et al. 1973; Abelev 1973; Talerman and Haije 1974; Bourgeaux et al. 1974).

Alpha-fetoprotein was first demonstrated as a specific constituent of normal human fetal serum by Bergstrand and Czar in 1956. In the human embryo, serum fetoprotein reaches its maximum concentration of about 3000 mg/l at about 12 to 13 weeks of gestation and then its level declines slowly until birth, when an average level of 55 mg/l is reached (Talerman and Haije 1974). After birth alpha-fetoprotein disappears from the serum. Abelev et al. (1963) first reported the existence of a similar protein in adult mice with primary hepatoma; Tatarinov (1966) confirmed this finding in adult humans with primary hepatoma and other researchers subsequently found the same globulin in patients with germ cell neoplasms (Hull et al. 1969; Mawas et al. 1971; Smith and O'Neill 1971).

Alpha-fetoprotein determinations have been found to be elevated in 15 of 115 patients (12 per cent) with germ cell tumors of the testes evaluated at Anderson Hospital (Bracken et al. 1975). The determinations were negative in all patients with seminoma (26 patients) and teratoma (9 patients), as well as for all patients with teratocarcinoma (6 patients) and embryonal carcinoma (7 patients) in whom the malignant disease was confined to the testis. Negative determinations were likewise present in 33 patients with embryonal carcinoma, 17 patients with teratocarcinoma and 2 patients with choriocarcinoma in whom metastatic disease was present. In the remaining 15 patients with metastatic embryonal carcinoma or teratocarcinoma serial determinations closely parallel the status of disease during and after therapy. Alpha-fetoprotein determinations represent an additional biological marker which can be used when elevated to assess the results of therapy and detect early recurrent disease.

Serum LDH

Serum lactic dehydrogenase (LDH) activity is frequently elevated in patients with malignant neoplastic disease, presumably related in part to the necrosis of tissue. In studying 150 cases with various malignant diseases, Zondag (1964) found a typical serum enzyme pattern with elevated LDH activity in the middle fraction. A special serum LDH-isoenzyme pattern with high activity in LD1 and LD2 fractions was observed in patients with testicular tumors. Additional investigations will be necessary to ascertain the value of these findings in the diagnosis and follow-up examinations of malignant testicular tumors.

Additional Studies

Attempts to find other specific laboratory studies to aid in the diagnosis of testicular malignant disease have not been successful. An increased sedimentation rate is non-specific and of little help. Investigation of urinary lactic acid dehydrogenase activity has shown it to be non-specific for all types of genitourinary disease. Ramkissoon et al. (1964) studied 44 patients with urinary tract symptoms and reported minimal elevation of urinary lactic acid dehydrogenase in one patient with a seminoma of the testis. Schmidt (1966) in performing similar determinations in 133 patients with urinary tract disease, found no increased LDH activity in the one patient with a testicular tumor.

Roswit et al. (1950) studied the possible role of radioactive phosphorus (P^{32}) as an aid in the diagnosis of testicular tumors and concluded that it might have value as an adjunct to present diagnostic methods. However, two errors in diagnoses were reported in the six patients evaluated for testicular enlargements.

Acevedo et al. (1973) have measured urinary excretion of nonesterified cholesterol (NEC) in 19 cases of testicular seminoma and eight patients with either choriocarcinoma, teratocarcinoma or embryonal carcinoma. All cases of seminoma revealed a normal urinary excretion of NEC regardless of the state of the disease, whereas a remarkable correlation between hyperexcretion of NEC and the presence of the other cell types was documented. In addition, the urinary excretion of NEC appeared to correlate with the effects of therapy and the clinical course of the disease in these latter cases. Unfortunately, this test is not specific for testicular neoplasms since it has been shown to be elevated in other conditions, i. e., prostatic hyperplasia, prostatic carcinoma, ovarian tumors, etc. Its value in diagnosis and monitoring the course of nonseminomatous testicular tumors must await further evaluation.

RADIOLOGICAL PROCEDURES

The radiological procedures considered essential for determining the extent of disease in patients with testicular tumors and which should be performed in all cases include: (1) chest roentgenograms, (2) excretory urograms and, (3) bilateral pedal lymphangiograms. In selected instances, inferior venacavography, selective renal venography and skeletal surveys may be required to complete the evaluation prior to planning therapy.

Chest Roentgenograms

A chest X-ray with supplemental lateral views included should be the initial radiographic procedure performed on every patient. Examination of the mediastinum may reveal lymph borne metastases. Solitary or multiple parenchymal lesions are not infrequently demonstrated (Figs. 5-1 and 5-2.) A round, dense and well demarcated shadow is characteristic. The roundness of these pulmonary lesions has been attributed to hematogenous spread with the expanding lesions maintaining the outline of the vein lumens in which their growth began (Dean 1951). Routine chest laminography is not required. In 76 patients with testicular malignancy who had a routine posteroanterior and lateral roentgenogram of the chest followed by chest laminography, laminograms failed to detect a single metastatic lesion not found on the routine chest X-ray (Woodhead et al. 1968). Chest laminography, however, may aid in clarifying the nature of suspicious or indistinct pulmonary lesions.

Excretory Urograms

Excretory urograms provide a safe and simple means for studying the retroperitoneal areas. Periaortic and perirenal lymph node involvement may be diagnosed by displacement or obstruction of the kidneys or ureters (Fig. 5-3). Serial examinations performed during subsequent visits are useful for evaluating the results of therapy or in detecting recurrence of disease.

Lymphangiography

The importance of this examination is discussed in detail in Chapter 4 by Doctors Wallace and Jing. Although lymphangiography has not gained universal acceptance as a routine diagnostic examination in cases of testicular malignant disease, evaluation of the procedure at Anderson Hospital has shown it to be extremely accurate in detecting metastatic spread.

Cavography

Inferior venacavography (Figs. 5-4 and 5-5) first introduced by dos

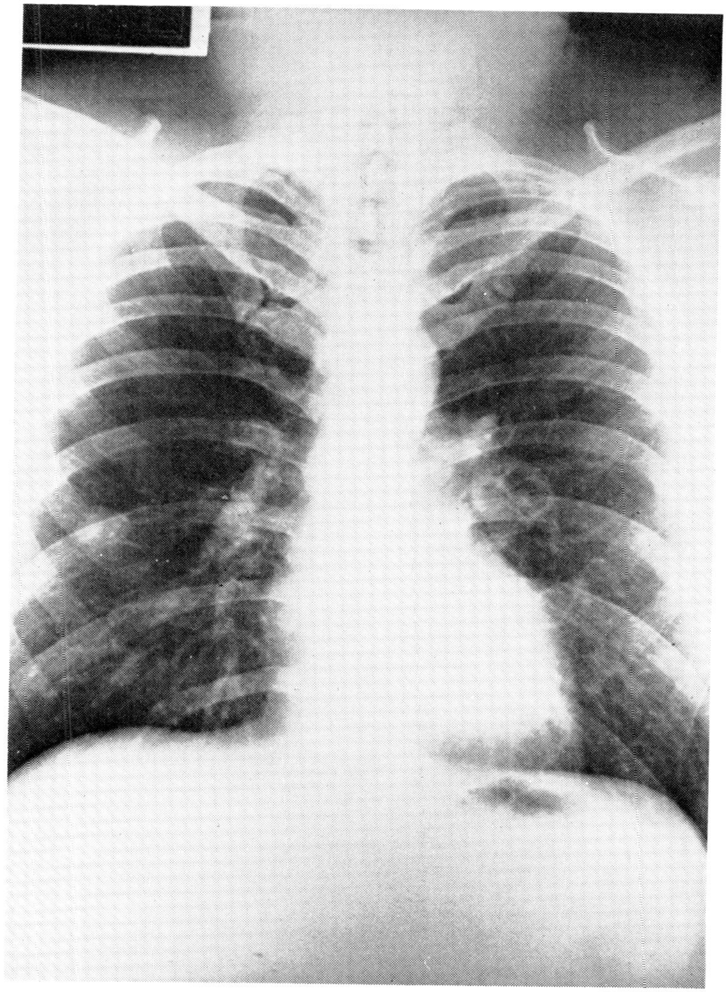

Fig. 5-1A. Solitary metastasis in the right lung.

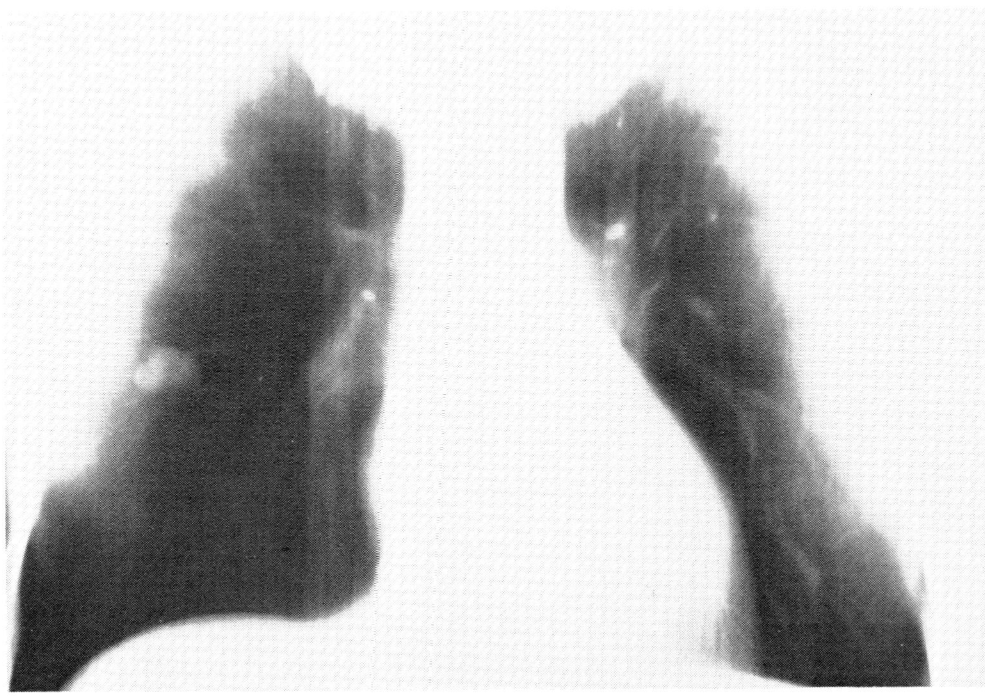

Fig. 5-1B. Chest laminography failed to demonstrate other pulmonary lesions.

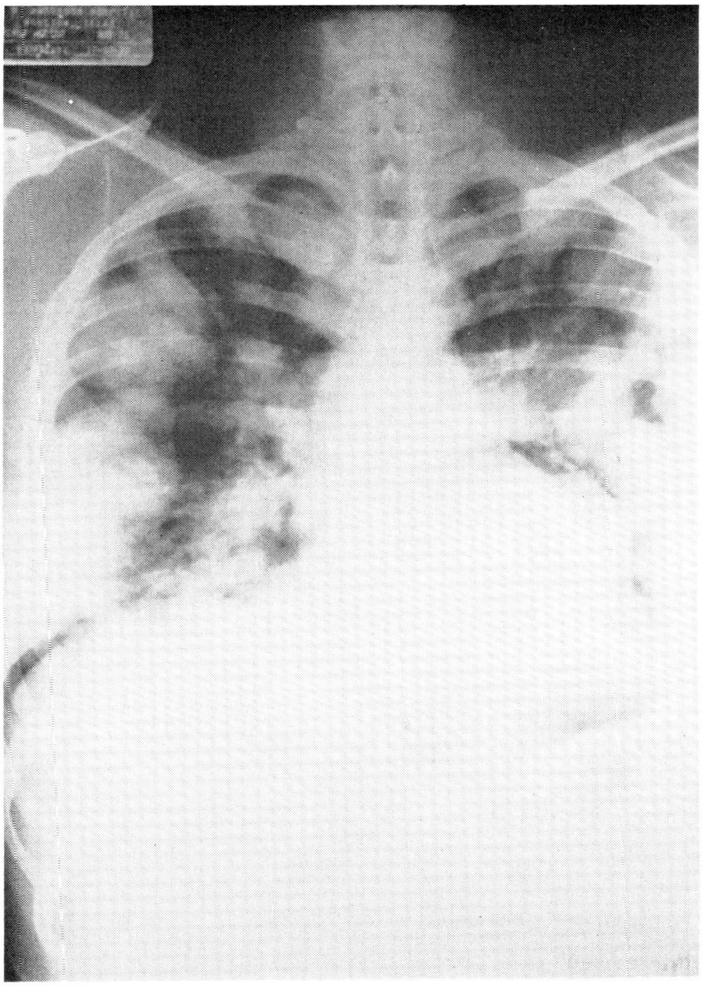

Fig. 5-2A. Multiple parenchymal lesions present on initial chest x-ray in a 25 year-old male presenting with a testicular mass.

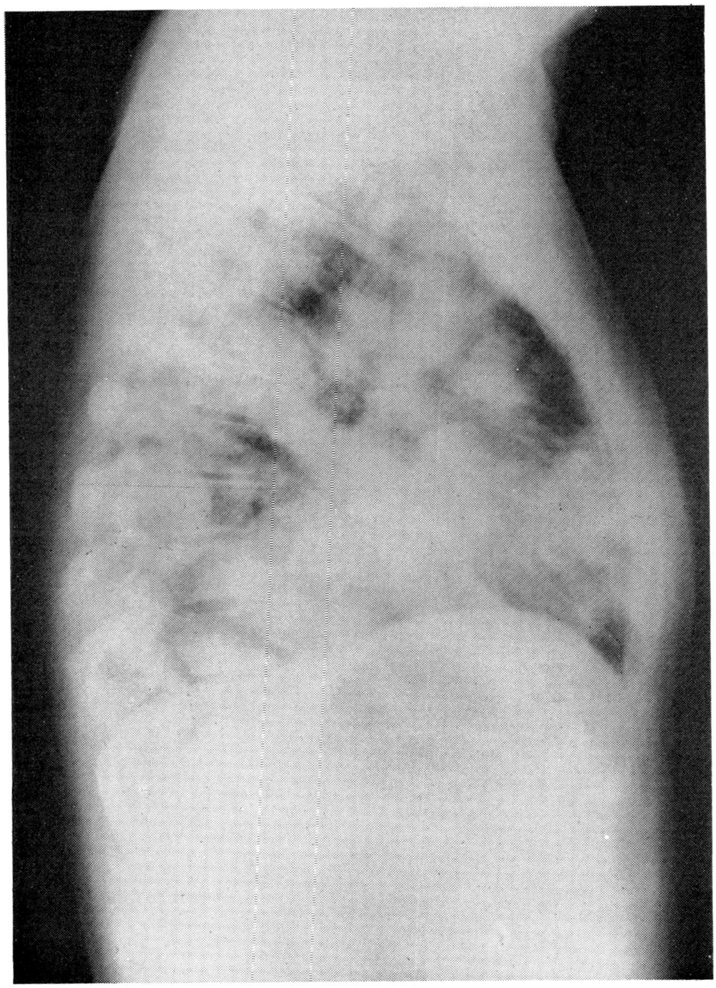

Fig. 5-2B. Multiple parenchymal lesions present on initial chest x-ray in a 25 year-old male presenting with a testicular mass.

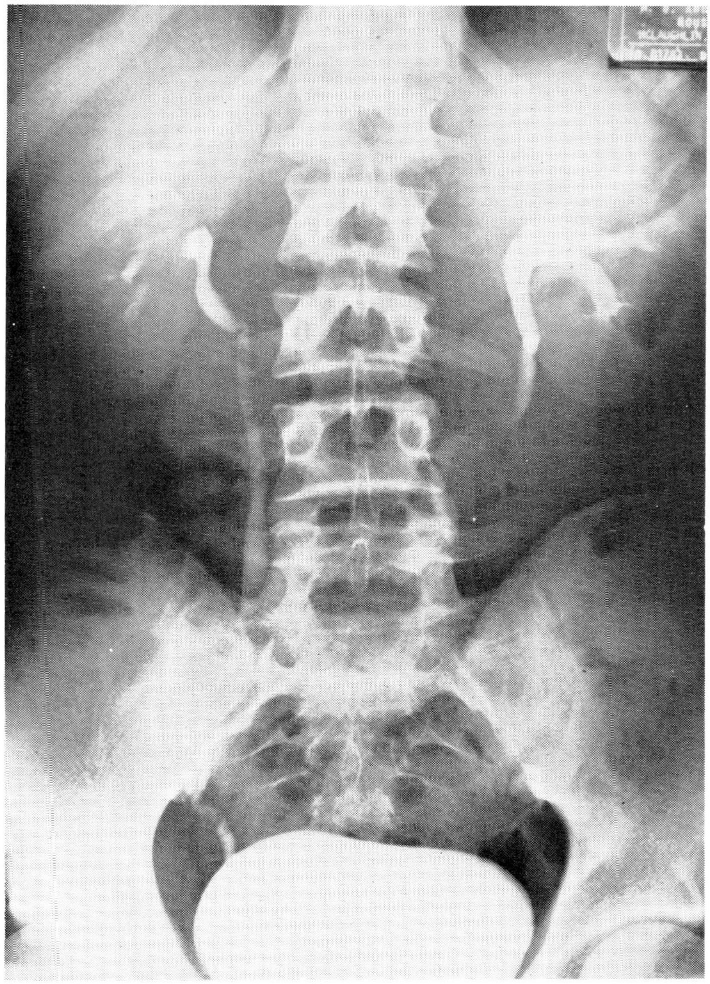

Fig. 5-3. Left ureteral deviation due to enlarged retroperitoneal lymph nodes in a patient with embryonal carcinoma of the testis.

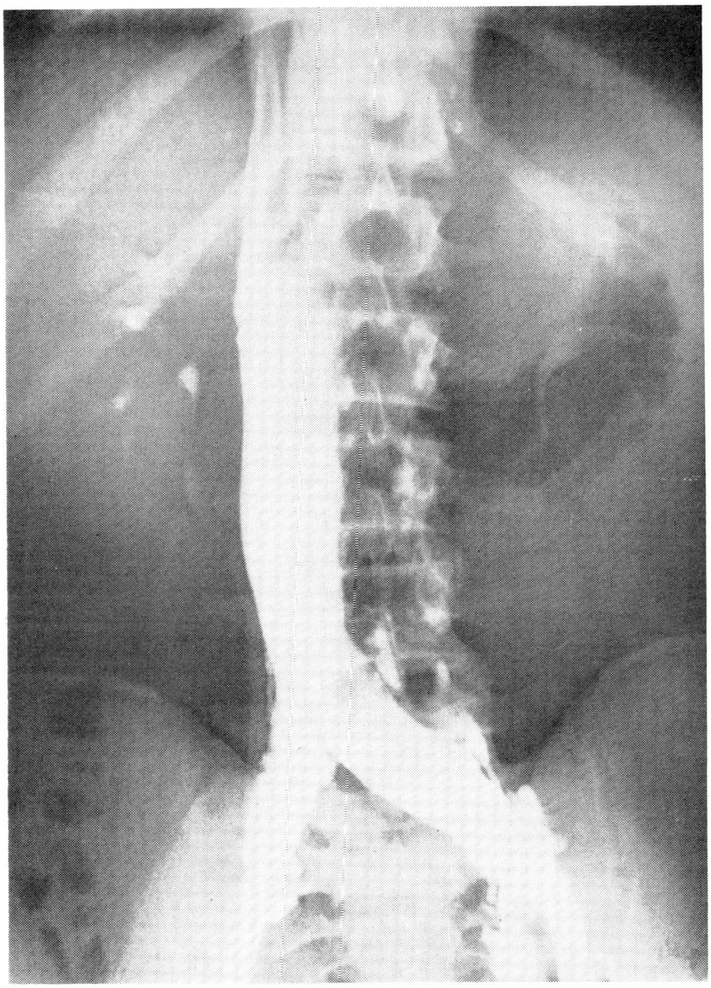

Fig. 5-4. Normal inferior venacavogram.

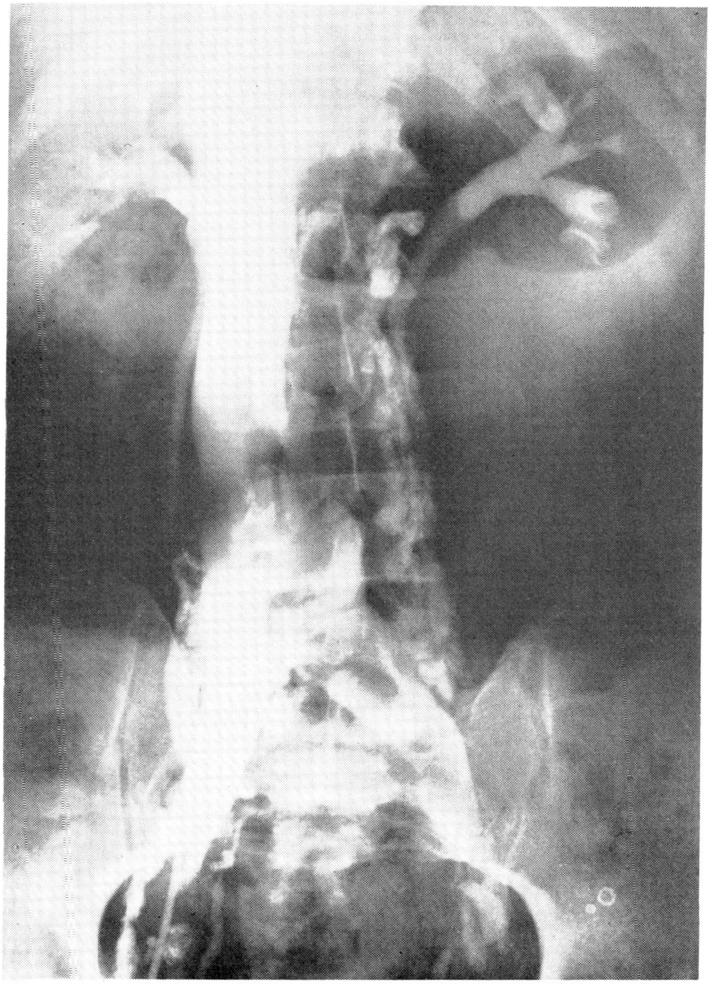

Fig. 5-5. Large retroperitoneal mass compressing inferior vena cava.

Santos (1935) has received only limited application in the evaluation of patients with malignant testicular disease. Kaufman and Burke (1956) and Kaufman et al. (1956) have emphasized its value in detecting retroperitoneal lymph node metastases from testicular tumors. They concluded that the demonstration of gross deformity or compression of the inferior vena cava by retroperitoneal lymph node metastases negates the performance of radical retroperitoneal lymph node dissection. Lockhart et al. (1960) recommended its routine use in all cases of testis tumors, believing that he could diagnose many adenopathies which otherwise could not be palpated or in which other radiographic procedures did not yield clear results. Ekman et al. (1965) reported its use in 31 cases of testis tumors; in 11 instances positive findings were noted and as a rule they considered these cases inoperable. In the two cases with abnormal venacavograms that underwent surgical exploration, the disease was considered inoperable. In twenty cases in whom negative reports were noted, 19 underwent lymphadenectomy and in 12 cases positive lymph nodes were subsequently proven on histologic examination. It was their impression that the procedure was useful in assessing operability but that it did not increase the possibility of determining the presence of small metastases.

Isotope scans

The recent introduction of radionucleotide lymph scanning has demonstrated ability to localize areas of metastatic disease from testicular carcinoma. Bailey et al. (1973) studied 27 consecutive patients with testicular carcinoma seen at Walter Reed Army Medical Center between August 1, 1971 and August 1, 1972 and concluded that gallium-67 citrate scans were more accurate than lymphangiography in detecting metastatic spread. Glassburn et al. (1972) reporting on the use of 198AU abdominal lymph scans have likewise demonstrated significant correlation between lymph node scans and biopsy or lymphangiographic findings. Our experience, however, suggests that at present these studies are less reliable than routine lymphangiography and require metastatic foci in excess of 2 cm diameter for localization. These studies do have practical application whenever lymphangiography is contraindicated due to iodine allergy, severe pulmonary insufficiency, unsuccessful attempts at lymphangiography or prior injury, trauma or disease of the lower extremities.

CHAPTER 6

TESTICULAR MALIGNANCIES AND THE LYMPHATIC SYSTEM

by

Sidney Wallace and Bao-Shan Jing

It is essential to have a thorough knowledge of the lymphatic system, the lymphatic channels, and the lymph nodes to adequately manage patients with testicular malignant disease (Rouviere 1938; Ruszniak et al. 1960; Yoffey and Courtice 1970). The opacification of the lymphatic system as a clinical procedure was introduced by Hudack and McMasters (1932). Following an intradermal injection of a vital blue dye, the visualization and eventual clearing of the dye, as well as the filling of the dermal and subcutaneous lymphatics was interpreted as a manifestation of the function of the lymphatic system. Servelle and Deysson (1951) injected percutaneously a radiopaque water-based iodine containing contrast material into dilated dermal lymphatic channels in patients with chylous edema. Kinmouth (1952) utilized lymphangiography as it is performed presently, by injecting intradermally a vital dye, cannulating a subcutaneous lymphatic and injecting intralymphatically a water-based radiopaque contrast material for the evaluation of edema of the lower extremities. Bruun and Engeset (1956) introduced an oil-based radiopaque agent into a fistulous tract which was contiguous with the lymphatic system opacifying the deeper lymphatics and nodes. In 1959, Shanbrom and Zheutlin, by intranodal injection of radiopaque media, opacified adjacent lymphatics and nodes. Hreschyshyn and Sheehan in 1960 employed the intralymphatic injection of an oil-based contrast material, Ethiodol, for the opacification of lymphatic channels and nodes. Wallace et al. (1961) further refined this procedure and applied the technique to a wide range of studies of lymphatic dynamics and nodal abnormalities.

TECHNIQUE : PEDAL LYMPHANGIOGRAPHY

The method to be described is a modification of Kinmouth's basic technique (Kinmouth 1952; Hreschyshyn and Sheehan 1961; Jackson et al. 1961; Wallace et al. 1961; Arvay and Picard 1964; Ruttiman and Del Buono 1964; Fuchs 1965; Maddison 1967; Tong 1969; Jing and Gianturco 1970). Alpha zurine 2G or Patent Blue V, 0.25 to 0.5 mg., is injected intradermally in the first interdigital web space on the dorsum of each foot (Fig. 6-1A). In the presence of edema, multiple interdigital web spaces are injected. The intradermal injection allows for almost immediate visualization of the intradermal lymphatics since these vessels are plentiful in the dermis. The absence of valves in these vessels allows for multidirectional flow with rapid opacification of the subcutaneous lymphatics. The centripetal flow in the subcutaneous channels is directed by the valves. A small longitudinal incision, 1.5 cm to 2 cm in length, is made approximately 5 cm proximal to the site of the intradermal injection. When a subcutaneous lymphatic containing the blue dye is visible through the skin, the incision can be made paralleling this vessel (Fig. 6-1B). A superficial lymphatic, immediately subcutaneous in position, is identified and dissected free of the surrounding tissue. A ligature placed proximally along the lymphatic temporarily occludes the vessel merely by elevating it. "Milking" action from the site of the intradermal injection toward the isolated channel maximally distends the lymphatic. The lymphatic is cannulated with a fine gauge needle, 27 or 30 gauge (Figs. 6-1C and 6-1D). Ethiodol, an ethylester of poppyseed oil containing 37 per cent iodine, is injected under low and constant pressure over approximately 1 to 1-1/2 hours. The injection can be accomplished in many ways utilizing an automatic injector, a screw clamp injector or gravitational pressure employing lead weights placed on the barrel of the syringe. Gravitational pressure is currently utilized in our department (Fig. 6-1E) (Dolan and Moore 1962; Jing and Gianturco 1970).

In adults, 6 to 10 ml of contrast material are required in each lower extremity to opacify the complete lymphatic drainage system to the level of the thoracic duct. The amount of radiopaque media necessary to opacify the lymphatic system should be kept to a minimum without, however, sacrificing the completeness of the opacification of the lymphatics and nodes. Radiographs taken during the injection will help to determine the amount of contrast media necessary. Any alteration in lymphatic dynamics, particularly lymphatico-venous anastomoses, can be appreciated only during the injection phase and may necessitate termination of the examination to minimize complications.

Examinations in children can be undertaken at almost any age; the youngest child in our series was 5 months of age. General anesthesia or deep analgesia are invariably necessary in children below 8 to 10 years of age. The feet are immobilized by taping them to a sand bag. The examination must be carefully monitored by fluoroscopy, image intensification or frequent radiographs, and the study should be terminated once the cisterna chyli is opacified. In a child, as little as 1.5 to 2 ml injected into each lower extremity may be adequate.

Roentgenograms are taken at the completion of the injection to demonstrate the lymphatic pathways (Figs. 6-2A and 6-2B). The patient should remain supine throughout the procedure for better visualization of the thoracic duct.

If the lymphatic channels are incompletely visualized the patient is asked to ambulate for 15 to 30 minutes and is then re-examined by a radiograph of the abdomen. The contrast material initially remaining in the lymphatics of the lower extremities will have traversed into the lymphatics of the retroperitoneal area as well as the thoracic duct. The radiopaque media usually leaves the vessels within 2 to 4 hours after the completion of the injection. As a matter of convenience, repeat radiographs are done in 24 hours to evaluate the lymph nodes (Figs. 6-2C and 6-2D). Normally, the nodes may be demonstrable for at least 4 weeks but may remain opacified for as long as 7 years. Roentgenograms for the observation of changes during this period may be obtained without further injection. Repeat examinations may be necessary and have been performed as many as 5 times on the same patient over a period of 8 years with no observable alteration in the lymphatic system attributable to the procedure.

The routine radiographic sequence includes: (1) examination of the lower extremities; (2) anteroposterior, lateral, and both obliques of the pelvis

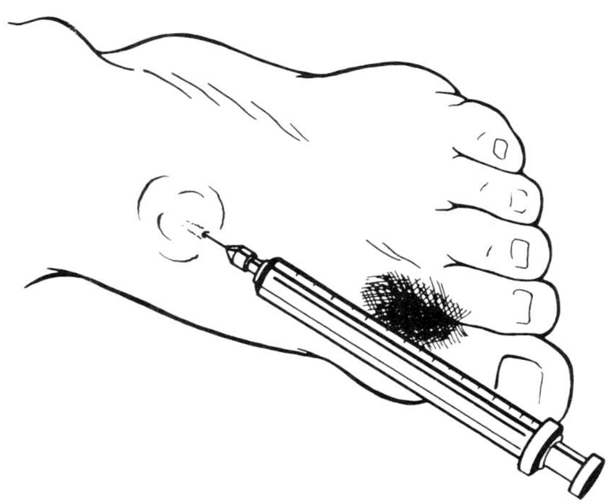

Fig. 6-1A. Technique. Particulate blue dye is injected intradermally into the lst interdigital web space. A large wheal of local anesthetic agent is made on the dorsum of the foot.

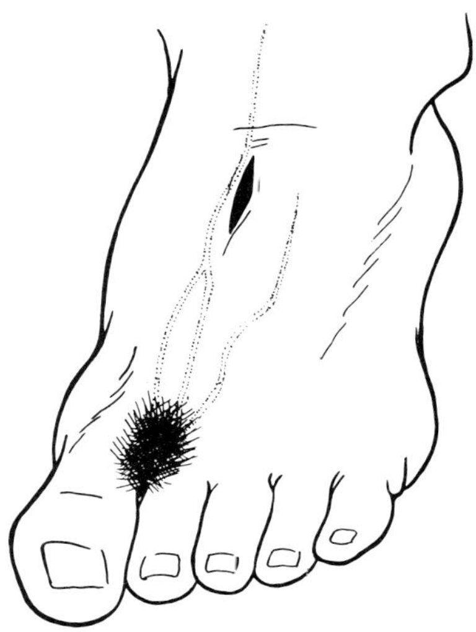

Fig. 6-1B. Technique. The incision parallels the lymphatic channels.

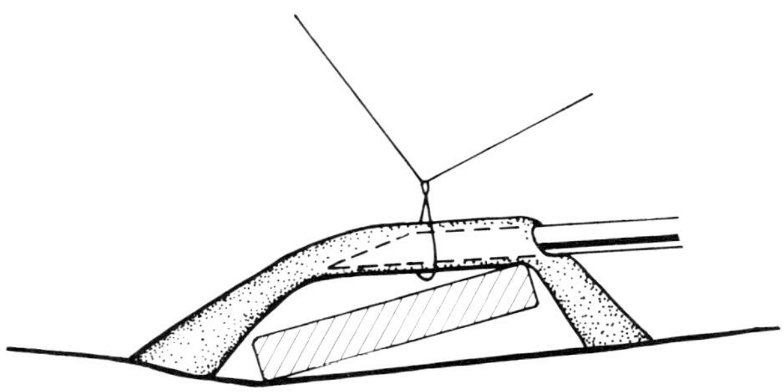

Fig. 6-1C. Technique. Cannulation of the lymphatic.

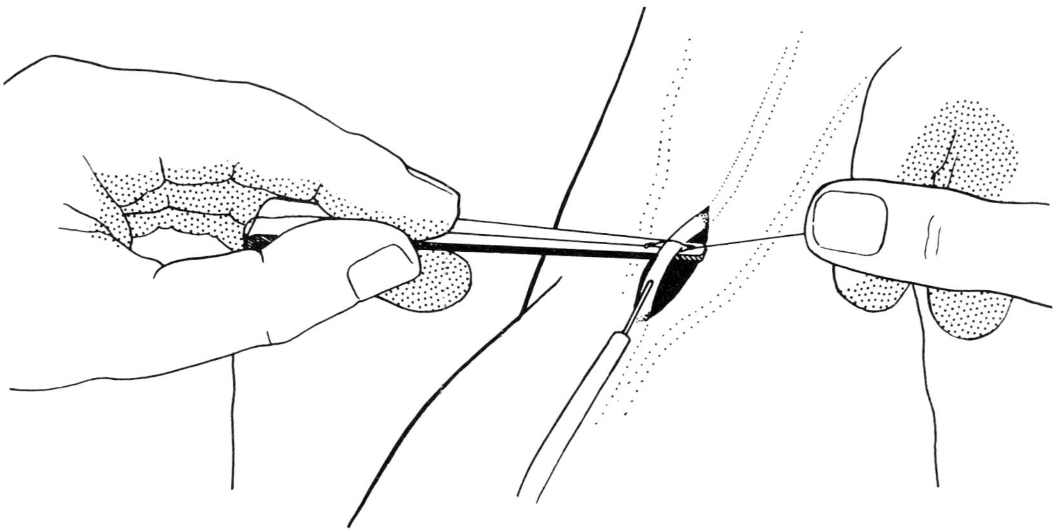

Fig. 6-1D. Technique. The needle is secured by a ligature.

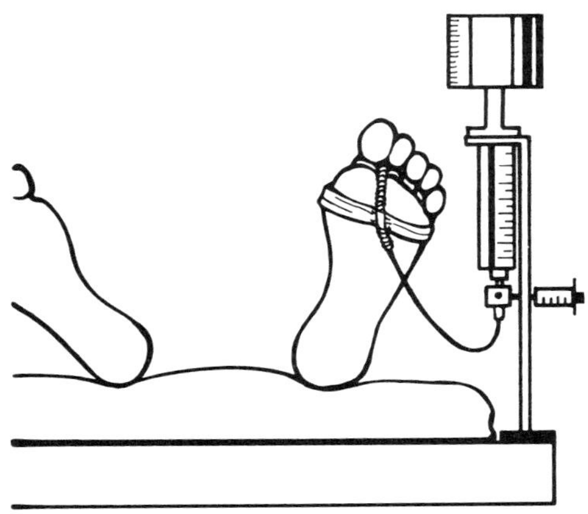

Fig. 6-1E. Technique. Gravitation pressure injection (Dolan & Moore 1962; Jing & Gianturco 1970).

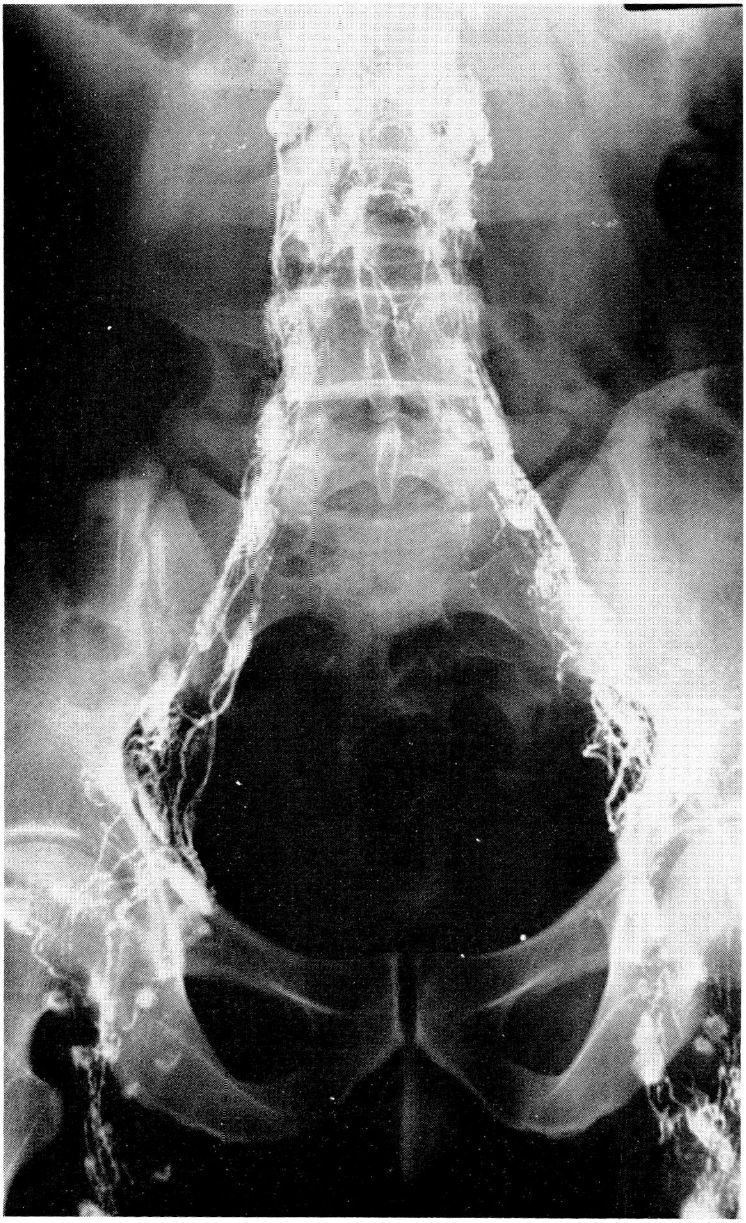

Fig. 6-2A. Normal lymphangiogram. Lymphatic Phase - anteroposterior projection.

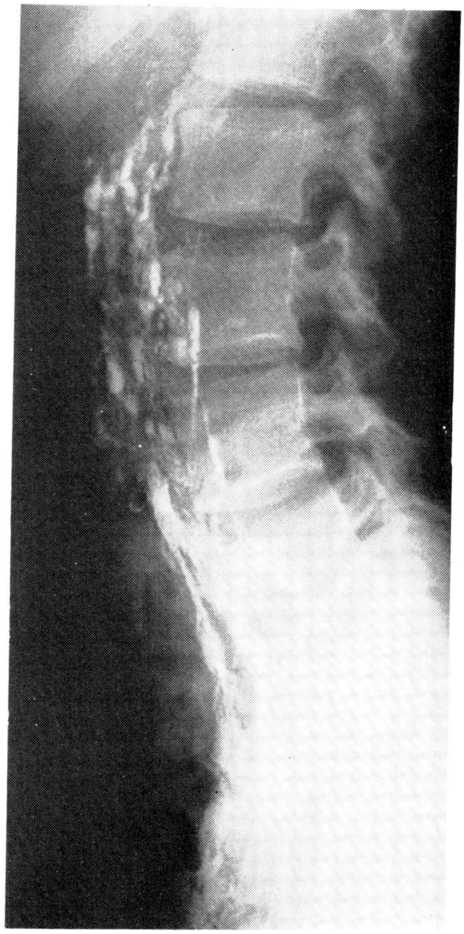

Fig. 6-2B. Normal lymphangiogram. Lymphatic Phase - lateral projection.

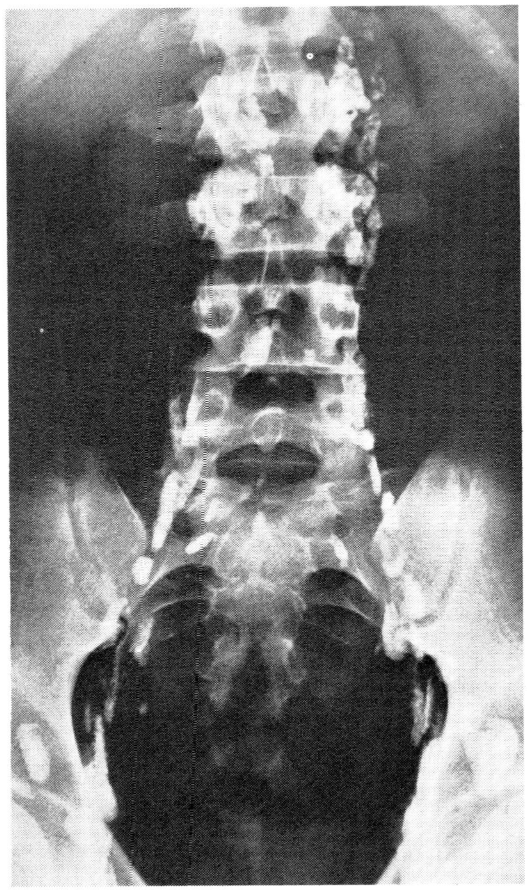

Fig. 6-2C. Normal lymphangiogram. Nodal Phase - anteroposterior projection.

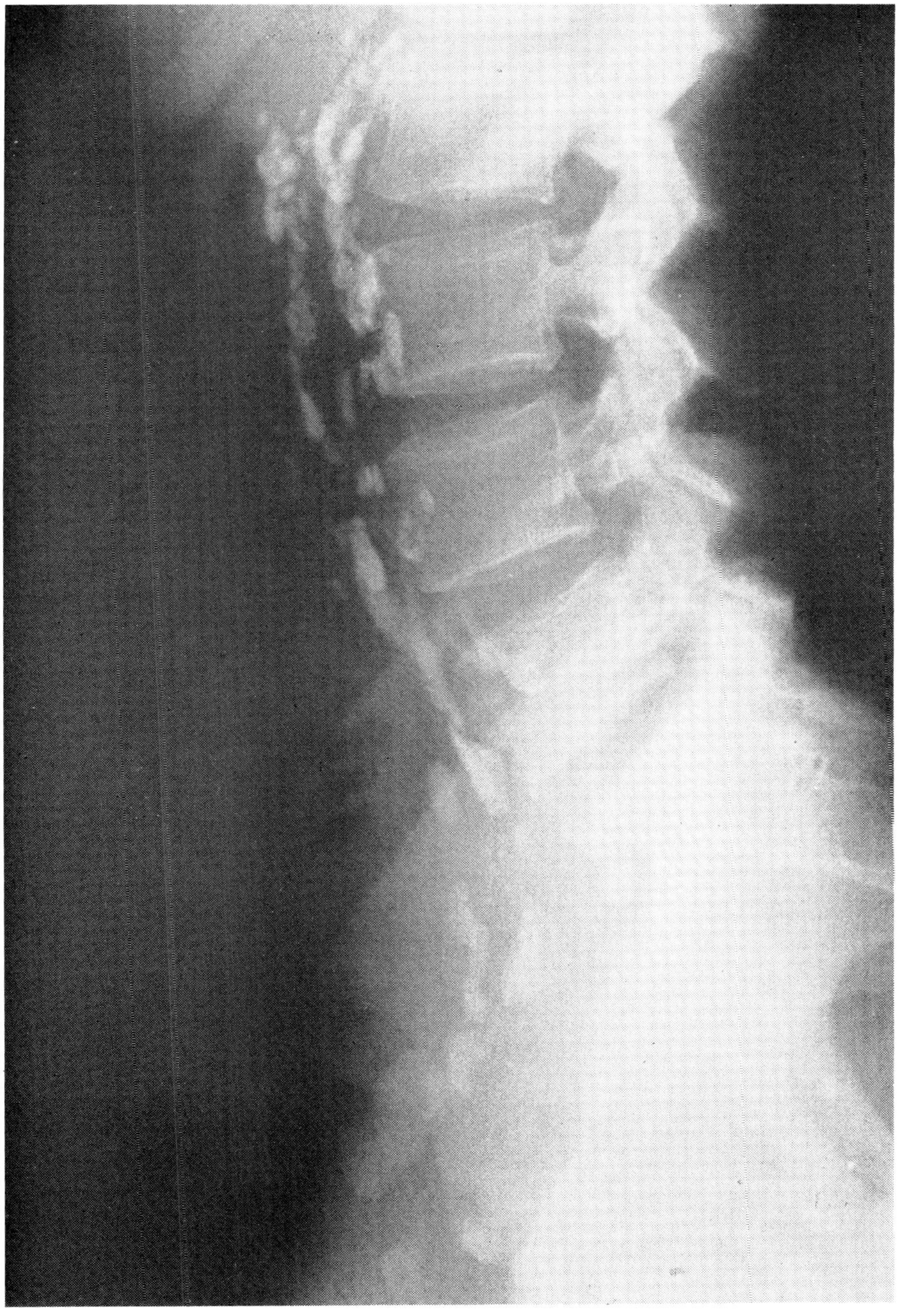

Fig. 6-2D. Normal lymphangiogram. Nodal Phase - lateral projection.

and abdomen; and (3) anteroposterior and lateral supine views of the chest. Multiple projections provide a three dimensional picture of the lymphatics and nodes. Tomography, in selected instances, may add significant informa- (De Roo 1964). A technically adequate examination is essential for proper interpretation.

NORMAL LYMPHATIC PATHWAYS AND NODES

The lymphatic pathways generally parallel the blood vessels. In the lower extremities, the superficial lymphatics follow the greater and lesser saphenous veins in the anterior and posterior compartments, respectively. The lymphatics of the anterior compartment are demonstrated following the injection of the lymphatics on the dorsum of the foot. The lymphatics of the posterior and deep compartment may be opacified by the injection of a superficial lymphatic on the lateral aspect of the heel or a deep perivascular lymphatic posterior to the medial malleolus adjacent to the posterior tibial artery. Occasionally, both anterior and posterior compartments may be visualized by the injection of a lymphatic on the dorsum of the foot due to a congenital variant.

The lymphatics throughout the lower extremities are of fine caliber and increase slightly in size beyond the inguinal area. The presence of valves is more obvious in the pelvis, producing a definite beaded appearance. The iliac channels are divided into three primary pathways, medial, middle, and lateral, which are best delineated in the oblique projections of the pelvis (Herman et al. 1964). Internal iliac lymphatics and nodes may at times be opacified but are usually incompletely filled. At the upper level of the sacrum, there is intercommunication of the lymphatics from each iliac area making up the para-aortic or retroperitoneal lymphatic plexus. These lumbar pathways join with the gastrointestinal trunk to form the cisterna chyli between L-2 and T-10 where it continues as the thoracic duct. Failure to demonstrate gastrointestinal and renal lymphatics is due to the centripetal flow in these channels to the thoracic duct.

The thoracic duct, the major lymphatic collecting channel, was described by Bartel in 1909 as originating from the junction of the lumbar and gastrointestinal trunk to form the cisterna at L-2 to T-10 (Figs. 6-3A, 6-3B, 6-3C and 6-3D). It then traverses along the thoracic spine crossing toward the left at T-5 to empty into the left subclavian vein at the venous angle. This description, however, is found in slightly less than 50 per cent of the patients (Ruszniak et al. 1960). Numerous anatomical variations of the thoracic duct are present, allowing for the opacification of mediastinal, hilar, paratracheal, supraclavicular, cervical, and axillary lymphatics and nodes (Rouviere 1938; Celis et al. 1956; Servelle 1963; Nusbaum et al. 1964; Wallace 1968). To and fro lymphatics from the thoracic duct allow filling of the mediastinal nodes. A right-sided lymphatic trunk, as a branch of the main thoracic duct, explains the perfusion of hilar, anterior mediastinal, and right supraclavicular nodes as part of the normal distribution (Figs. 6-3E and 6-3F). The persistence of a double thoracic duct, as well as the many variations are easily explained by the progression of events in the embryology of the major collecting trunk.

TECHNIQUE: TESTICULAR LYMPHANGIOGRAPHY

Opacification of the testicular lymphatic drainage can be accomplished by an intratesticular or intralymphatic approach (Sterns and Gordon 1960; Busch and Sayegh 1963; Brizzi et al. 1965; Busch et al. 1965; Cook et al. 1965; Chiappa et al. 1966; Leducq et al. 1966; Sayegh et al. 1966; Walqvist et al.

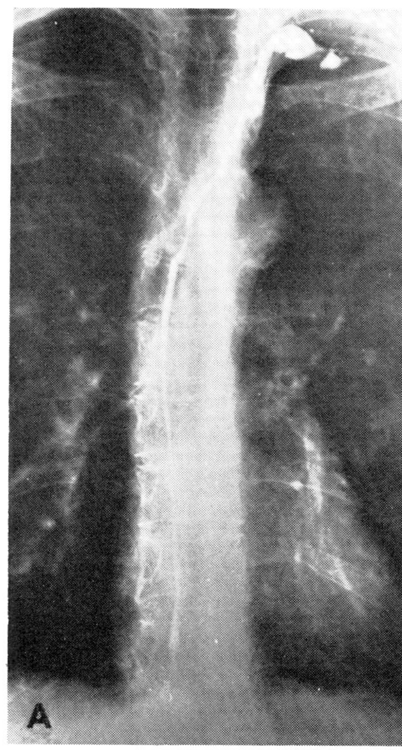

Fig. 6-3A. Thoracic duct. Classical distribution of the thoracic duct.

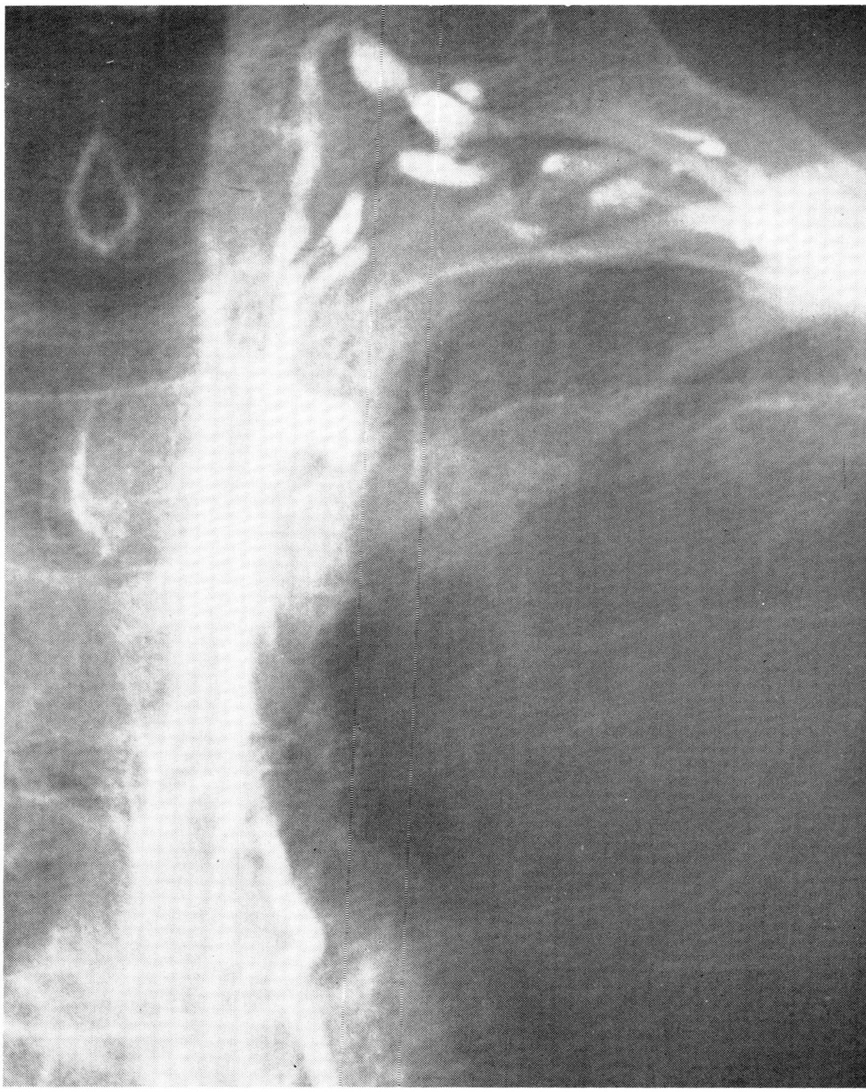

Fig. 6-3B. Thoracic duct. Double thoracic duct emptying on the left side, normal variation.

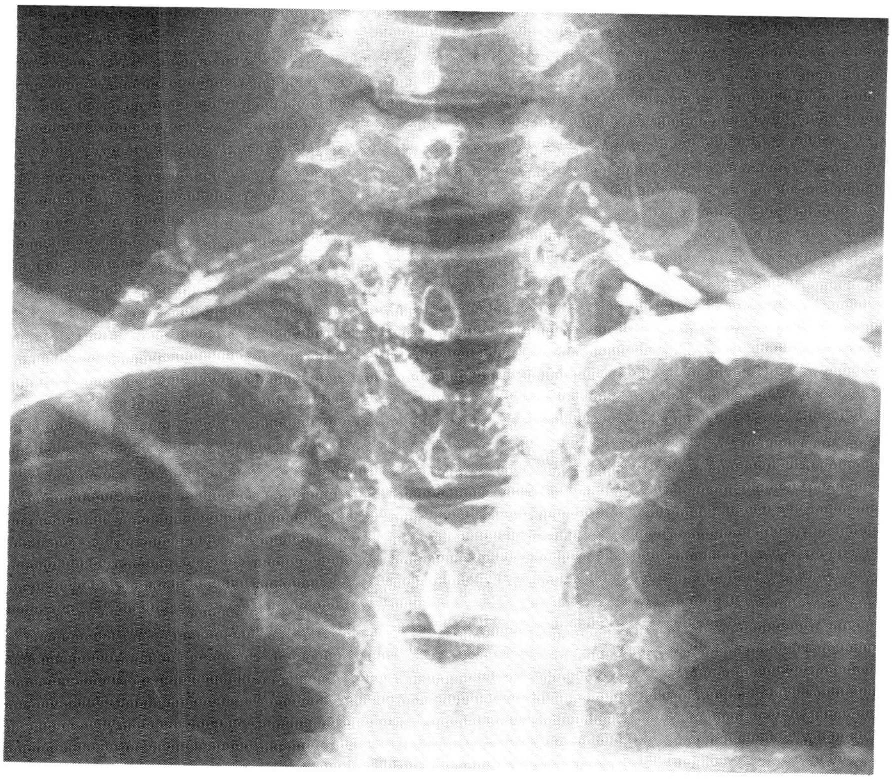

Fig. 6-3C. Thoracic duct. Bilateral communication with the subclavian veins, normal variation.

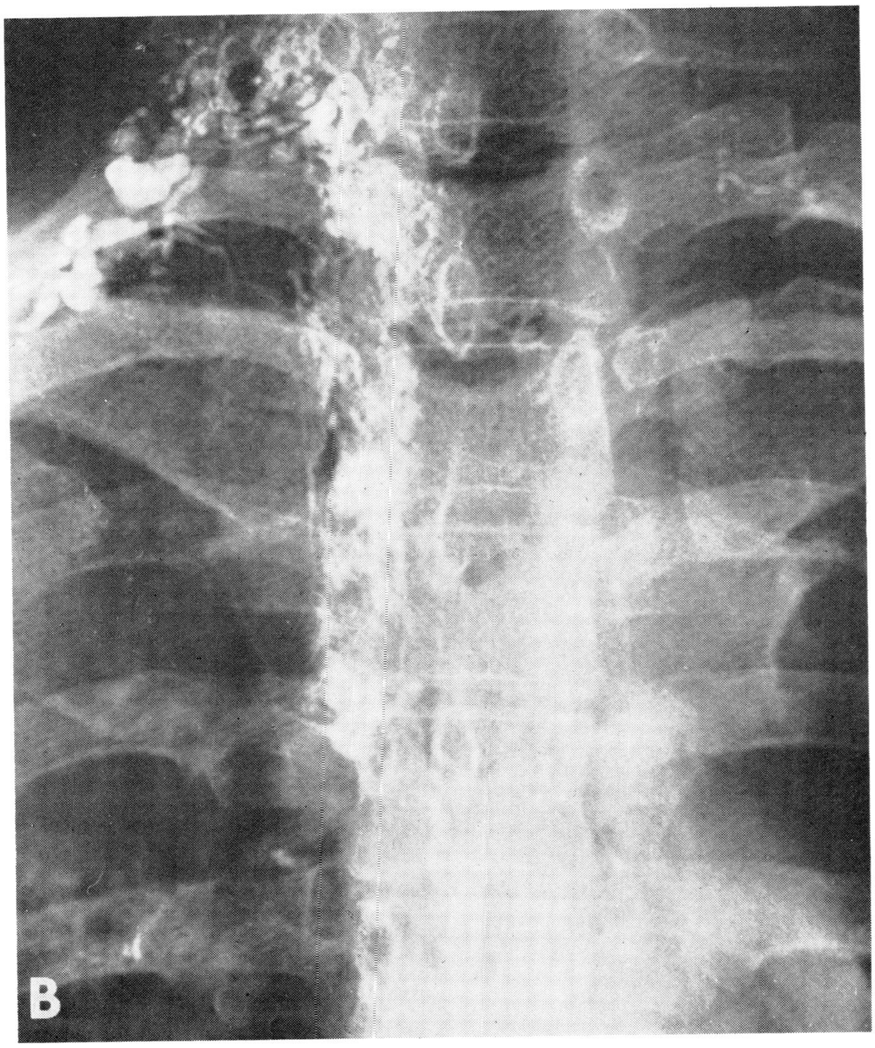

Fig. 6-3D. Thoracic duct. The thoracic duct terminated as a plexus emptying into the right subclavian vein. A smaller channel is seen on the left. A normal variation.

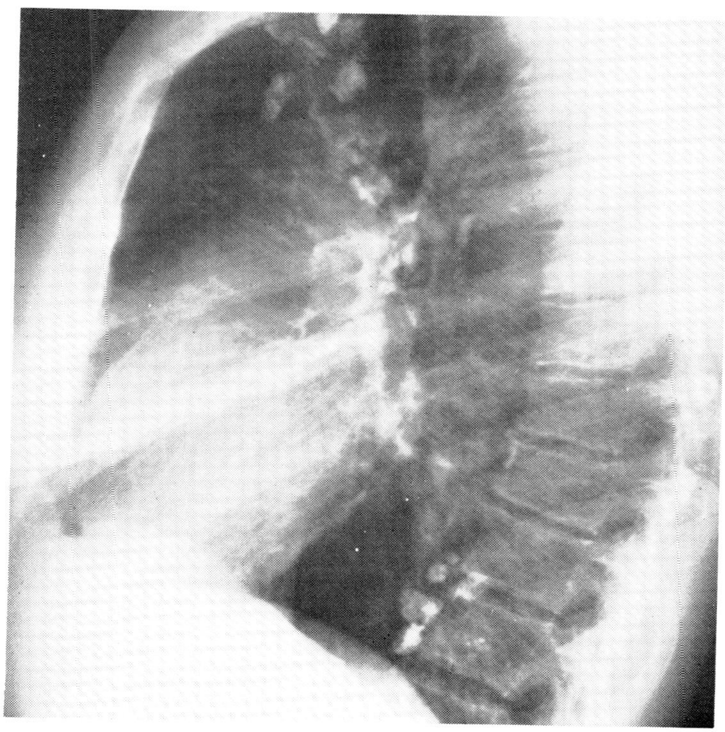

Fig. 6-3E. Thoracic duct. Opacification of mediastinal and supraclavicular nodes, a manifestation of a normal variation of the thoracic duct.

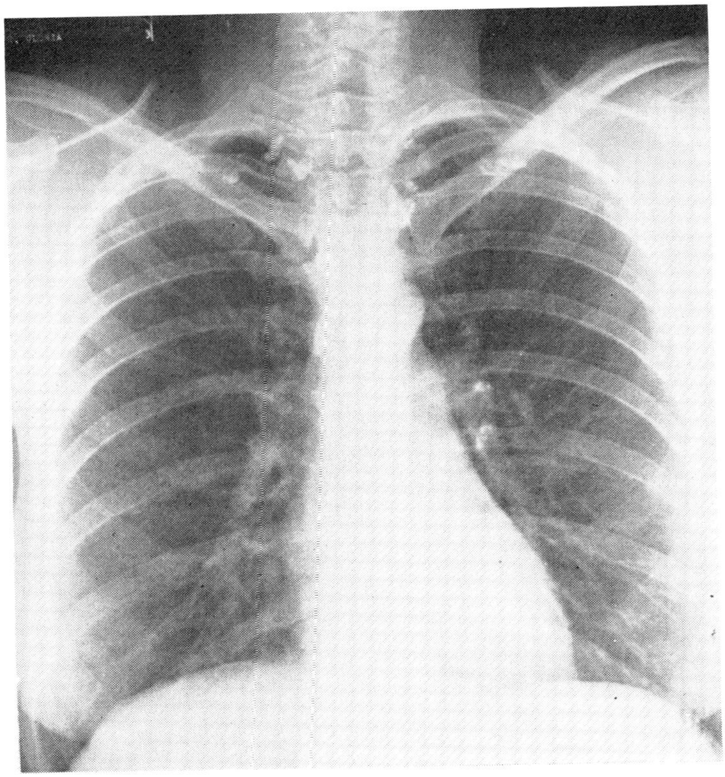

Fig. 6-3F. Thoracic duct. Opacification of mediastinal and supraclavicular nodes, a manifestation of a normal variation of the thoracic duct.

1966; Markland 1968). The disposition of contrast media into the testicle has been reported but the yield is limited; the intralymphatic instillation of radiopaque material is preferred which necessitates a more extensive surgical procedure. Approximately 0.25 to 0.5 ml of the vital dye is injected directly into the testicle. In the presence of a neoplasm in the testicle, this method should be undertaken with caution because of the possibility of spreading malignant tumor cells. The study is best performed in patients with testicular malignant disease without the use of a vital dye (Maddison 1967). Following the dissection of the spermatic cord, a ligature is placed around the spermatic cord, obstructing the 8 to 10 major lymph trunks. Gentle "milking" action from the region of the testicle toward the ligature will produce distention of the lymphatics. If a vital dye has been used, the lymphatics will become visible with the blue material. In the absence of the dye, the dilated lymphatics of the cord can be identified as colorless, glistening, beaded, thin-walled channels. A lymphatic is isolated, dissected, and cannulated by a needle or catheter. These channels are in general larger than the pedal lymphatics but more fragile, necessitating slow and cautious injection to minimize rupture and extravasation. Approximately 3 to 5 ml of contrast material is injected over a period of 30 minutes to 1 hour.

Radiographs must be taken during the procedure to adequately demonstrate the lymphatics and nodes. Anteroposterior, oblique and lateral views can be exposed following the completion of the surgery. Further roentgenograms are done in 24 hours to better appreciate nodal architecture.

This technique undoubtedly prolongs the operative procedure. However, the additional information is of considerable importance.

TESTICULAR LYMPHATIC DRAINAGE

Testicular lymphatics accompany the internal spermatic artery and vein and drain into the lumbar glands which lie between the level of the aortic bifurcation and the renal vein (Rouviere 1938). In 10 per cent of patients, these trunks end in the node at the angle between the right renal vein and the inferior vena cava. The left testicular lymphatics drain into the para-aortic nodes near the left renal vein in approximately two-thirds of the patients. They may also end in glands at the level of the bifurcation of the aorta or even into the common iliac nodes.

Lymphatics from the epididymis may accompany the testicular lymphatics to the lumbar nodes or terminate in the external iliac nodes along with the lymphatics draining the tunica vaginalis.

Clinical investigation utilizing direct testicular lymphangiography by Busch and Sayegh (1963), Busch et al. (1965), Cook et al. (1965), Sayegh et al. (1966), and Chiappa et al. (1966) have confirmed Rouviere's findings (Fig. 6-4). They demonstrated testicular lymphatic channels terminating in a sentinel node at the level of L-1 to L-2 on the left and L-1 to L-3 on the right, slightly lateral to the lumbar nodes usually opacified by pedal lymphangiography. From the right testis there may be direct filling of the lateral nodes above or below the right renal vein or direct filling of the left lateral nodes. There may be immediate crossover of the right testicular lymphatics to the contralateral nodes. Busch and Sayegh (1963) and Arvay and Picard (1964) demonstrated direct communication between the lumbar nodes and the mediastinal nodes independent of the thoracic duct. In the final analysis, important nodes that are not opacified by the pedal route can be filled by testicular lymphangiography. Therefore,

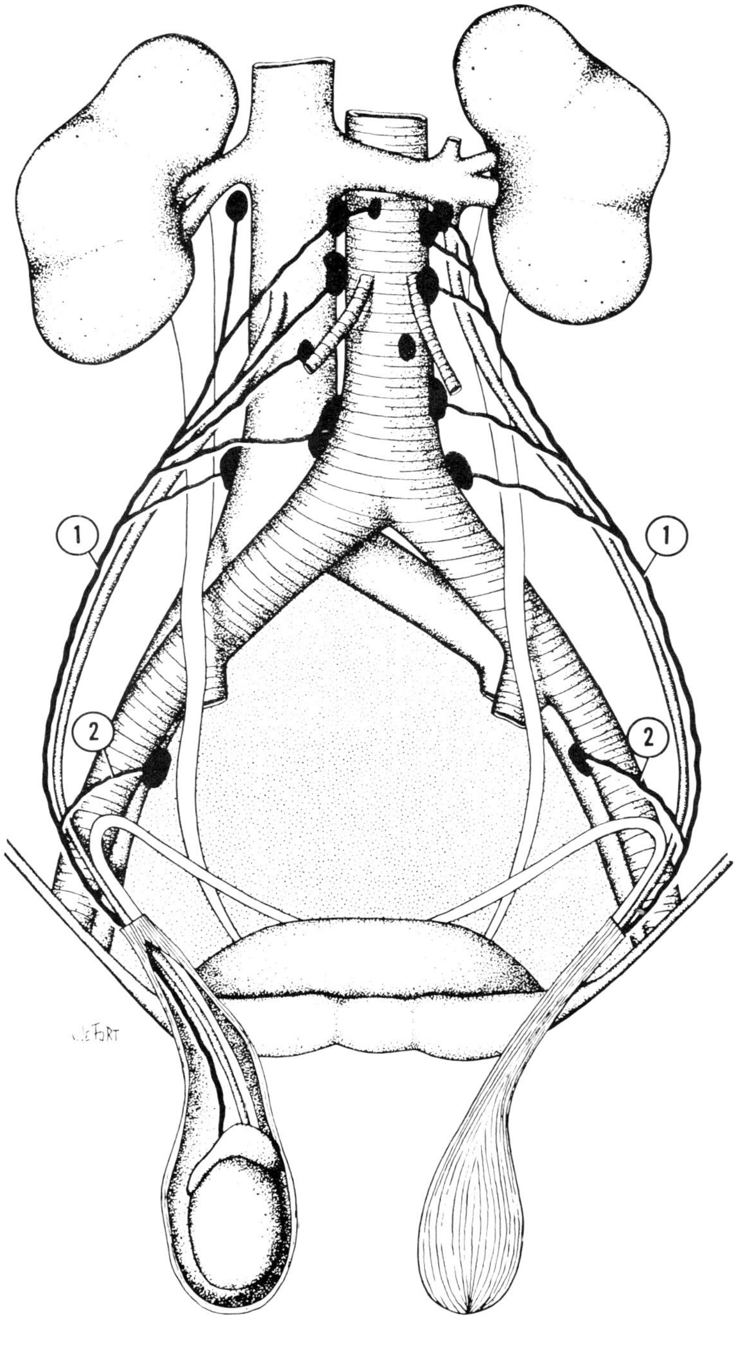

Fig. 6-4A. Testicular lymphatic distribution. Normal testicular lymphatic drainage. (1) Testicular lymphatics. (2) Drainage from epididymis, tunica vaginalis and ductus deferens.

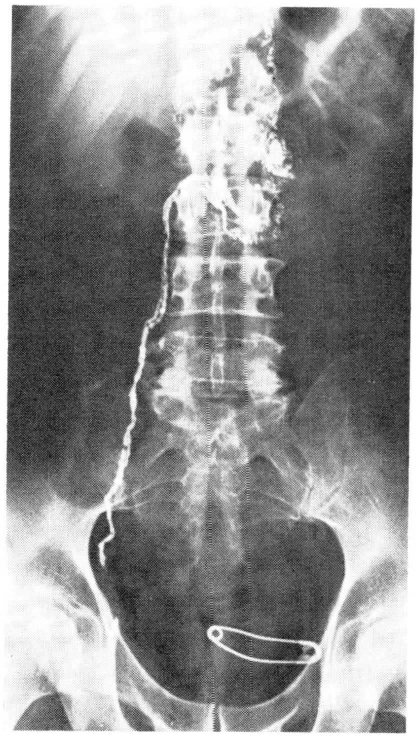
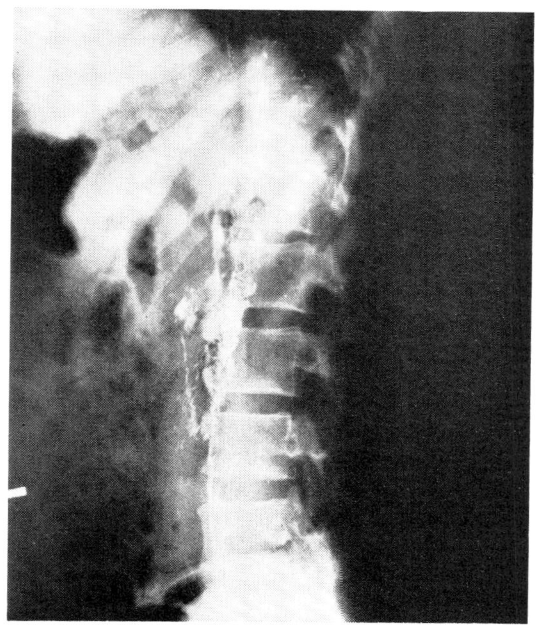

Fig. 6-4. Testicular lymphatic distribution. B, Right testicular lymphangiogram, anteroposterior projection. C, Lateral view (Busch and Sayegh 1963.).

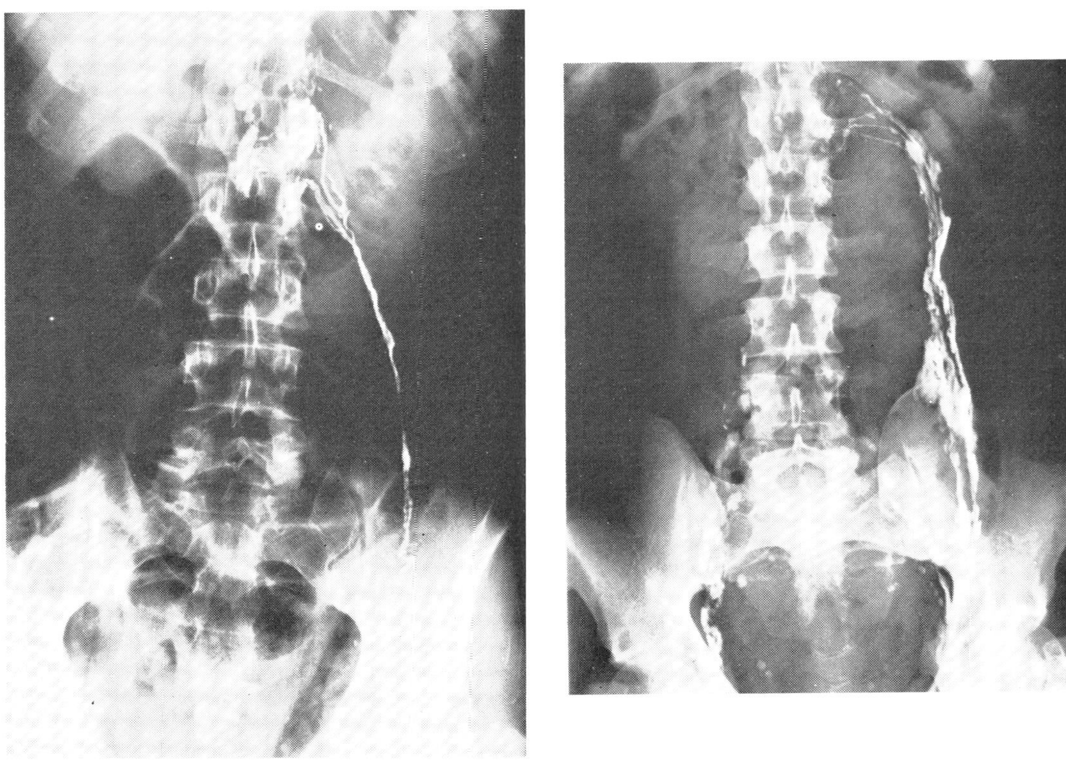

Fig. 6-4. Testicular lymphatic distribution. D, Left testicular lymphangiogram, anteroposterior projection (Busch and Sayegh 1963). E, Left testicular lymphangiogram in a patient with a horse-shoe kidney.

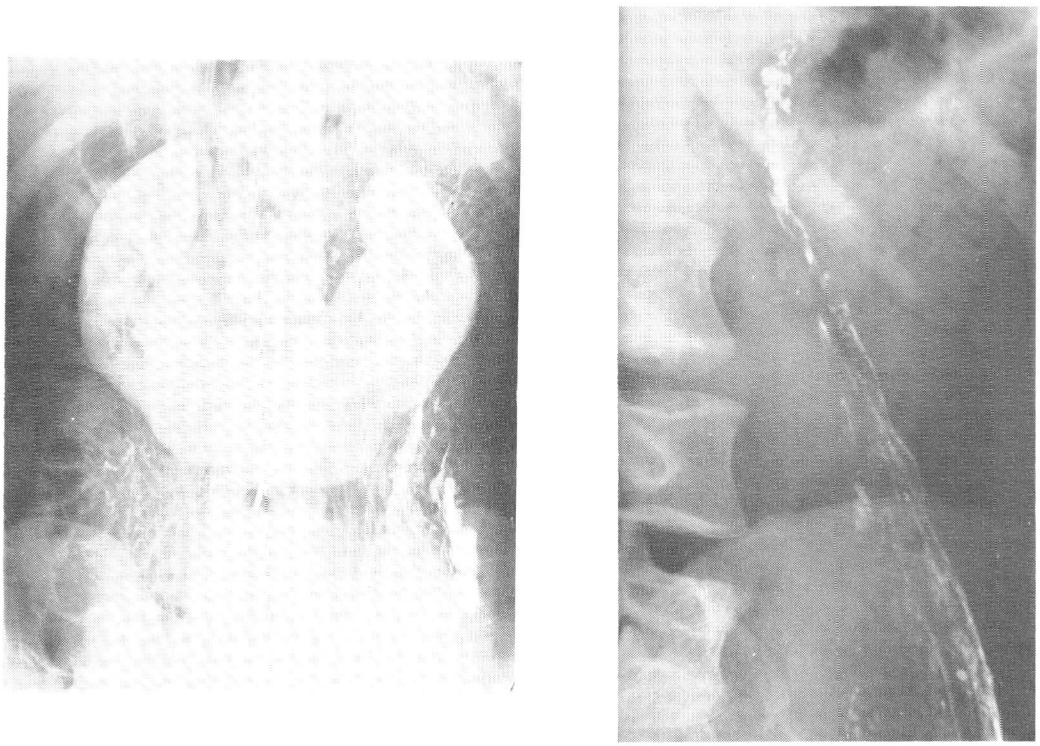

Fig. 6-4. Testicular lymphatic distribution. F, Arteriogram of the horse-shoe kidney in the above patient. Note the relationship of the opacified nodes to the kidney. G, Testicular lymphangiogram. Note the lateral distribution and flow to first echelon node.

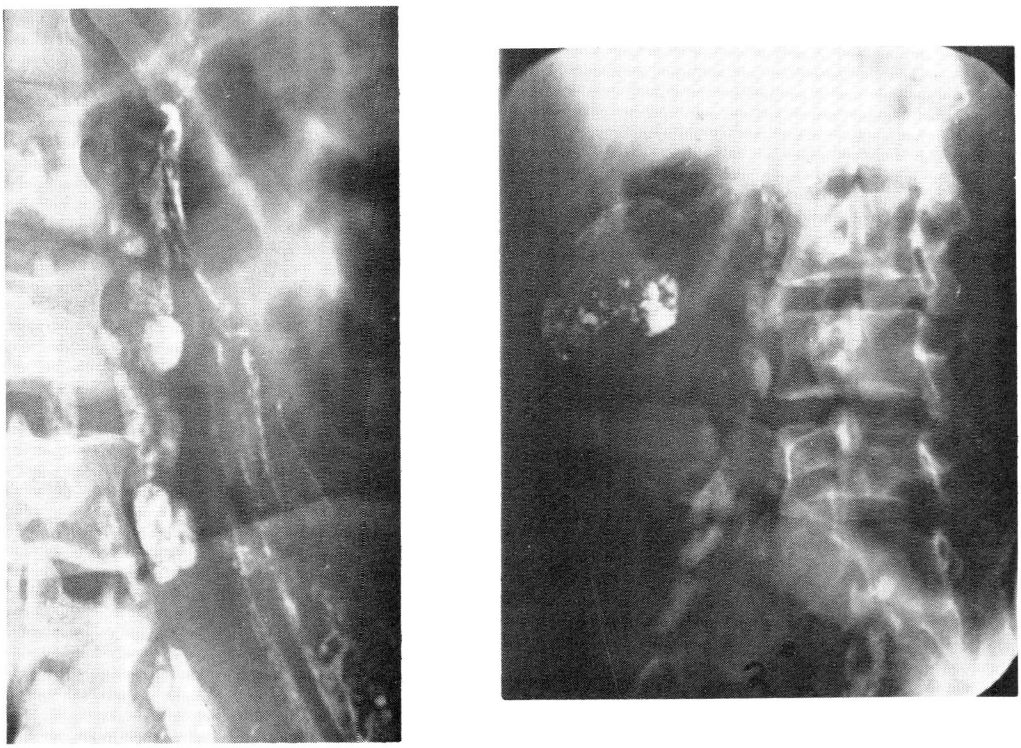

Fig. 6-4. Testicular lymphatic distribution. H, Pedal lymphangiogram on the same patient as G. Note the relationship of the nodal groups. I, Seninomatous metastasis to the first echelon node demonstrated by testicular lymphangiography. This involved node was not opacified by pedal lymphangiography (Cook et al. 1965).

the combined approach should be used whenever possible (Busch and Sayegh 1963; Arvay and Picard 1964; Busch et al. 1965; Cook et al. 1965; Chiappa et al. 1966).

Engeset (1964) demonstrated radiographically the testicular lymphatics in rats and, by injecting tumor cells, showed that variations of lymphatic distribution were largely responsible for the sequence of metastases. Distribution #1 illustrates the mechanism for sentinel node metastases prior to lung; #2, sentinel and lung metastases occurring concurrently and #3, pulmonary metastases preceding or present in the absence oı sentinel node involvement (Fig. 6-5). Thus far, in human testicular lymphangiography with the injection of one or perhaps two testicular lymphatic trunks, analogous categories have not been found.

COMPLICATIONS

The risks of lymphangiography have been minimal in comparison to the amount of useful information obtained (Rutledge et al. 1959; Jackson et al. 1961; Arvay and Picard 1964; De Roo 1964; Fraimow et al. 1964; Koehler et al. 1964; Ruttiman and Del Buono 1964; Fuchs 1965; Gold et al. 1965; Ruttiman 1967; Koehler 1968; Ujiki et al. 1968; Lameer 1969; Dodd et al. 1970; Rasmussen 1970). However, the complications that can occur are as follows:

I. Local

Infection: Infection can be minimized by sterile technique, a minimum of trauma, and vigorous lavage of the incision after completion of the procedure.

When the examination is undertaken on a diabetic, the diabetes should be under control. In the presence of severe peripheral vascular disease and/or diabetes the risks of an incision must be seriously considered.

Sterile Fluid Collections: Cleansing will also decrease the incidence of contrast induced sterile fluid collections. Postoperative lymph collections may occur at the incision but ligation of lymphatics at the end of the procedure is seldom necessary. These collections resolve spontaneously or may be handled by drainage and a compression dressing.

Edema: In patients with preexisting edema the examination may temporarily increase the edema. This may be due to delayed emptying of the oil-based contrast material from the available functioning lymphatic channels in the presence of an existing lymphatic obstruction.

Lymphangitis: This is an extremely rare occurrence in lymphangiography with the use of oil-based materials. It has been reported more frequently when chlorophyl and emulsifying agents have been added to the Ethiodol.

II. Systemic

Blue Discoloration: The injection of the vital blue dye results in blue urine for at least 24 to 48 hours. This material is cleared by the kidneys without obvious problems. Generalized blue discoloration of the skin is produced when too much vital dye has been injected.

Chills, Fever, Malaise: The etiology of these frequent complaints may be a foreign protean reaction. Symptomatic therapy with aspirin, fluids, and bedrest will usually suffice.

Hypersensitivity: Allergic reactions may be precipitated by the vital dye, the local anesthetic or the iodine-containing oil-based contrast material. Other vital dyes, such as Evans blue, are available but a lymphatic can be isolated at times without the aid of vital dyes (Maddison 1967). Alternative local anesthetic agents can be utilized.

Urticaria may occur at the site of the dermal injection, along the dis-

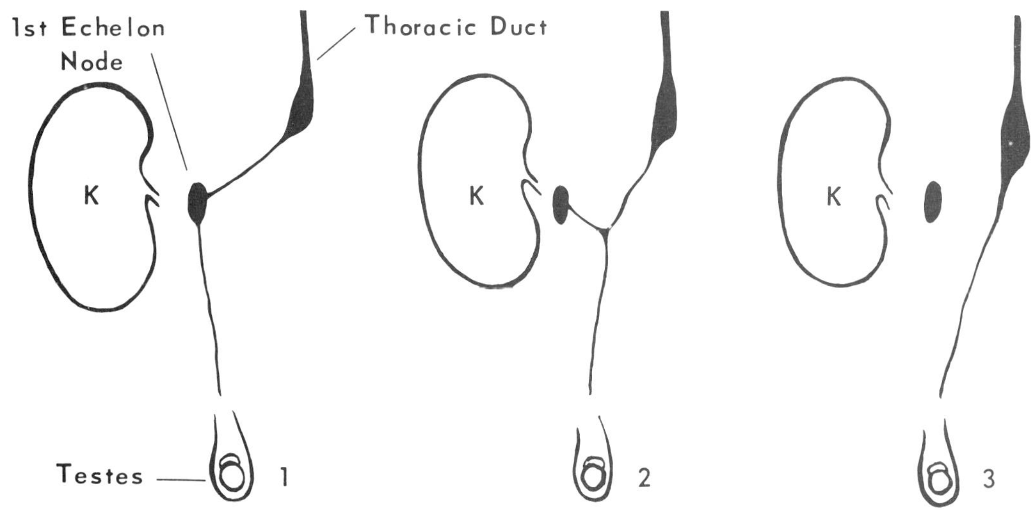

From Arnfinn Engeset, M. D. "An Experimental Study of the Lymph Node Barrier - Injection of Walker Carcinoma 256 in the Lymph vessels"
Extrait de Acta Union Internationale Contre Le Cancer Vo. XV #3–4, 1959

Fig. 6-5. Variations in lymphatic distribution in part determine modes of metastases.

tribution of the blue filled lymphatics, or become diffuse. Occasionally, there will be blue discoloration of the urticarial patches.

These reactions may occur after the initiation of the injection of Ethiodol and force termination of the procedure because of the difficulty in determining the specific allergan. Antihistamine therapy will usually suffice.

One of our patients experienced severe asthma, almost status asthmaticus, which was controlled only by steroids. The problem persisted for one week.

Peripheral vascular collapse may be due to an allergic reaction to any of these agents. Delayed reaction, days after the examination, has been reported (Koehler 1968) and may be due to fatty acid toxicity resulting from the break-down products of the oil-based media.

Pulmonary Embolization: The major complication of lymphangiography is pulmonary embolization (Fraimow et al. 1964; Gold et al. 1965). All patients will experience oil embolization because of the direct continuity of the lymphatics to the venous system. Pulmonary diffusion capacity is invariably impaired as measured by the single breath carbon-monoxide method. The diffusion impairment occurs 2 to 4 hours after the injection and may persist for days or weeks. Punctate radiopacities distributed throughout the lungs are best seen on the 24-hour roentgenogram (Fig. 6-6). On occasion, more diffuse patchy densities may be present. Hemoptysis is rare.

Pulmonary embolization is seldom a clinical problem when the amount of contrast media utilized is limited. Preliminary evaluation of the pulmonary status by a history and chest roentgenogram is usually sufficient. Any evidence of pulmonary functional impairment, especially when related to pulmonary fibrosis, should negate lymphangiography. When there is any doubt concerning the patient's pulmonmonary status, function studies should precede lymphangiography.

Systemic Embolization: Systemic embolization has been reported including the rare cases of cerebral emboli (Koehler 1968; Rasmussen 1970). This suggests shunting to the systemic circulation by passing or overcoming the pulmonary barrier. Lymphangiography is obviously contraindicated with a known cardiac shunt. The risks of overcoming the lung barrier may be minimized by limiting the amount of material injected. The demonstration of a lymphatico-venous anastomosis should terminate the procedure.

Lipogranulomas: Oil-based contrast material injected into lymph nodes creates an inflammatory process - lipogranulomas. This reaction is at a maximum within 1 to 2 weeks and then gradually subsides. The engorgement of nodes resulting from the inflammatory process produces some enlargement of the contrast filled nodes. With complete subsidence of the reaction there is a decrease in the size of the nodes in 1 to 2 months. This should not be mistaken for a response to any therapeutic regimen. There have been no proven long-term complications precipitated by the contrast material in the nodes, lymphatics, or lungs.

Tumor Dissemination: The propagation of metastatic emboli by the instillation of oil-based contrast material is a risk which needs further experimental investigation. The experiments by Zeidman et al. (1955) indicate that the contrast material does not permeate through carcinomatous tissue in the node. Ujiki et al. (1968), however, have recently demonstrated a progression of metastases to the next echelon nodes in animals examined by lymphangiography in contrast to those who have not been so studied. The significance of this findings must still be determined in patients.

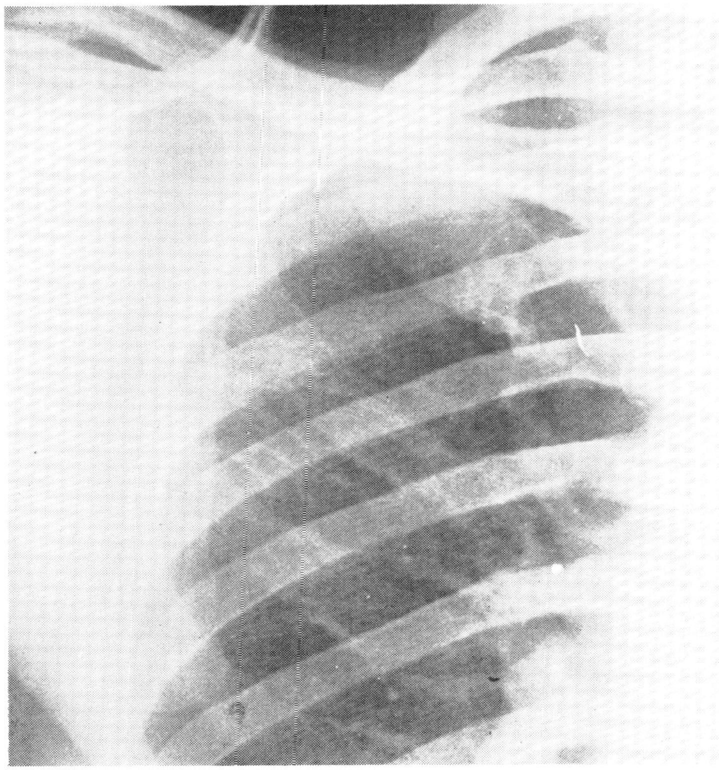

Fig. 6-6. Pulmonary embolization of the oil-based contrast material.

LYMPHATIC DYNAMICS

The lymphatic system is the third major component of the body's vascular network. Lymphatic dynamics are governed by the same physiologic principles that regulate the blood vascular system but they function with a decelerated velocity. Abnormalities in any one of the body's fluid compartments precipitate changes in the others in an attempt to maintain homeostasis.

The classic concept of the lymphatic system limits it to the morphologic definition of those endothelial-lined pathways which transport fluid overload from the blood vascular system centripetally, eventually communicating with the venous system, and acting as a safety valve to maintain continuity of the intravascular fluid pool. The lymphatic network is located primarily on the surfaces of the body and viscera. Less numerous endothelial-lined lymphatic pathways, close to the arteries and veins, permeate the parenchyma of the organs and musculoskeletal system.

An essential function of this portion of the vascular system is the conservation and restoration of large molecular particles, primarily proteins. If this functional definition is considered, other avenues of fluid transport need to be included (Wallace 1970). The interstitial spaces, the body's potential cavities (pleural, pericardial, and peritoneal), the perivascular and perineural spaces, the subserosal and subadventitial spaces can be thought of as a paralymphatic (Ottaviani 1947) or prelymphatic (Foldi 1971) system. These pathways are probably as extensive as the endothelial-lined lymphatic system but are less well defined and supply the necessary avenues of transport from the cellular level to the endothelial-lined lymphatics. This system is analogous to the most primitive mode of fluid transport in invertebrates and plants.

The lymphatic and pre-lymphatic compartments are probably continuous and eventually drain into the venous system via lymphatico-venous anastomoses. The major site of communication is at the junction of the primary collecting trunk, the thoracic duct and the subclavian vein. Numerous anastomoses functioning in a reverse capacity are available throughout the body. Lymphatico-venous communications are probably governed by humoral and neurogenic stimuli which regulate the pressure gradients and thus determine directional flow (Valeyeva 1961; Threefoot et al. 1963).

Interruption of the lymphatic circulation results in the utilization of collateral channels to circumvent the obstruction and re-establish continuity (Herman et al. 1964). If these alternate pathways are inadequate, there is an accumulation of relatively static fluid.

The lymphatic network, so vital in the maintenance of fluid equilibrium, also provides available avenues for the transport and dispersion of tumor emboli. Patterns of lymphatic metastases depend to a great extent upon the distribution of normal lymphatic vessels and lymph nodes, the variations from normal, and the alternate pathways employed in the event of obstruction. Lymphangiography, although only quasi-physiologic because of the pressure of injection, permits a radiographic portrayal of these dynamic principles (Wallace 1968).

A. Mechanical Obstruction

Interruption of lymphatic vessels is usually followed by retraction and thromboses of the transected ends (Reichert 1926; Bellman and Oden 1956). As long as the ends are in close proximity, rapid regeneration and recannulization will re-establish continuity in 4 to 8 days. In the interim, the collateral pathways are those in the immediate vicinity of the obstruction which are available and patent (Blalock et al. 1937). Belan et al. (1963) and Malek (1959) have shown that lymphatico-venous anastomoses can serve temporarily as alternate routes but cease to function once the normal pathways are available. With disruption of a larger segment, approximation may be impossible and alternate pathways must permanently accomodate the increased fluid load. If these channels are inadequate to circumvent the occlusion, protein accumulates in the interstitial tissues with resulting edema. The availability of alternate routes increases as the obstruction becomes more centrally located. The compensating flow patterns include lymphatico-lymphatic, lymphatico-prelymphatic and lymphatico-venous anastomoses.

The lymphatics of each compartment of the lower limb are functionally separate. Only on rare occasions, e.g. congenital variations, will the superficial and deep lymphatic circulation opacify simultaneously after the injection of a superficial lymphatic on the dorsum of the foot. However, with interruption of the anterior channels, the superficial vessels in the posterior group may be opacified. Alternate deep pathways used after obstruction of the anterior vessels may be seen paralleling the deep arteries and veins. Dermal lymphatics will also function as collateral pathways in the event of obstruction of subcutaneous channels. If adequate collateral circulation exists, edema does not occur.

When lymphatic pathways are interrupted, extensive collateral circulation is available. As long as these channels are present and patent they will reroute the lymph flow in an effort to maintain continuity. This phenomenon is illustrated in the pelvis, the retroperitoneal area, and the thoracic duct (Fig. 6-7A).

Clinically, these principles are important and must be understood when contemplating a radical node dissection. A preoperative lymphangiographic examination demonstrating lymphatic obstruction may suggest that the surgical procedure cannot adequately encompass the possible metastatic foci. Lymphatic channels are invariably interrupted after radical surgery (Fig. 6-7B). The direction of lymph flow and perhaps the sequence of any subsequent metastases are influenced by the entirely new dynamic environment. Any subsequent dissection must consider the entirely new circumstances produced by the surgical procedure.

Metastases, therefore, are not usually bizarre but progress in an orderly fashion dependent upon the lymphatic distribution. Once the normal channels are interrupted, use of the available pathways results in complex and extensive patterns. These patterns are not predictable and their diversity indicates the futility of radical dissection in the presence of lymphatic obstruction.

B. Lymphocysts and Lymphatic Fistulae

After injury to the larger lymphatics, including the thoracic duct, there is free egress of lymph. If this lymph is confined, a pseudocyst or lymphocyst is formed. The incidence and magnitude of these postoperative complications depend on multiple factors - the caliber of the transsected lymphatics, the intralymphatic pressure, the velocity of lymph flow and the completeness of lymphatic ligation, the availability of residual functioning channels, and the adequacy of collateral pathways. A lymphocyst occurs shortly after surgical intervention which helps in differentiating it from recurrent disease. The fluid that accumulates in the "cyst" is not static. Aspiration of this collection is usually followed by fairly rapid re-accumulation, demonstrating this dynamic activity.

Lymphocysts are encountered most frequently as a complication of radical lymph node dissections (Rutledge et al. 1959; Dodd et al. 1970). If the confined collection is in a stra-

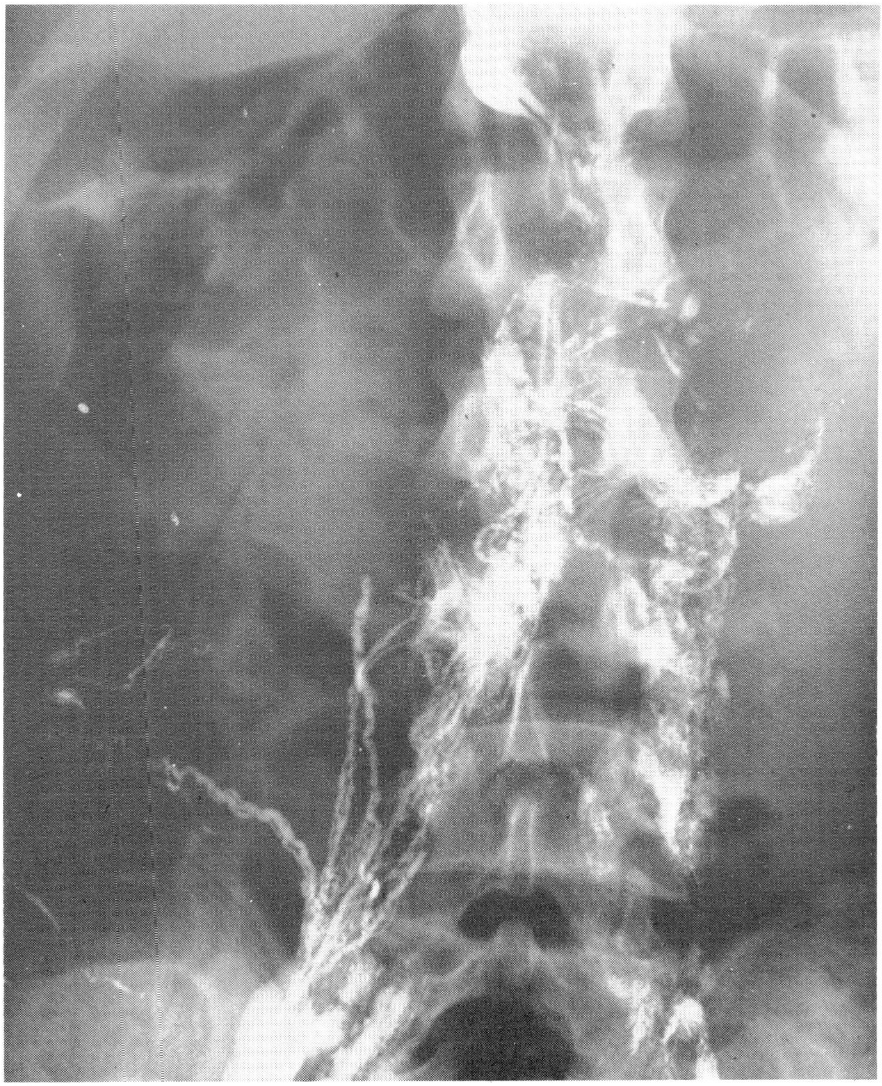

Fig. 6-7. Mechanical obstruction. A, Obstruction by metastatic carcinoma from the testicle. Collateral pathways are opacified.

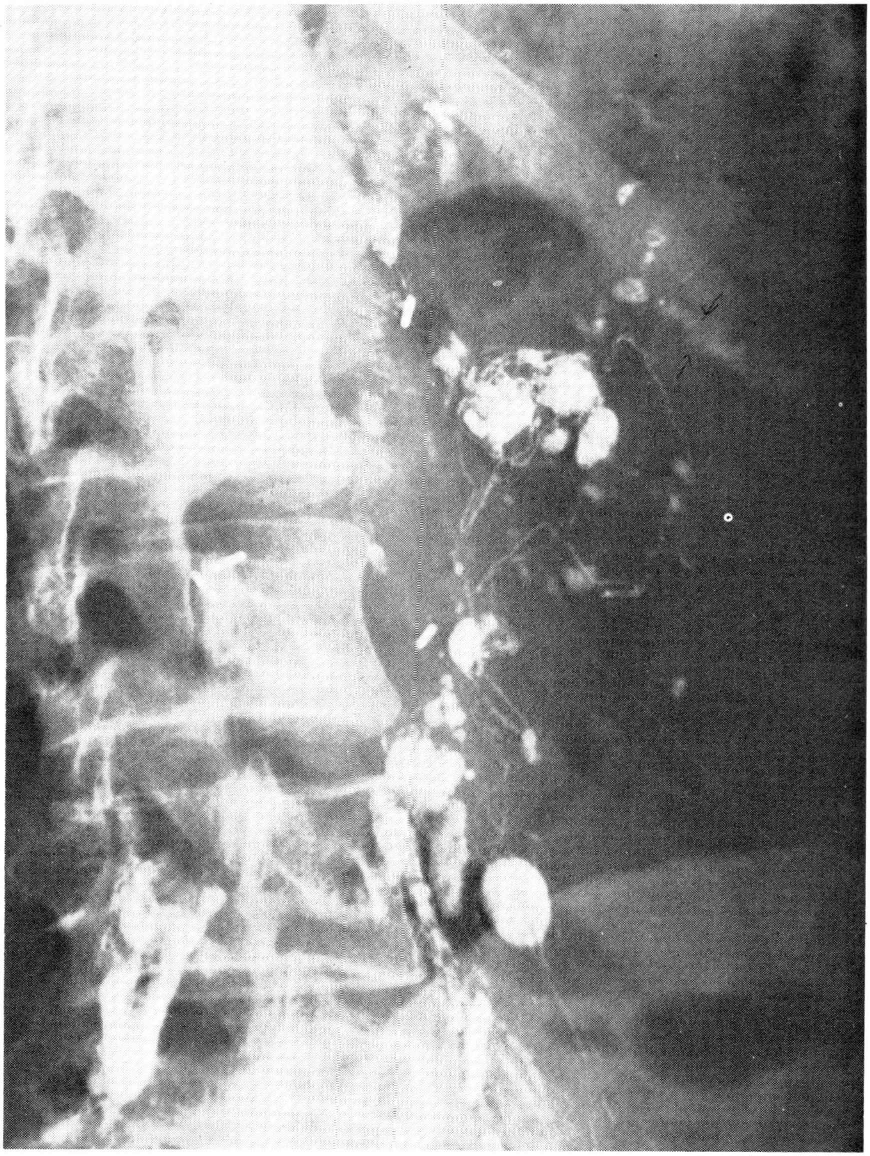

Fig. 6-7. Mechanical obstruction. B, Lymphatic obstruction following retroperitoneal node dissection.

tegic position it will cause clinical problems. A lymphocyst of any magnitude along the course of a ureter may produce distortion or obstruction (Fig. 6-8).

When the volume of the confined fluid is great enough, it may present signs and symptoms of a mass; that is, pressure on the adjacent organs. The medial displacement of phleboliths in the pelvis may suggest the existence of a lymphocyst. Obstruction of the pelvic veins and edema of the lower limbs may be secondary to this complication.

The surgeon is, therefore, faced with a dilemma when performing a radical pelvic node dissection. If all the lymphatics are ligated, obstruction of lymph flow may result in edema of the lower limbs. On the other hand, transsection and free egress of lymph from the endothelial channels may precipitate the formation of lymphocysts. Incomplete dissection will usually result in sufficient channels to maintain flow bypassing any interruption. Lymphocyst formation depends on the extent of the dissection and the scrupulous ligation of the transsected lymphatic channels.

The escape of lymph into a potential cavity, viscus, or through the skin after transsection of the lymphatic channels may cause the formation of a fistulous tract. Considerable circulating fluid may be lost through a lymphatic fistulae. Neoplastic invasion of lymphatic pathways may also cause a lymphatic fistulae.

C. Chylous Reflux

Chylous reflux is the reflux of chyle from the intestinal lymphatics into the skeletal lymphatic pathways. It presents one of the most dramatic examples of altered lymphatic flow patterns and illustrates both the use of collateral circulation and the production of fistulous tracts as a method of decompressing the lymphatic system in the face of obstruction (Fig. 6-9). This phenomenon may result from either congenital or acquired obstruction of the lymphatic system. Servelle (1963) has described in detail the possible mechanisms involved.

The congenital incompetence of lymphatic valves, primarily in the thoracic duct, results in stasis and reflux of chyle; that is, a physiologic obstruction with reversal of flow. In many children with this condition the thoracic duct is visualized throughout its entire extent during lymphangiography. However, lymphangiography as performed at the present time is not completely physiologic. The injection is given with a constant head of pressure which may overcome the incompetency of the valves and, for all practical purposes, creates a competent system.

The acquired variety of chylous reflux may be associated with any process producing chronic thoracic duct obstruction. Proximal to the point of obstruction, there is dilation of the lymphatics with secondary incompetence of the lymphatic valves producing retrograde flow, a picture dynamically identical to the congenital type. This results in an increase in the intralymphatic pressure and eventual rupture of these channels with the production of lymphatic fistulae and an egress of chyle. Filariasis is the most frequent parasitic etiologic agent in the production of chylous reflux. This results in an intralymphatic inflammatory process with obstruction and utilization of collateral circulation. Tuberculosis, neoplasm, trauma, fibrosis, etc. may produce the same phenomenon.

Clinical manifestations such as chyluria (Kittridge et al. 1963; Swanson 1963; Picard 1967; Ahrens and Goldrick 1971), chylometria and chylous edema (Servelle and Deysson 1951) depend on the site of the obstruction, the anatomical variations, and the collateral pathways used. In chyluria, the kidney is the prime target organ. Chyluria is seen most frequently during pregnancy

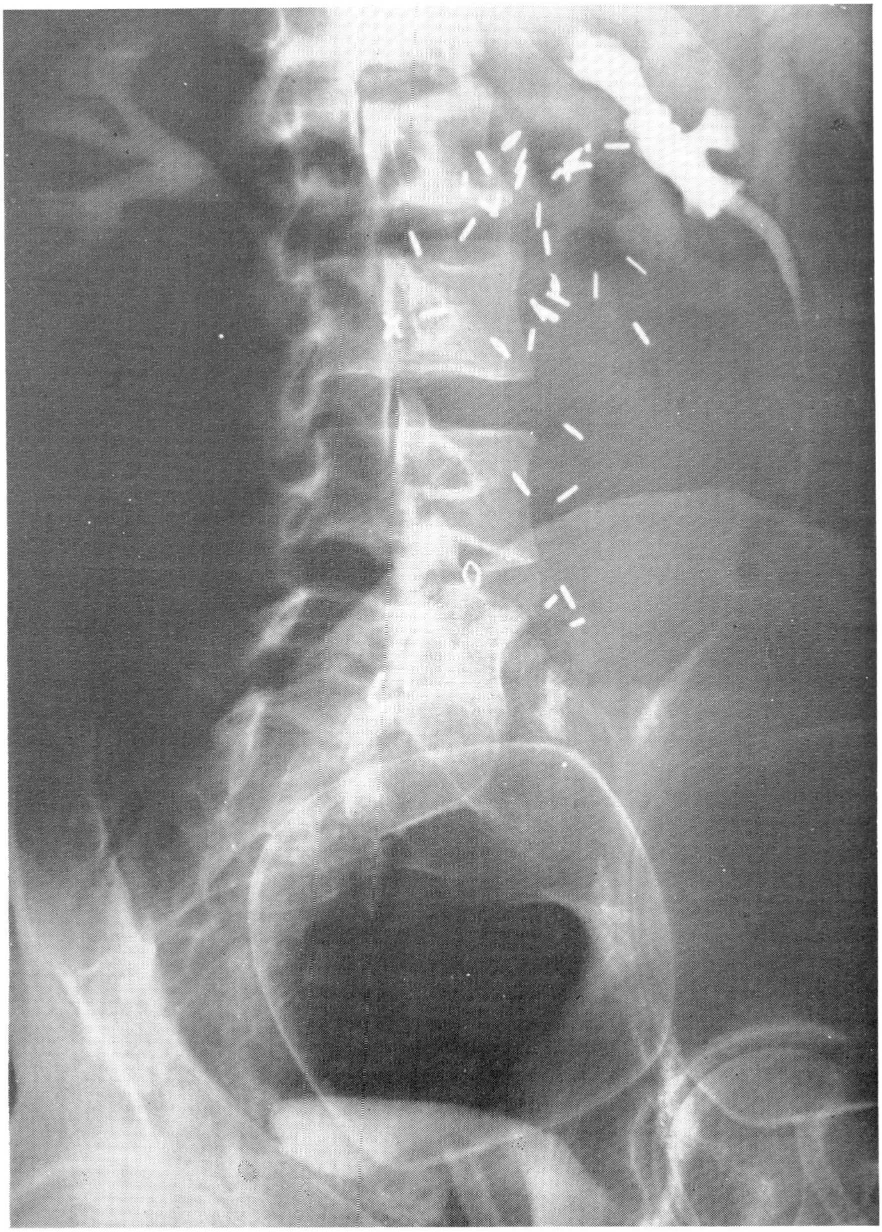

Fig. 6-8. Postoperative lymphocyst. A, Displacement of the left ureter is noted shortly after retroperitoneal node dissection for embryonal carcinoma of the testicle.

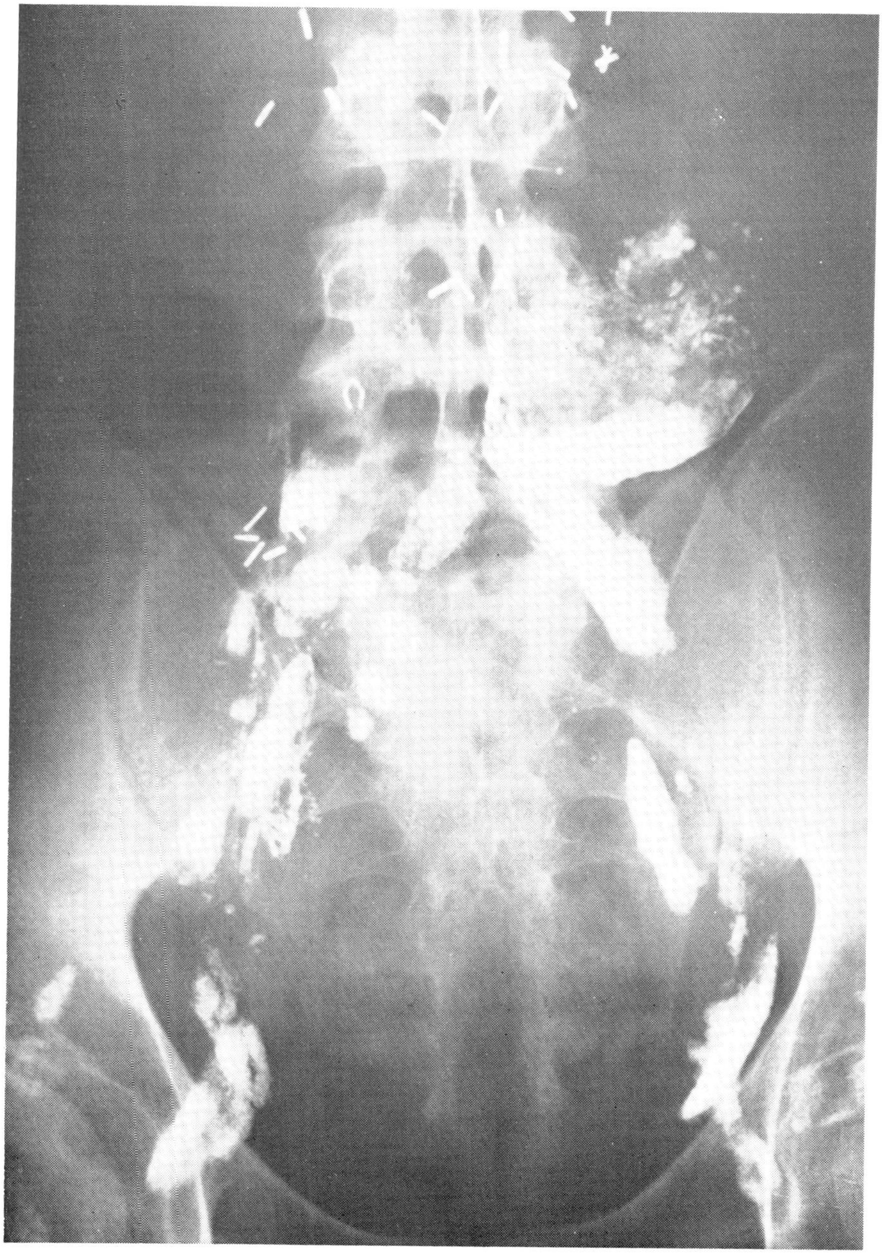

Fig. 6-8. Postoperative lymphocyst. B, Lymphangiogram demonstrates the distortion of the ureter to be due to a lymphocyst (same patient as 8A).

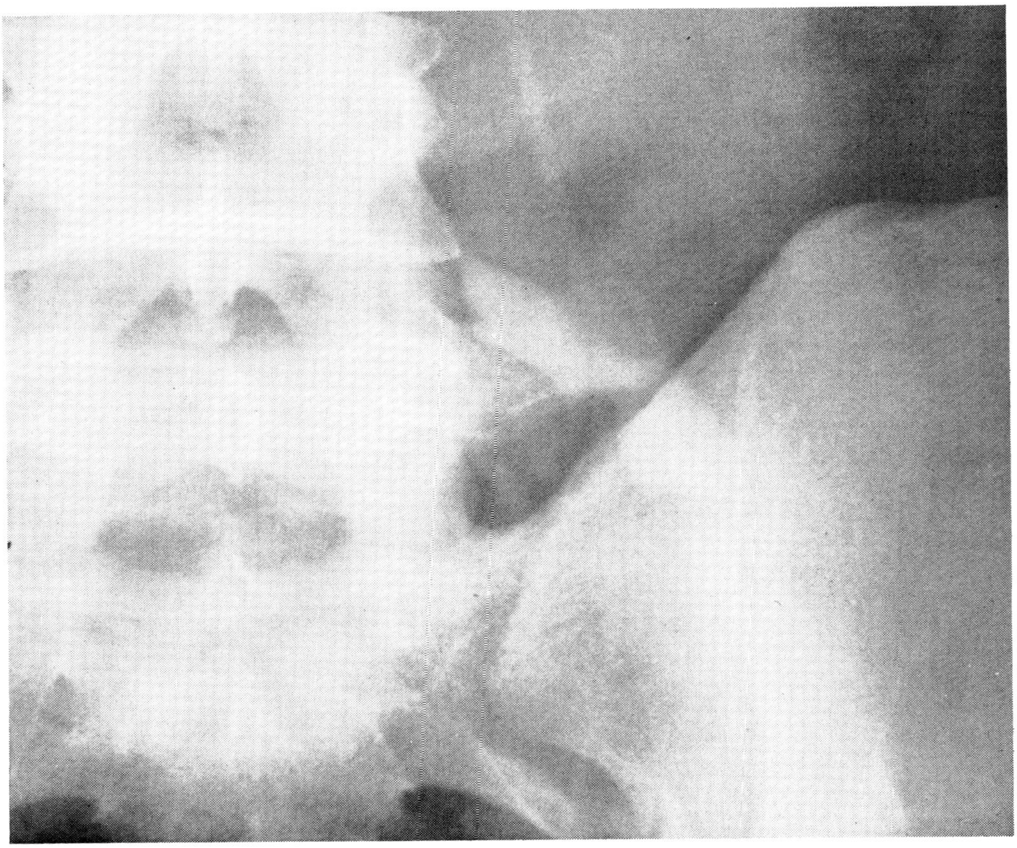

Fig. 6-8. Postoperative lymphocyst. C, Calcification of a postoperative lymphocyst 7 years after surgery.

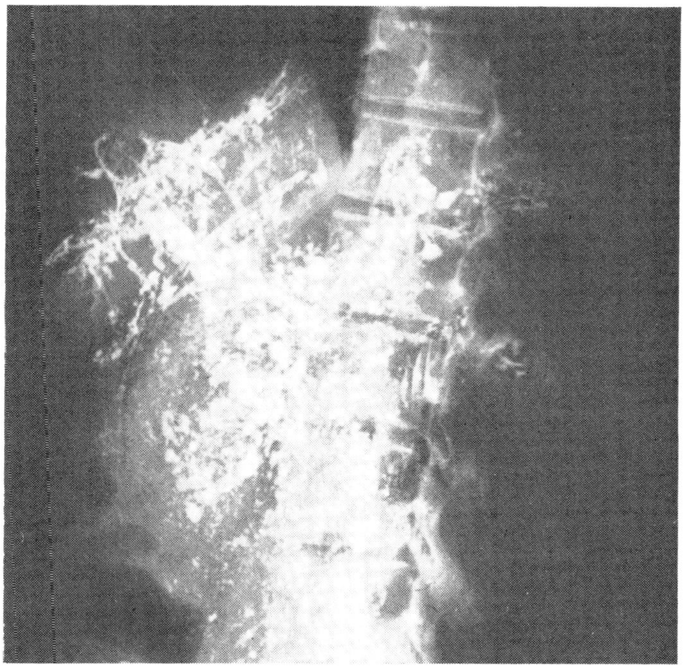

Fig. 6-9. Chylous reflux. A, Protein losing enteropathy due to fistulous tracts from the lymphatics to the biliary tract and small bowel (Bismuth et al. 1963).

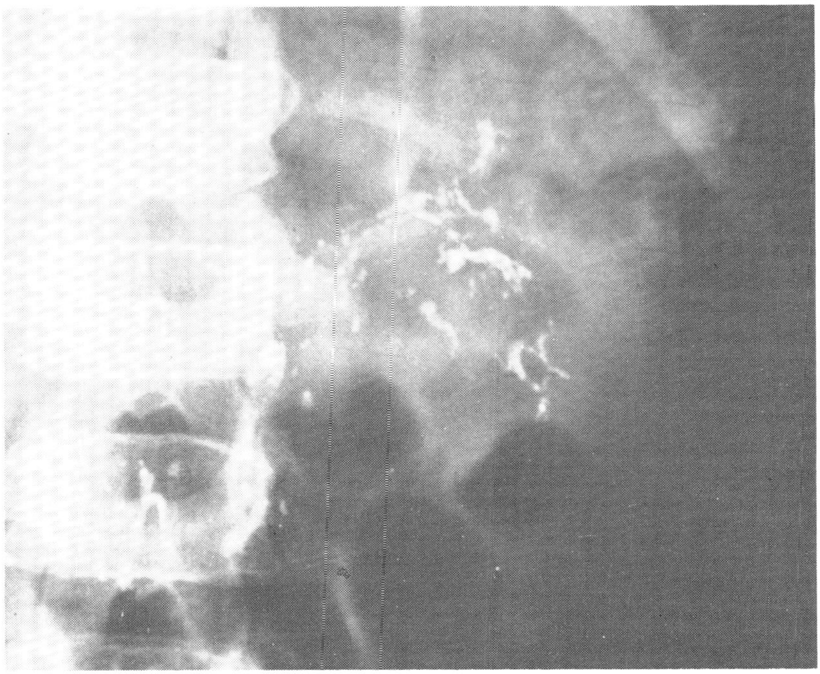

Fig. 6-9. Chylous reflux. B, Chyluria - reflux into the renal lymphatics (Swanson 1963; Ahrens and Goldrick 1971).

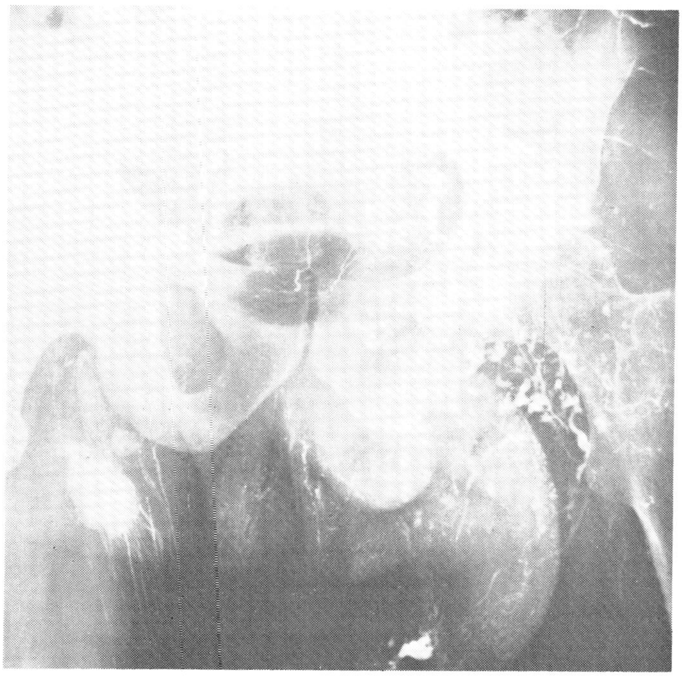

Fig. 6-9. Chylous reflux. C, Chylous edema - dilated collateral lymphatics in the pelvis and scrotum (Henner, Dallas). Scrotal chylous edema - the opacified vesicles which, when punctured, contained chyle (Henner, Dallas).

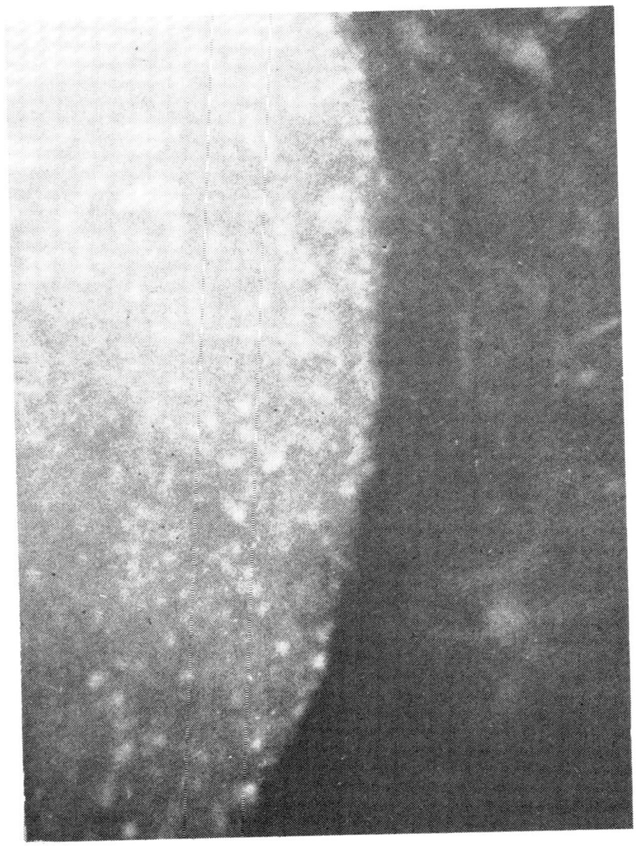

Fig. 6-9. Chylous reflux. D, Chylous edema - dilated collateral lymphatics in the pelvis and scrotum (Henner, Dallas). Scrotal chylous edema - the opacified vesicles which, when punctured, contained chyle (Henner, Dallas).

and may result from a mechanical obstruction produced by the enlarging uterus. It may be transient, disappearing after delivery. Proteinuria noted during pregnancy may be due to chyluria. Even when the patient is not pregnant, chyluria may be intermittent. The exact mechanisms are not totally understood.

The mechanisms involved in the production of some forms of protein-losing enteropathy are closely allied with chylous reflux (Bismuth et al. 1963). Contrast material on occasion can be seen entering into the small bowel demonstrating a communication between the lymphatic channels and the visceral lumen.

D. Prelymphatic or Paralymphatic Pathways

The paralymphatic or prelymphatic pathways include all of the non-endothelial lined pathways which are available for the transport of large molecular particles, especially proteins, and are presumed to be in continuity with the endothelial lined lymphatic vessels (Wallace 1968; Wallace 1970; Foldi 1971). Included in this category are the potential spaces in the interstitial tissues, pleural, pericardial, and peritoneal cavities, the subserosal and submucosal spaces, and the perineural and perivascular spaces.

E. Visceral Lymphatic Pathways

With obstruction of skeletal lymphatics, lymph flow may be rerouted via visceral channels (Wallace 1970). The lymphatic plexuses of the subserosal and submucosal layers are available for collateral circulation. On occasion, contrast material seems to accumulate circumferentially in the wall of the viscus (Fig. 6-10A). The radiopaque material may be in a potential space which is probably available for fluid transport, as well as, for tumor emboli.

F. Perineural and Perivascular Spaces

There are sheath-like structures surrounding vessels and nerves which produce actual or potential spaces between the vessel or nerve wall and the enveloping membrane (Ruszniak et al. 1960; Foldi 1971; Wallace 1968). Considerable controversy has arisen concerning the existence of these spaces as well as their functioning capacity. The Virchow-Robin spaces surrounding cerebral vessels have been considered artifacts by many. Larson et al. (1966) were unable to demonstrate any connection between the perineural spaces and the lymphatic system. However, as far as we are concerned, perineural and paravascular spaces probably communicate with endothelial-lined lymphatic vessels.

A tubular cuff of contrast material has been observed which clearly follows the distribution of major vessels. Sequential roentgenograms have indicated that this cuff is not extravasation. The caliber and distribution of the column are suggestive of contrast material within the perivascular or perineural sheath (Fig. 6-10B). The clinical importance of this pathway in the dissemination of tumor has been emphasized (Dodd et al. 1970). Since the perineural space provides a relatively unopposed pathway along which tumor cells may propagate, it would seem logical that they may be utilized as collateral pathways for fluid transport in the presence of obstruction.

G. Lymphatico-venous Anastomoses

Lymphatico-venous anastomoses complete the vascular circuit (Job 1918; Malek 1959; Ruszniak et al. 1960; Wallace 1968). The major central lymphatics are formed by budding from the veins which create the potential for these lymphatico-venous communications. The classic example of lymphatico-venous anastomoses occurs

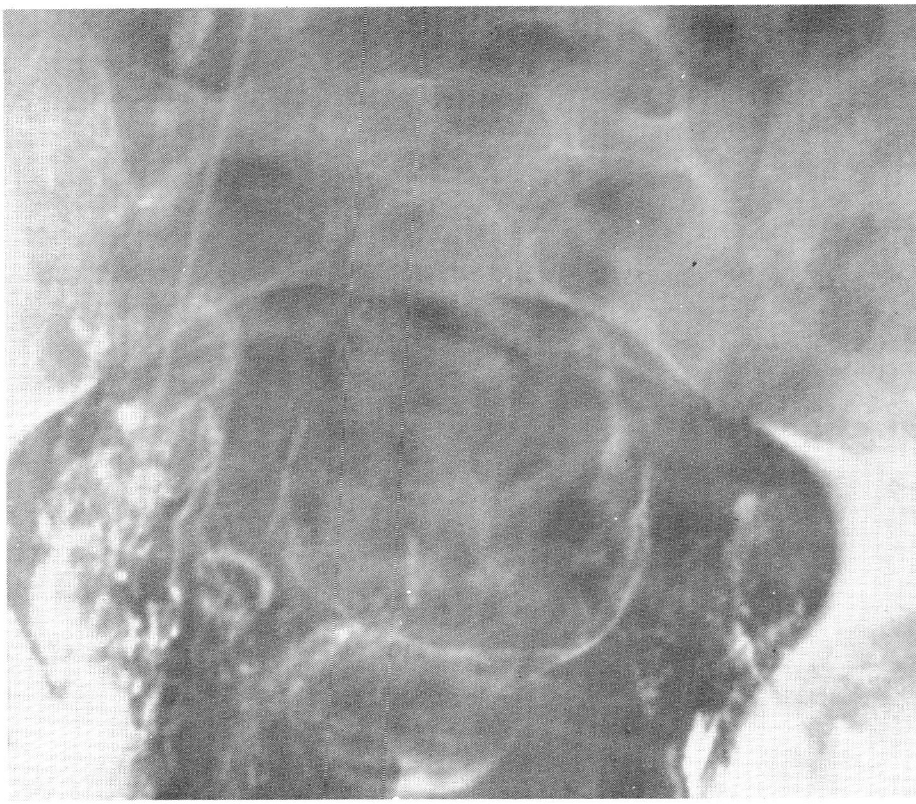

Fig. 6-10. Paralymphatic pathways. A, Visceral space obstruction of the iliac lymphatics with opacification of the wall of a pelvis viscus.

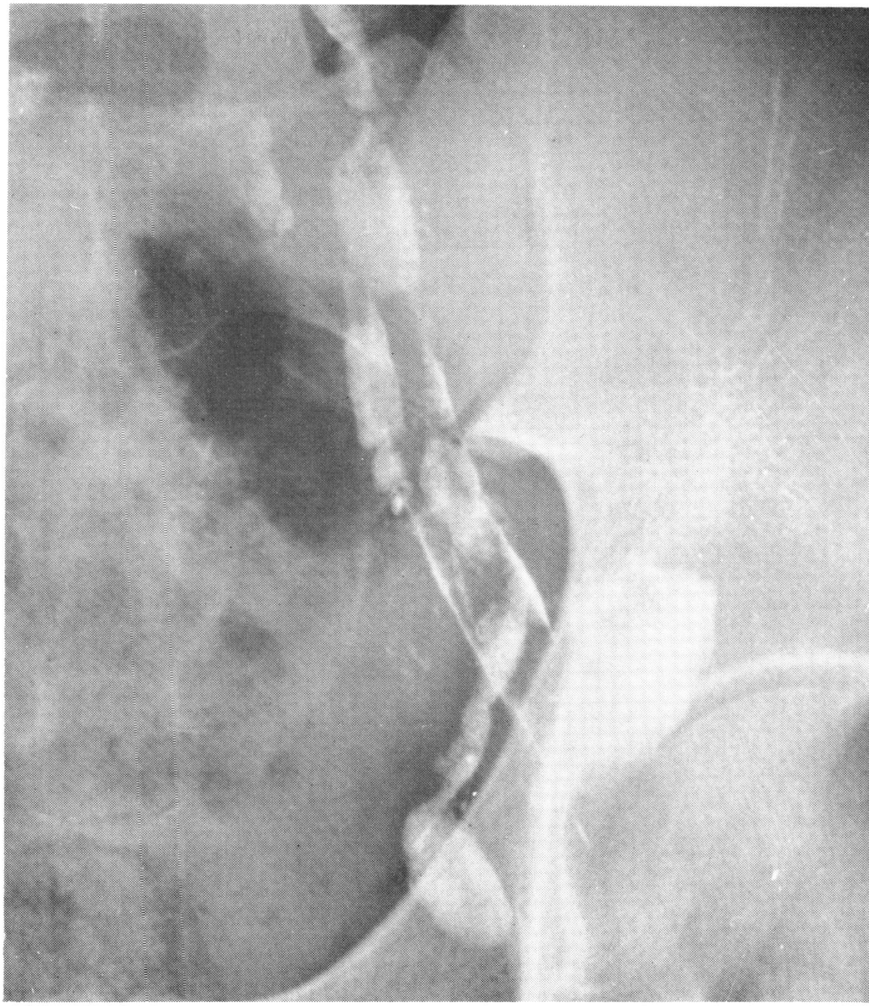

Fig. 6-10. Paralymphatic pathways. B, Perivascular space - a cuff of contrast material surrounds the iliac artery.

at the junction of the thoracic duct with the subclavian vein at the venous angle. Until recently, this was considered to be the only such communication. Threefoot et al. (1963) have confirmed the existence of these communications after ligations of the thoracic duct in animals. The visualization of lymphatico-venous anastomoses occurred approximately 2 weeks after ligation. With the addition of hexamethonium these communications appeared more rapidly. These findings suggest that hydrodynamic, humoral, and neurogenic stimuli govern the utilization of these communications (Valeyeva 1961). Threefoot et al. (1963) also noted that in patients with chronic renal disease there was an increase in the number of lymphatico-venous anastomoses.

With the clinical use of lymphangiography, lymphatico-venous anastomoses have been demonstrated with increasing frequency. These channels, to be visualized, must be large enough to accept the bolus of contrast material. Recently, lymphatico-venous communications have been visualized in cases of lymphatic obstruction. Radiographic portrayal of the event must be done during the injection of contrast material. The speed of flow within the lymphatics is minimal in comparison to that in veins. Once the oil droplets gain access to the veins, they rapidly disappear. With the help of the constant forward pressure exerted during lymphangiography, this event can be captured. This is facilitated if there is a partial concomitant obstruction in the venous system which decelerates venous flow, allowing contrast material to accumulate in a larger bolus.

The different gradations in the visualization of lymphatico-venous anastomoses are illustrated in the following cases (Fig. 6-11).

In keeping with Threefoot's findings of an increased frequency of lymphatico-venous anastomoses to the inferior vena cava at the level of the renal veins, a lymphatico-inferior vena caval communication was opacified in a patient with retroperitoneal metastases from a seminoma (Wolfel 1965). The portal venous radicals were filled during lymphangiography in another patient with lymphatico-portal anastomoses. Obstruction of retroperitoneal lymphatics, as well as the inferior vena cava itself, allows the utilization of the collateral venous pathways to the portal system and eventual deposition of the oil-based contrast material in the liver venous radicals.

An understanding of lymphatic dynamics is essential in the adequate management of patients with testicular neoplasms.

LYMPHANGIOGRAPHIC INTERPRETATION

Interpretation of the lymphangiogram depends upon careful scrutiny of both lymphatic and nodal phases (Wallace and Jackson 1968; Bourquin 1969). Under normal circumstances, there is an inverse relationship between the size and number of nodes; the larger the nodes, the fewer their number. The size varies considerably. The inguinal nodes are slightly larger than the pelvic nodes, which are in turn slightly larger than the retroperitoneal nodes. A reversal of this relationship bears further investigation. Alteration in size, number, and architecture occurs in diseased stages. Interpretation of lymphangiograms (Table IX-XIII) may be categorized as:

1. Positive-unequivocal evidence of disease.
2. Suspicious - requires further verification by complementary techniques such as pyelography, venography and arteriography. Follow-up radiographs at monthly intervals or even repeat lymphangiography may demonstrate sufficient change to allow a positive diagnosis.
3. Irregular changes - con-

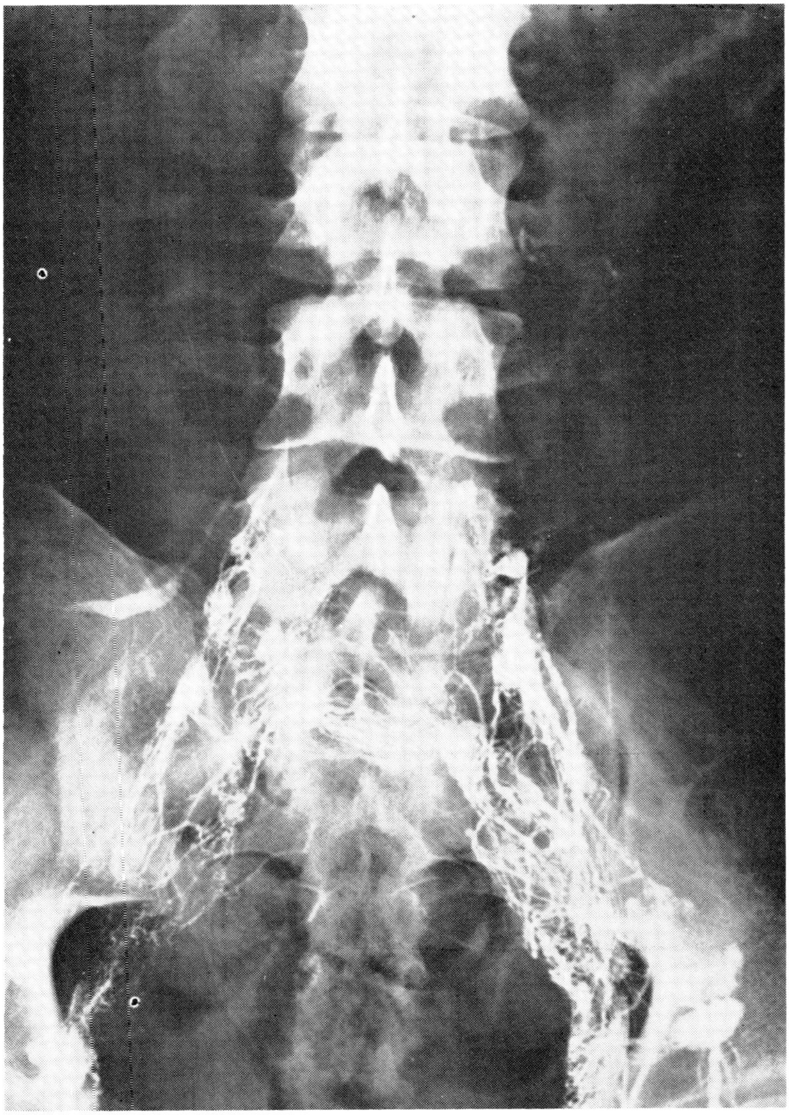

Fig. 6-11. Lymphatico-venous anastomoses. A, Lymphatico-portal vein anastomosis. This patient demonstrates para-aortic lymphatic obstruction by metastatic nodes from a carcinoma of the testicle. Lymphatico-venous anastomoses are opacified with subsequent filling of the liver.

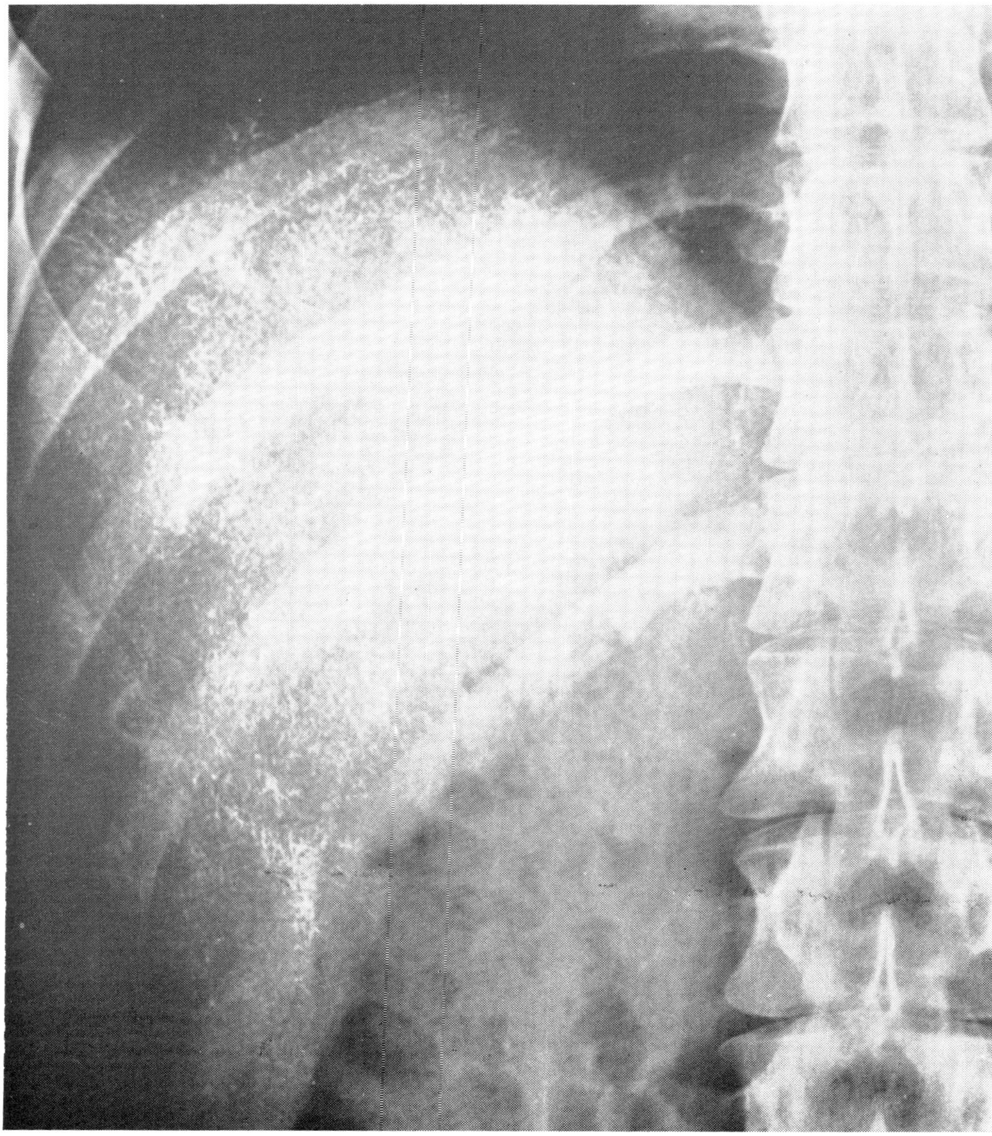

Fig. 6-11. Lymphatico-venous anastomoses. B, Lymphatico-portal vein anastomosis. This patient demonstrates para-aortic lymphatic obstruction by metastatic nodes from a carcinoma of the testicle. Lymphatico-venous anastomoses are opacified with subsequent filling of the liver.

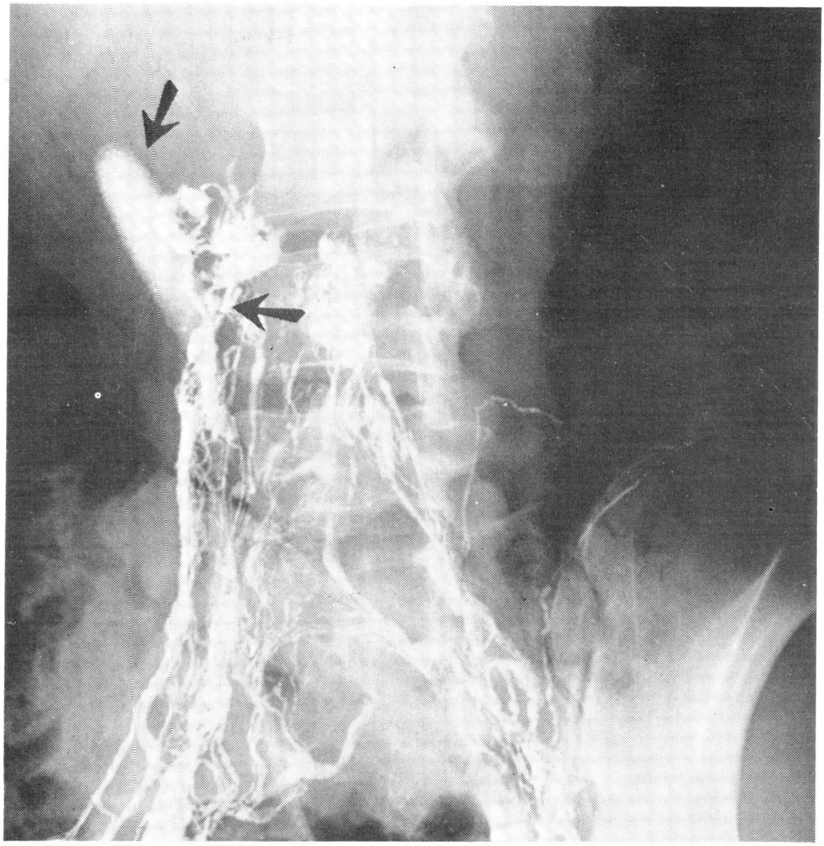

Fig. 6-11. Lymphatico-venous anastomoses. C, Lymphatico-inferior vena caval anastomosis. Seminomatous involvement of the para-aortic nodes resulting in lymphatic obstruction and utilization of lymphatico inferior vena caval anastomoses (↑) as collateral pathways (Wolfel 1965).

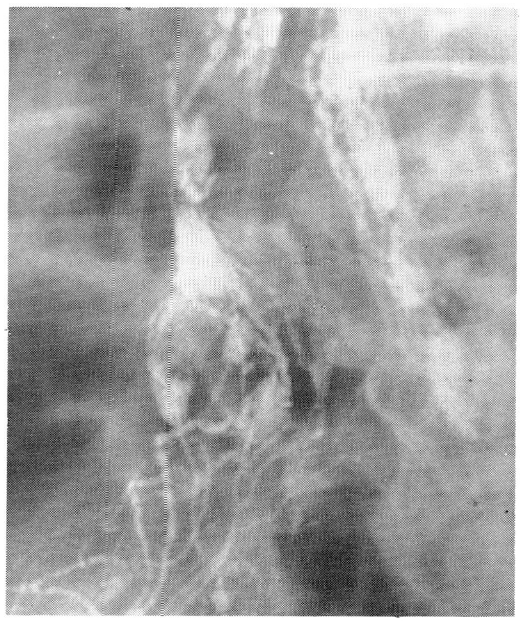

Fig. 6-11. Lymphatico-venous anastomoses. D, Lymphatico-venous anastomoses. Following retroperitoneal node dissection, lymphatic obstruction caused opacification of these alternate channels.

TABLE IX

CRITERIA - ABNORMAL LYMPHANGIOGRAM LYMPHATIC PHASE

1. Filling defect in a node not traversed by lymphatics.

2. Lymphatic obstruction and/or distortion.

3. Collateral circulation -
   Lymphatico - lymphatic
   Lymphatico - venous
   Lymphatico - prelymphatic

4. Lack of normal number of lymphatic channels.

5. Stasis of contrast material in lymphatics on 24 hour examination.

TABLE X

CRITERIA - ABNORMAL LYMPHANGIOGRAM NODAL PHASE

1. Filling defect (partial replacement with crescent deformity)

2. Complete replacement

3. Rounded node

TABLE XI

SECONDARY EVIDENCE OF METASTATIC DISEASE

1. Total replacement of nodes with lymphatic distortion or obstruction.
2. Lymphatic obstruction without collateral circulation.
3. Lymphatic obstruction with collateral circulation.

All above to be correlated with:

History and physical examinations
Urography
Venography
Arteriography

TABLE XII

INTERPRETATION

1. Definite evidence of metastasis
2. Suspicious*
3. Irregular nodes*
4. No definite evidence of metastasis*

*Considered negative in patient's management

TABLE XIII

DEFINITE EVIDENCE OF NODAL METASTASIS

Filling defect in a node

Not traversed by lymphatics

notes a negative study with some minor reservations which may be resolved by serial roentgenograms at regular intervals.

4. Negative - the limitation of this technique must always be appreciated.

The positive demonstration of disease has excellent correlation (Hreschyshyn and Sheehan 1960; Jackson et al. 1961; MacDonald 1962; Schaffer et al. 1962; Kittridge et al. 1963; Schaffer et al. 1963; Arvay and Picard 1964; Pomerantz and Kise 1964; Ruttiman and Del Buono 1964; Fuchs 1965; Wiljasalo 1965; Davidson 1967; Tetoni et al. 1967; Patriquin 1969; Wiljasalo 1969). A negative study on the other hand means little because microscopic changes are beyond the competence of the lymphangiogram.

False-positive interpretation of lymph node metastases has provoked considerable criticism of lymphangiography. A proper evaluation must have a three-dimensional approach since a false impression of a nodal defect may be produced by superimposition. Each node has a hilar defect, the proper identification of which is made only by paying close attention to the lymphatic phase (Fig. 6-12). Of particular importance is an understanding of the problems that arise in the evaluation of inguinal nodes. In general, they should be evaluated only when they function as the primary site of drainage from lesions of the lower limb and perineum. A high percentage of false-positives may be expected because of fatty replacement of nodal parenchyma in this area (Fig. 6-13). Fibrosis may on occasion be present as a result of repeated insults from minor infections or injuries to the lower limbs. In general, these spurious defects will be traversed by lymphatic channels which may be traced in the lymphatic phase.

False-positive interpretations may also be the result of inflammation. Acute inflammation is usually depicted lymphangiographically by enlargement of the nodes with maintenance of the normal architecture (Fig. 6-14A). The acute reaction to the lymphangiogram itself may result in a temporary enlargement of the nodes opacified. Local defects produced by small abscesses may simulate carcinoma. Chronic inflammatory disease may lead to confusion in the diagnosis of malignant lesions. The reactive hyperplasia of collagen disease presents a picture not unlike leukemia. Granulomatous disease can lead to confusion. Sarcoidosis (Akisada et al. 1969), tuberculosis, Hodgkin's disease and reticulum cell sarcoma have many similarities. Tuberculosis with cavitation and destruction of a portion of the node is difficult to differentiate from carcinoma (Figs. 6-14B and 6-14C). Despite these problems of interpretation, much valuable information is offered by this examination in the establishment of a differential diagnosis.

Carcinoma: In evaluating the case of a patient with a known carcinoma the involved nodes should lie along the primary and secondary echelon of lymphatic drainage. Variations in normal lymphatic anatomy are frequent and assessment of the lymphatic phase is essential to determine the pre-existing anomalous channels which will significantly affect the distribution of metastases. Carcinomatous spread usually occurs at the local site of drainage from a known primary. Changes at a distance from the primary site without evidence of bypass channels or lymphatic obstruction with collateral circulation should be viewed with great caution. Tumor emboli travel along the lymphatic channels, gaining access to the marginal sinus. At this point, their progress is impeded; they enlarge and obstruct the marginal sinus. Lymphatics do not traverse the area replaced by carcinoma but are distorted or obstructed by the carcinomatous focus (Figs. 6-15A and 6-15B). This may also be manifested by stasis of the

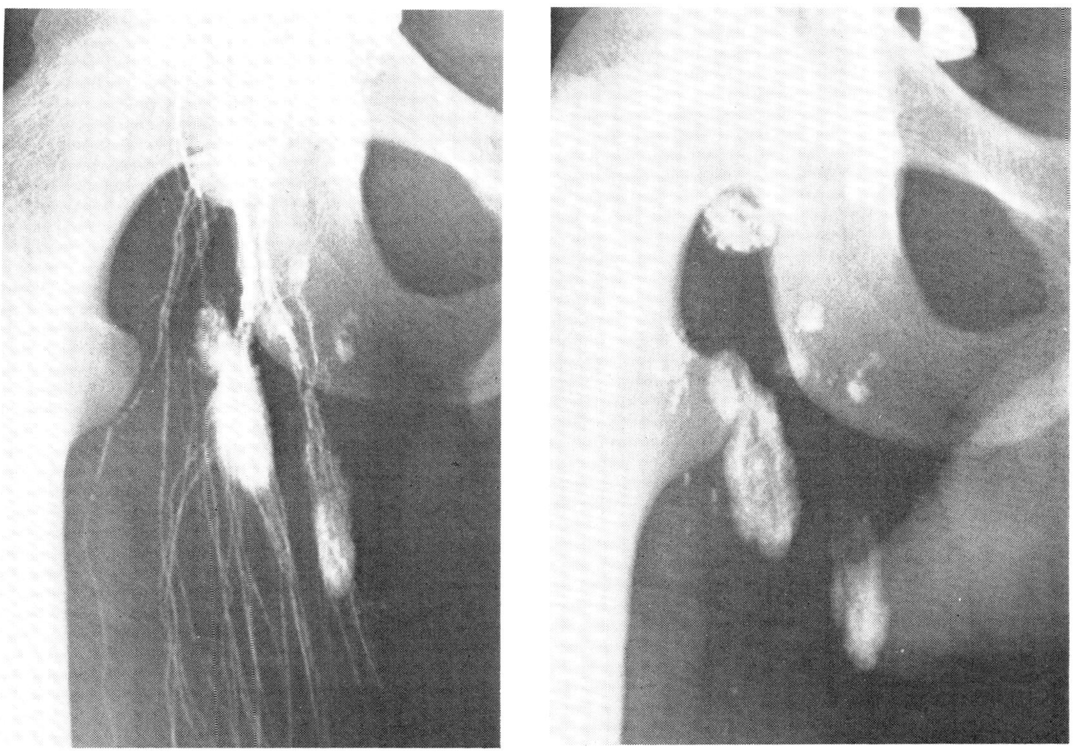

Fig. 6-12. Normal lymph nodes. A, Lymphatic phase. B, Nodal phase.

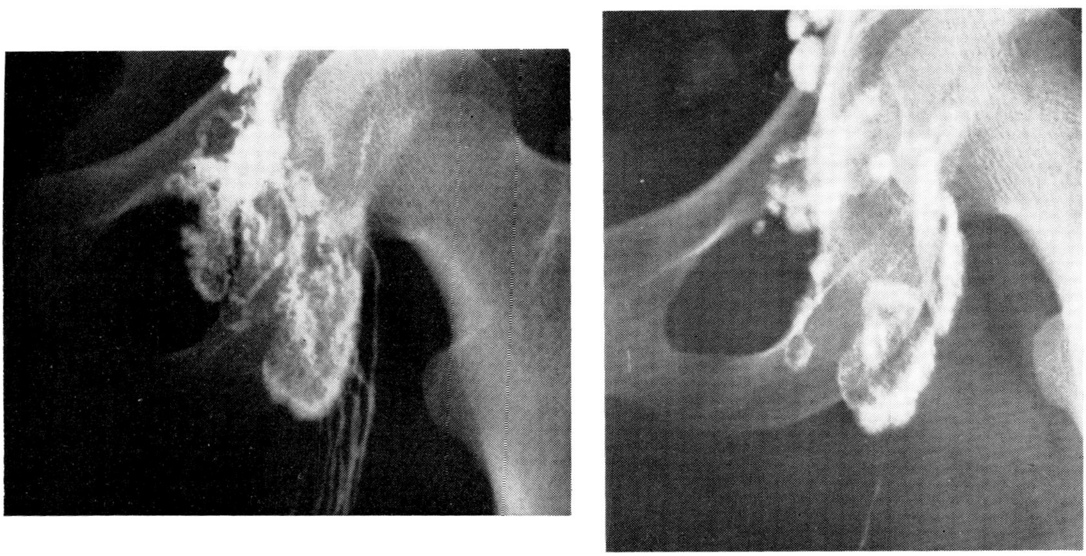

Fig. 6-13. Fatty replacement within a lymph node. A, Lymphatic phase. B, Nodal phase. The lymphatics traverse the area of fatty replacement.

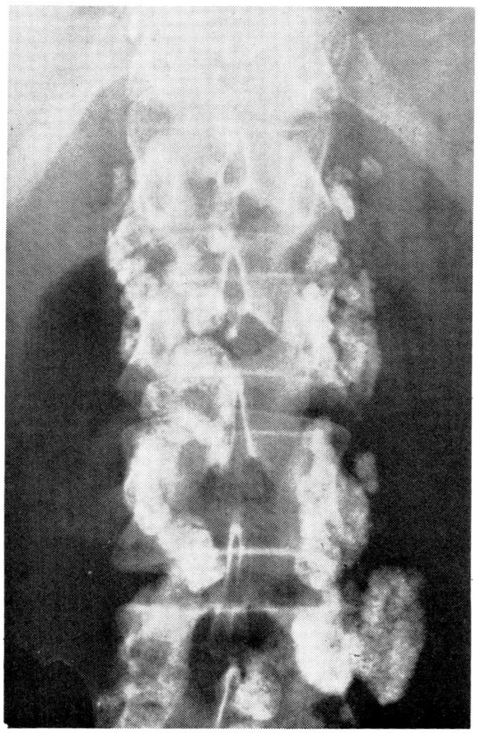

Fig. 6-14. Inflamatory disease. A, enlarged para-aortic nodes in a patient with pancreatitis.

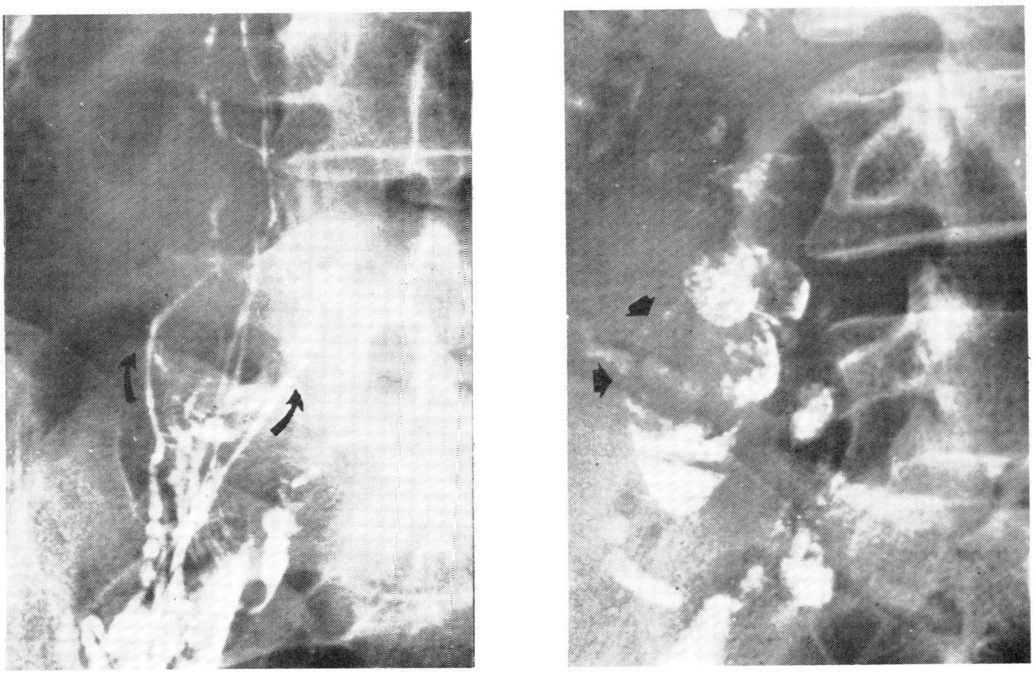

Fig. 6-14. Inflamatory disease. B and C, Tuberculosis. These changes simulate carcinoma.

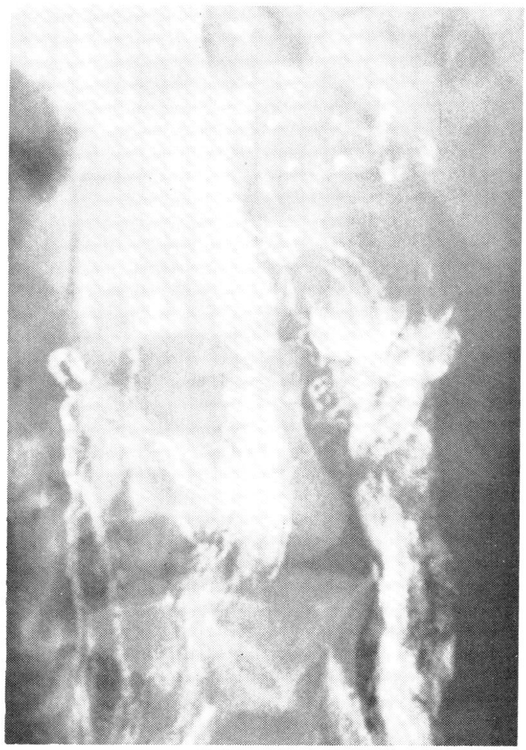

Fig. 6-15. Metastatic carcinoma. A, Lymphatic phase. The lymphatics do not traverse the defects produced by the metastatic involvement of the para-aortic nodes in a patient with carcinoma of the testis.

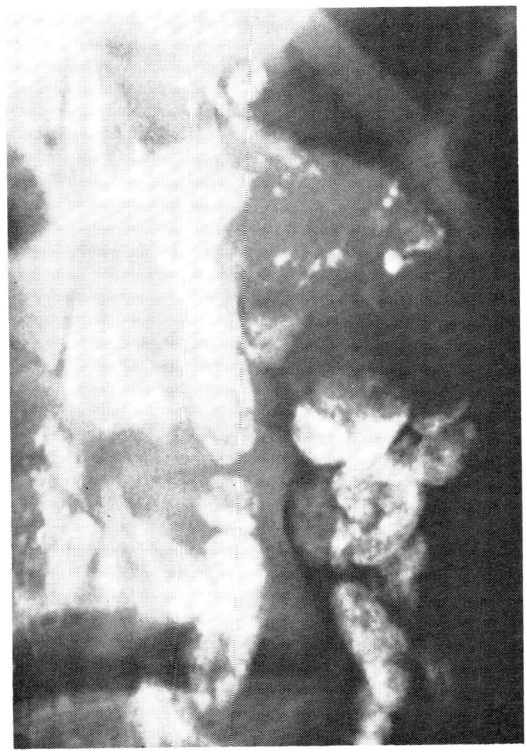

Fig. 6-15. Metastatic carcinoma. B, Nodal phase. The crescent deformity is produced by the metastasis and represents a partially replaced node.

channels as seen in the delayed roentgenograms or those taken 24 hours later. Failure of opacification of the lymphatics may indicate disease, even in the absence of obvious nodal involvement. When lymphatic pathways become obstructed by proliferating tumor, collateral circulation may be the only residual evidence of massive replacement of nodal tissue (Fig. 6-15C).

The lymphangiographic pattern of the node depends on the opacification of the residual functioning tissue. Deposition of tumor in the marginal sinus results in irregularities along the periphery of the node causing a moth-eaten appearance, frequently a crescent deformity (Figs. 6-16A and 6-16B). Undoubtedly, tumor emboli eventually gain access to the interstices of the node but the major alteration is in the margin. A three-dimensional view of the node is necessary for more accurate evaluation. Tomography may offer great assistance in the delineation of the architectural pattern in the node (De Roos 1964) (Figs. 6-16C and 6-16D). Initially, there may be a small increase in the size of the involved nodes. The configuration of the diseased node is more rounded in contrast to the normal oval or kidney shape of the node (Wiljasalo 1965). As the process progresses, the node is eventually totally replaced and therefore is not opacified. The absence of a node in an area with normal lymphatic channels is probably due to something other than malignant tumor. This finding may be verified by the use of complementary procedures such as venography and pyelography which will be discussed.

The major differential diagnosis is not carcinoma versus lymphoma but versus a false-positive defect, fatty replacement, fibrosis, etc. In contrast to false-positive defects, lymphatic channels do not usually traverse the area replaced by carcinoma (Zeidman et al. 1955).

Lymphomas: The strongest support for lymphangiography as a diagnostic tool has been in diagnosing and treating lymphomatous diseases. The radiographic picture of these diseases of the lymphoid tissue is due to a primary change in the intrinsic nodal architecture. In contrast to the findings of metastatic carcinoma, the margin of the node is for the most part intact until the late stage of the disease. The necessity of evaluating the lymphatic phase in this group remains important. The lymphatics remain patent longer and traverse the parenchyma and the tumor tissue until they are distorted and compressed. Certain patterns of growth or destruction by lymphomatous diseases are seen repeatedly allowing for a specific diagnosis (Wiljasalo 1969) (Figs. 6-17A and 6-17B). The criteria must be established by each radiologist in cooperation with his pathologist. The lymphangiographic interpretation is made from the evaluation of many nodes in contrast to the single node usually available to the pathologist. As the disease advances the ability to differentiate node patterns is virtually impossible. There is usually an increase in the size and number of nodes opacified.

Melanoma and Nodal Sarcomas: Two patterns have been reported in metastatic melanoma. The more frequent picture is that of well-circumscribed deposits in enlarged nodes in the local area of drainage. Lymphatics do not permeate these involved areas but are distorted or obstructed by them (Fig. 6-18). Occasionally, there is marked disorganization which may be associated with irregular destruction throughout the node and a more aggressive clinical picture.

Other sarcomas occasionally metastasize to lymph nodes. Their patterns are frequently similar to that seen in a localized variety of melanoma.

COMPLEMENTARY PROCEDURES

Venography may be of considerable assistance in establishing the eti-

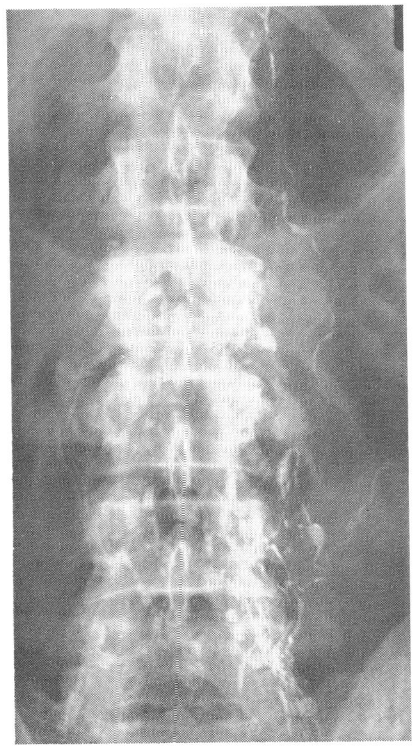

Fig. 6-15. Metastatic carcinoma. C, The lymphatics are displaced by totally replaced nodes in this patient with metastases from a seminoma of the testis.

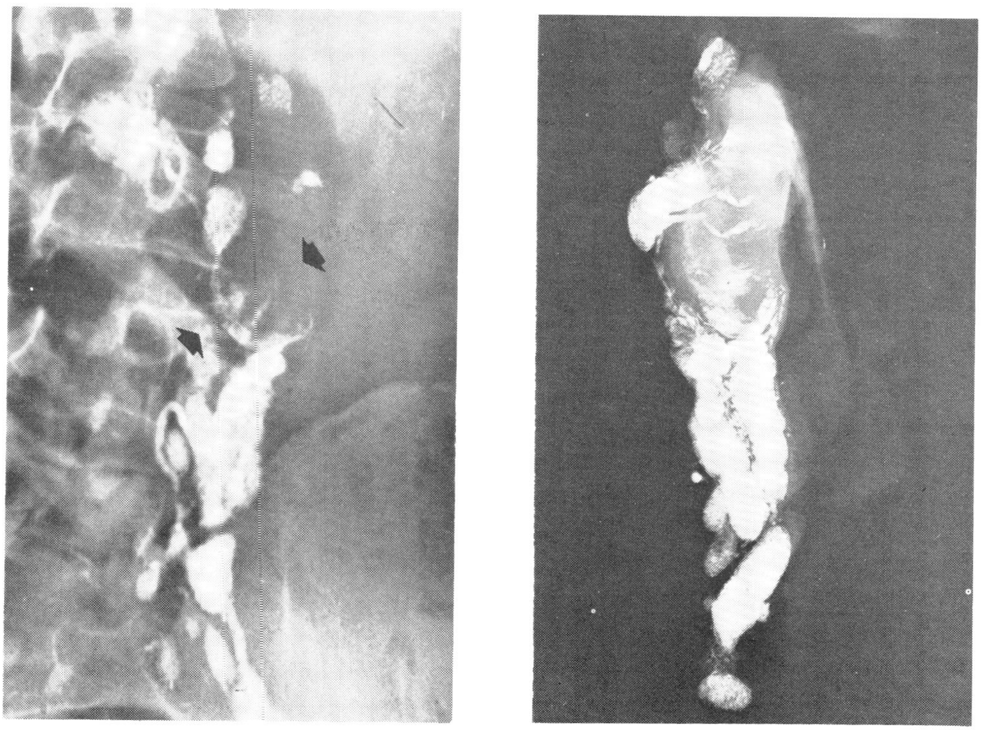

Fig. 6-16. Metastatic carcinoma of the testis. A and B, Crescent deformity produced by metastatic carcinoma from the testis. The nodes when removed confirmed the partial replacement by carcinoma.

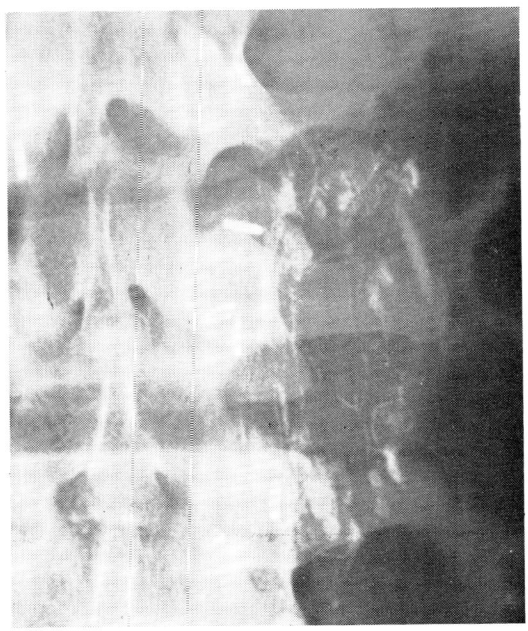

Fig. 6-16. Metastatic carcinoma of the testis. C, Tomography was of some assistance. In the better delineation of the abnormal node in this patient with metastasis from a seminoma of the testis.

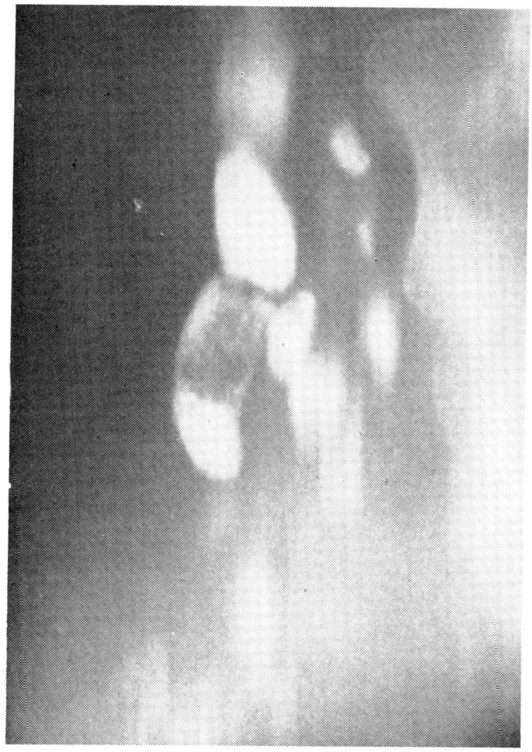

Fig. 6-16. Metastatic carcinoma of the testis. D, Tomography was of some assistance in the better delineation of the abnormal node in this patient with metastasis from a seminoma of the testis.

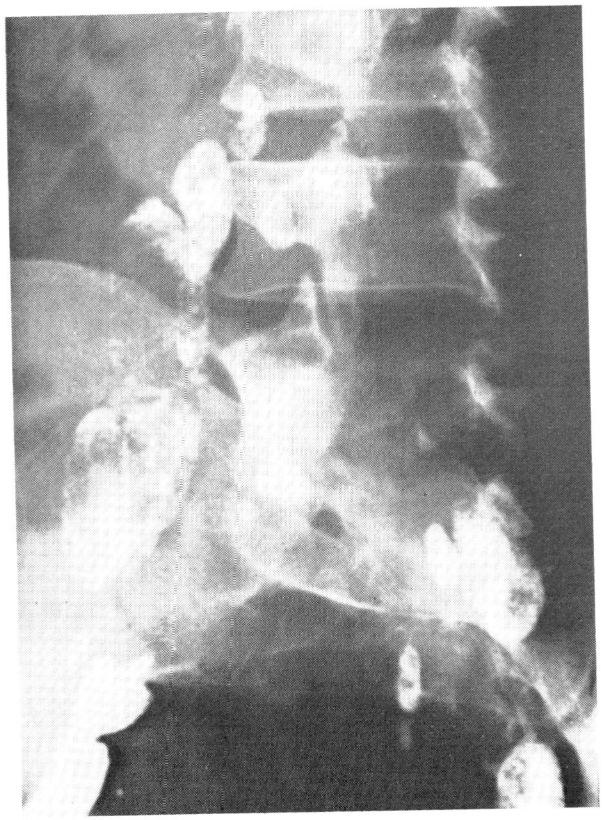

Fig. 6-17. Malignant lymphoma. A, Hodgkin's disease.

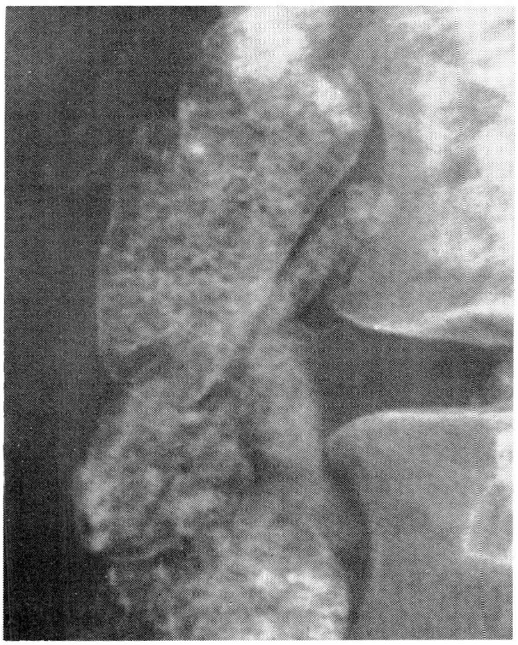

Fig. 6-17. Malignant lymphoma. B, Lymphocytic lymphoma.

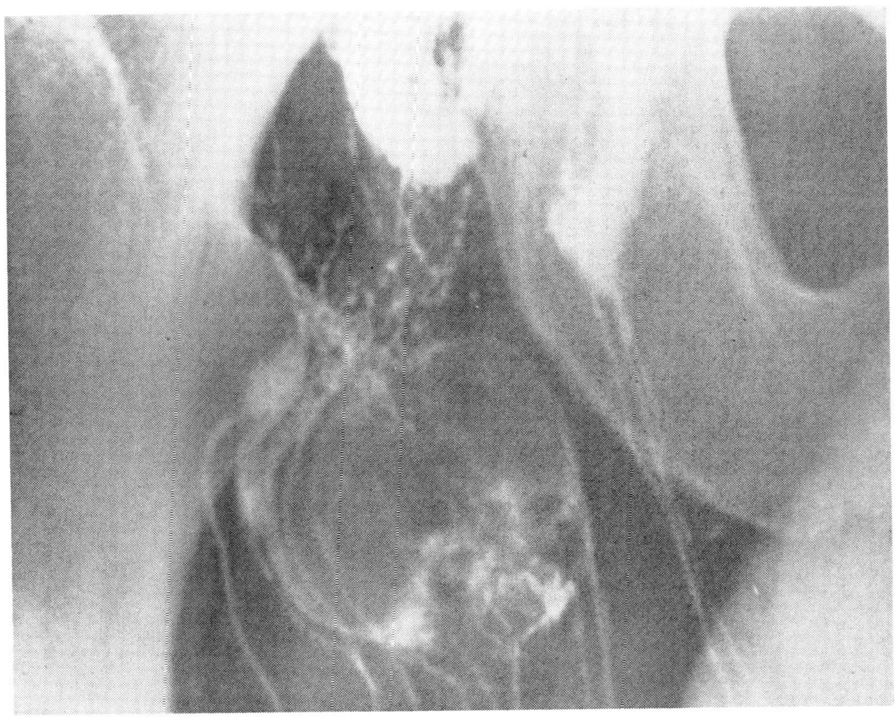

Fig. 6-18. Metastatic malignant melanoma. A, Lymphatic phase.

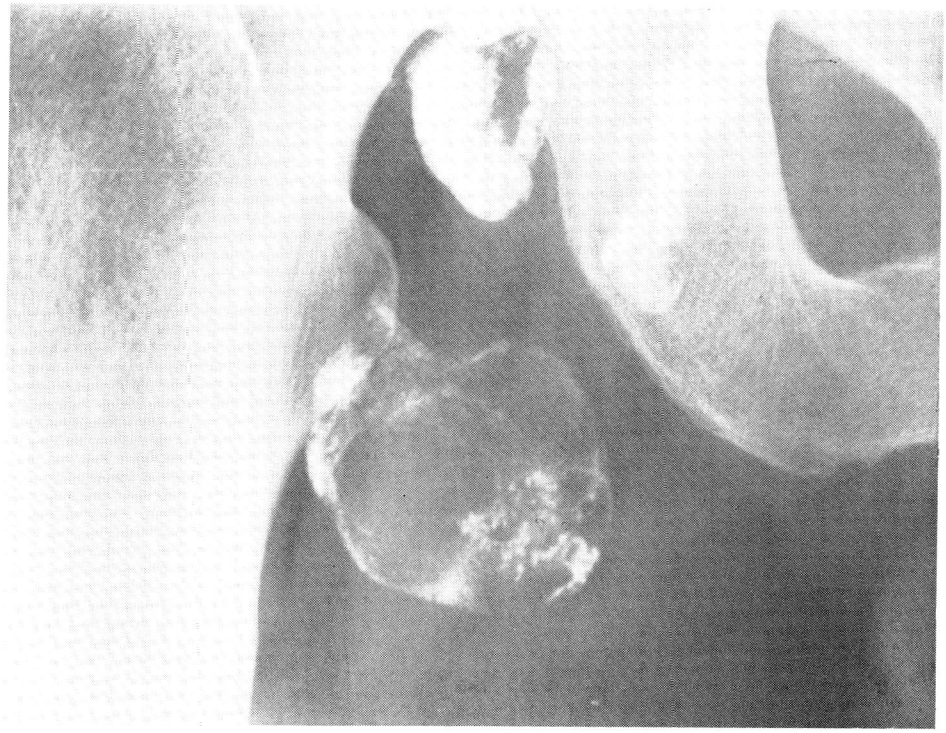

Fig. 6-18. Metastatic malignant melanoma. B, Nodal phase.

ology of lymphatic obstruction (Baum et al. 1963; Mahaffy 1964). This depends upon demonstration of the masses which distort or obstruct the adjacent vein. Difficulties may be encountered in the presence of thrombophlebitis. The natural limitations of this procedure are obvious and are dictated by the size and position of the involved nodes. Inferior vena cavography can evaluate only the right side of the retroperitoneal space (Fig. 6-19). However, in the region above L-2 where the lumbar trunks usually drain into cisterna chyli, thus bypassing any nodes above this level, vena cavography is of utmost importance.

After radiotherapy or chemotherapy, the problem of differentiation becomes more acute. These therapeutic approaches reduce the number and size of the nodes usually without significant effect on the lymphatic vessels (Lenzi and Bassani 1963; Engeset 1964). Rarely, after radiotherapy, additional pathways are demonstrated and are probably the result of fibrosis and minor obstruction of lymphatic channels. Venography done under these circumstances will reveal no evidence of a mass.

Pyelography is another complementary procedure in the evaluation of the retroperitoneal area. It may confirm the existence of totally replaced nodes by impression or obstruction of the urinary tract (Fig. 6-20). Suspected nodes can be more definitely implicated if they produce an associated change in the urinary tract.

PERCUTANEOUS RETROPERITONEAL LYMPH NODE BIOPSY

A percutaneous approach for retroperitoneal lymph node biopsy has considerable potential provided the technique can be accomplished with minimal complications and risks to the patient. In experimental studies we have modified the percutaneous technique described by Nordrstrom and Ruttman and have adapted them to the retroperitoneal area. Prior to biopsy the retroperitoneal nodes are opacified by pedal lymphangiography in the usual manner. Access to the retroperitoneal space is achieved from the inguinal area. A track is created utilizing cervical dilators and maintained by a teflon catheter. The retroperitoneal area is then insufflated with gas. Under fluoroscopic guidance, a long teflon sheathed metallic probe followed by a biopsy forceps are passed beneath the inguinal ligament along the perivascular plane and directed to the opacified lymph nodes. Biopsies are taken and documented radiographically and histologically (Fig. 6-21). To date, biopsies have been performed on cadavers and in living dogs without incident and suggests that the procedure with future refinements may hold promise as an additional diagnostic tool.

APPLICATIONS OF LYMPHANGIOGRAPHY IN TESTICULAR MALIGNANCIES

Detection of Nodal Metastases

Nodal metastases from testicular malignant disease show several different architectural patterns (Fig. 6-22). Involved nodes are more spherical than normal and may have a crescent deformity with the lymphatics failing to penetrate the marginal defects (carcinoma pattern). Occasionally, they may have a disrupted internal architecture with a relatively intact marginal sinus (lymphoma pattern). The latter picture is more frequently seen in some seminomas, lymphomas, and rhabdomyosarcomas of the testicle. At times, the metastatic nodes show both carcinoma and lymphoma-type patterns; a mixed variety. Only abnormal findings are of real value. A normal, suspicious or equivocal finding is considered to be normal in the management of the patient. Microscopic foci of tumor are beyond the

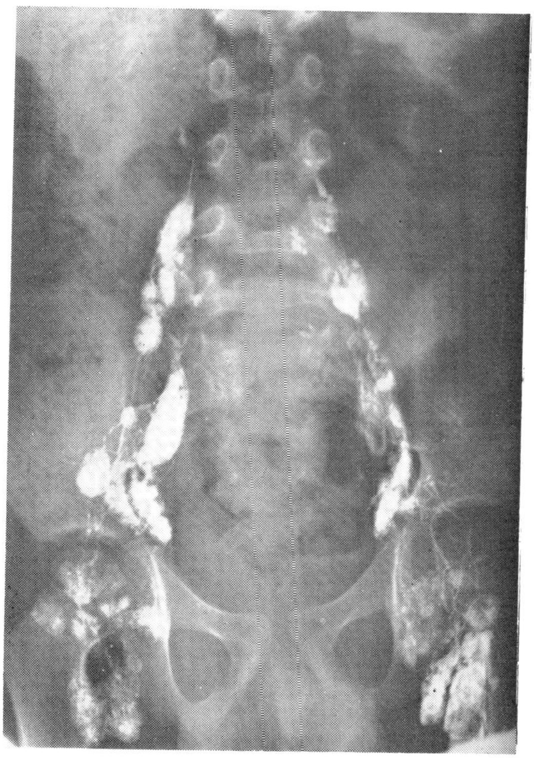

Fig. 6-19. A, This child with an embryonal carcinoma of the right testis showed minimal distortion of the upper retroperitoneal lymphatics on the right.

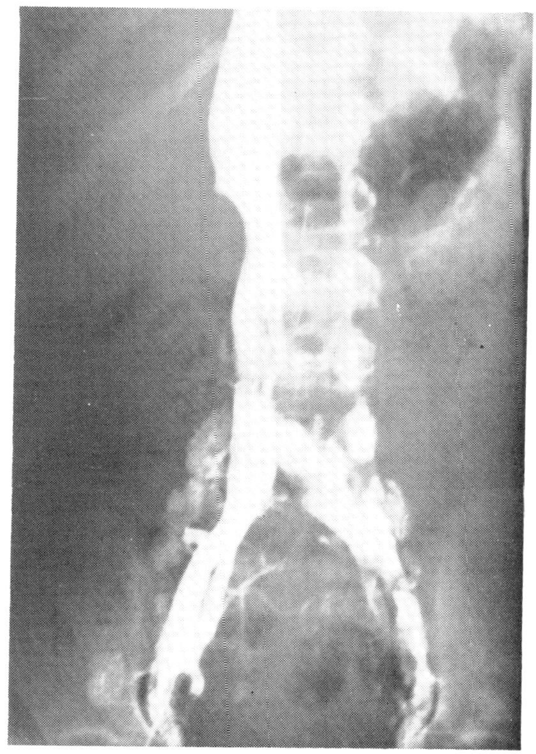

Fig. 6-19. Inferior venacavography. B, The inferior venacavogram demonstrated the presence of a large laterally placed mass.

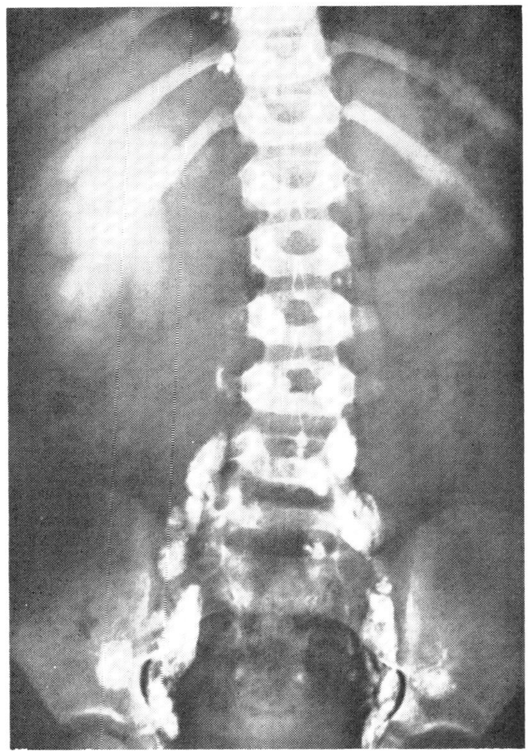

Fig. 6-19. C, The follow-up pyelogram revealed an obstructed ureter.

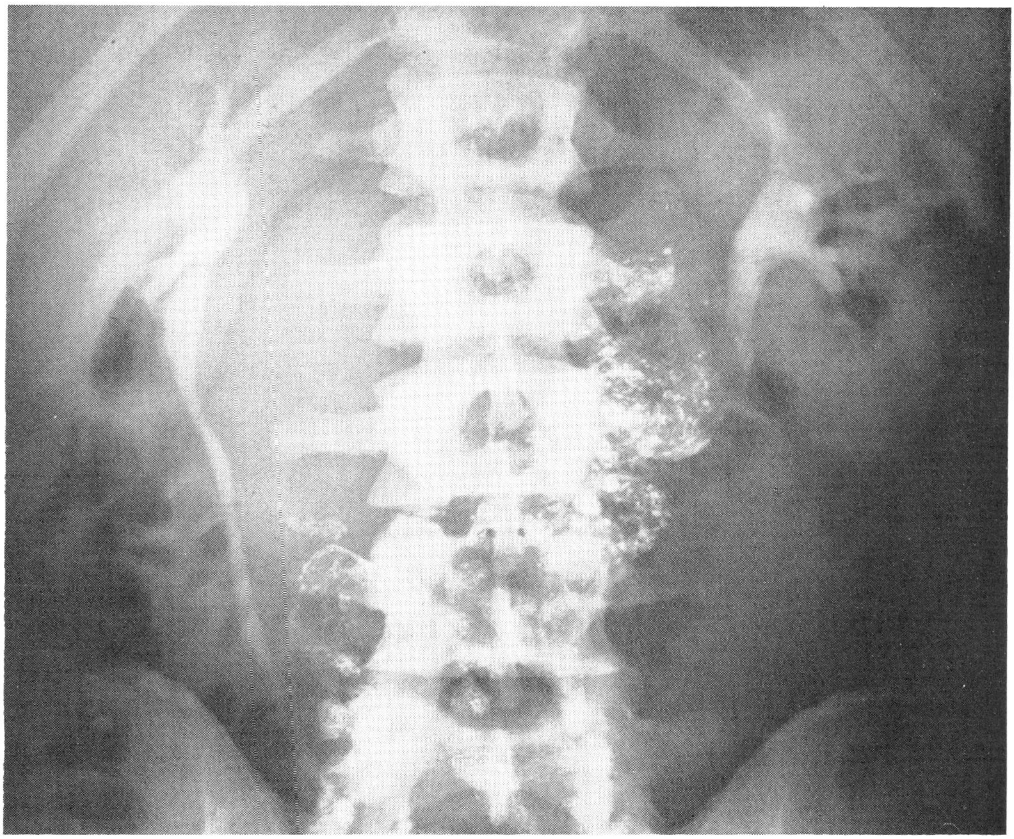

Fig. 6-20. Pyelography. Displacement of the ureters is produced by metastatic teratocarcinoma of the testis. The pyelogram aids in delineating the extent of the disease when the nodes are totally replaced as seen on the right side.

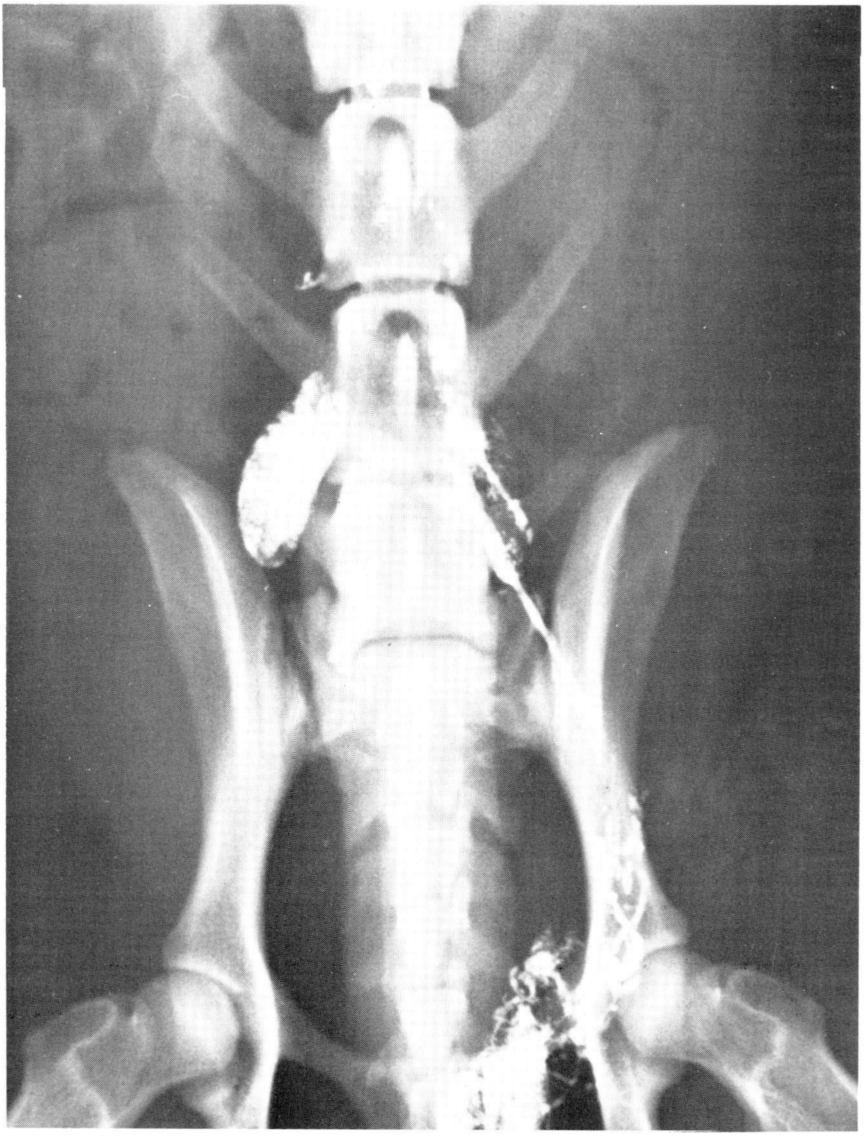

Fig. 6-21A. Large right periaortic lymph node in a dog.

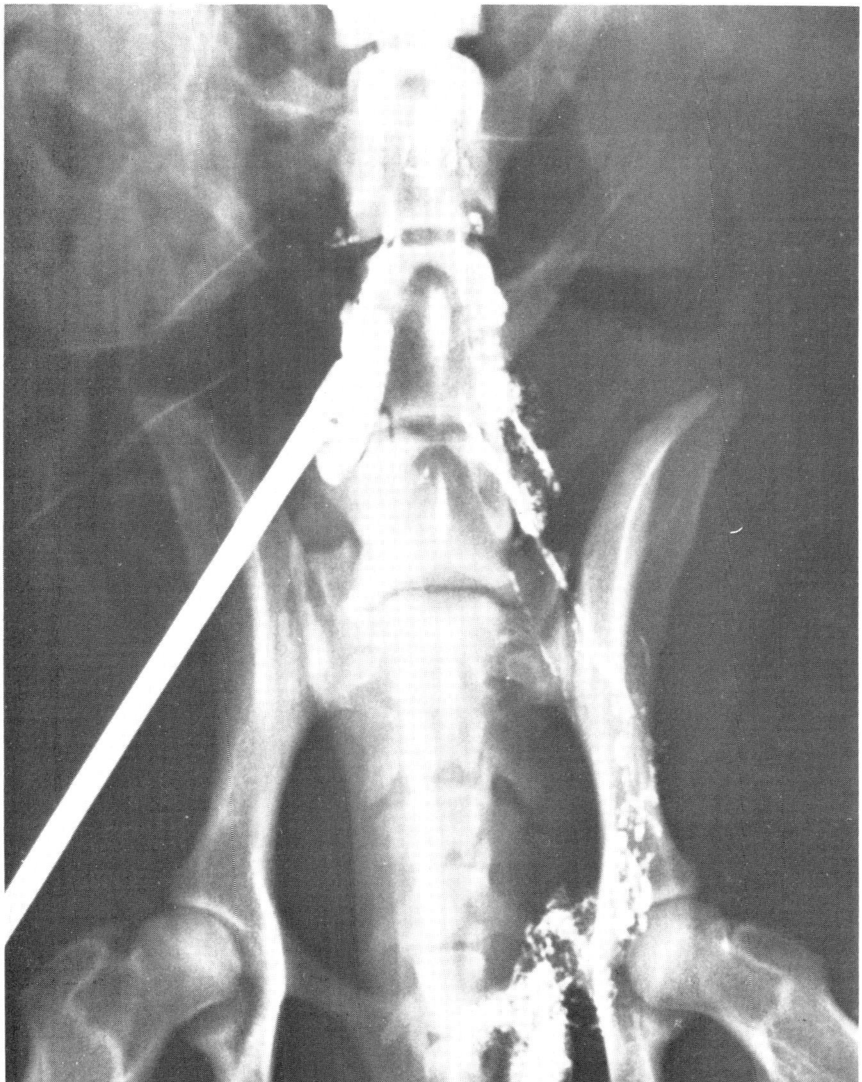

Fig. 6-21B. Percutaneous retroperitoneal lymph node biopsy forceps in place.

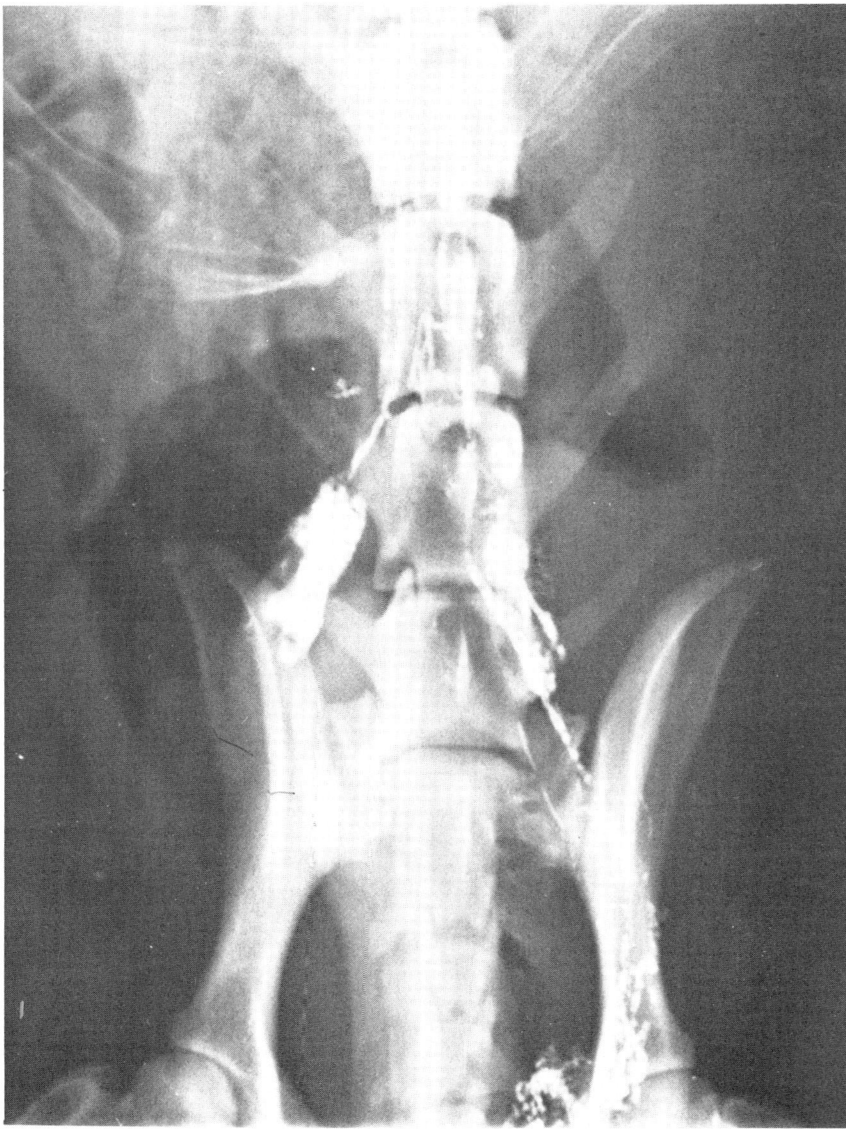

Fig. 6-21C. Post percutaneous lymph node biopsy film showing filling defect in node at site of biopsy.

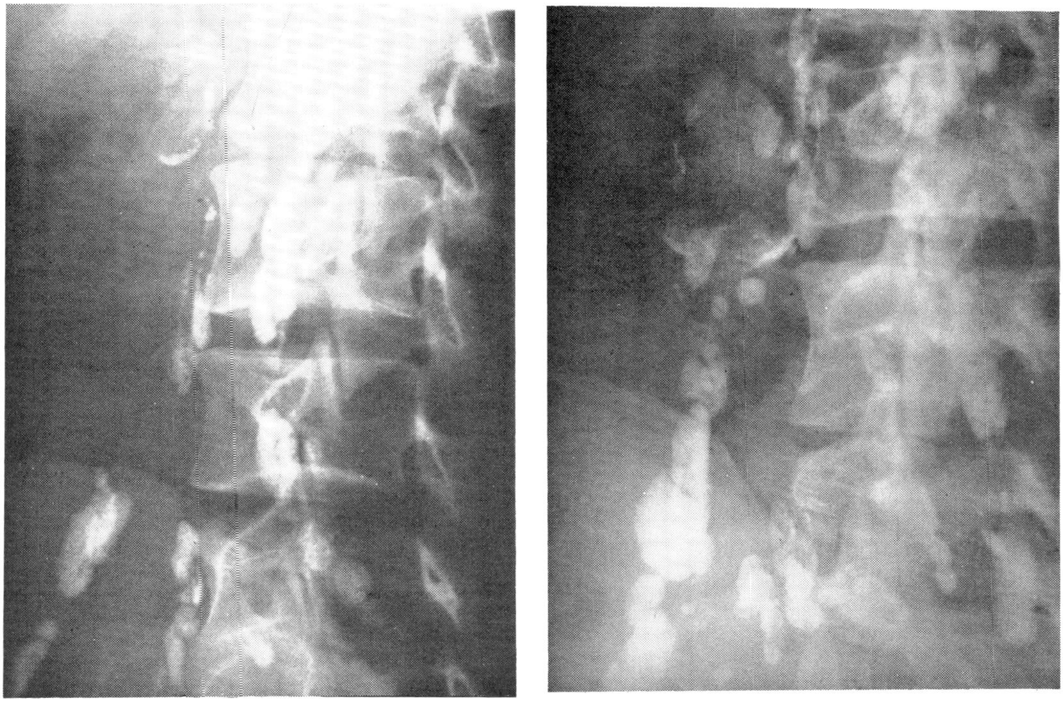

Fig. 6-22. Metastases from testicular malignancies. A, Embryonal carcinoma. B, Seminoma (carcinoma type pattern).

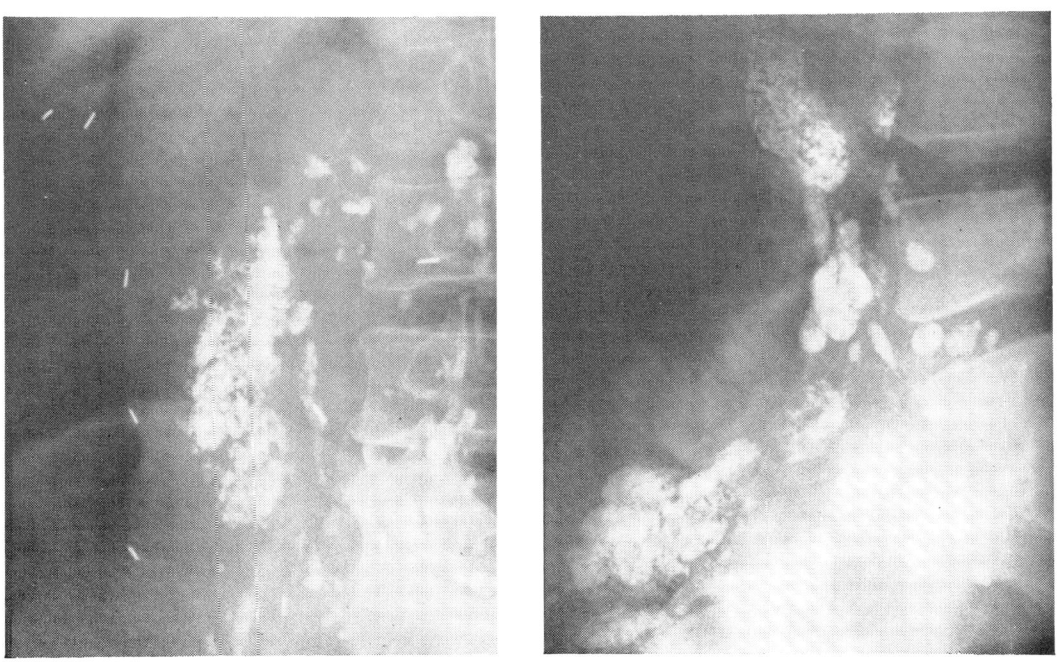

Fig. 6-22. Metastases from testicular malignancies. C, Seminoma (lymphoma type pattern). D, Rhabdomyosarcoma.

competence of this examination since metastases less than 3 mm in diameter cannot be detected by lymphangiography.

An Aid to Radiation Therapy

In testicular malignancies, the lymphangiogram often helps to delineate the location and extent of the metastatic lesion. It, therefore, facilitates an accurate placement of radiation portals. After a lymphangiogram, the contrast medium is retained in the lymph nodes for a considerable period of time. Therefore, the course of the disease can be followed closely and the effectiveness of radiation therapy can be evaluated accurately (Fig. 6-23). When lymph nodes which are considered positive for metastatic disease on lymphangiography are irradiated and subsequently excised, careful histologic examination is required to prove prior existence of malignant disease. Our experience suggests that not infrequently all that will remain of the malignant process is a small area of fibrosis and scarring (Fig. 6-24). This process has never been encountered in normal nodes and may be considered prima fascie evidence of prior metastatic spread.

Evaluation of Effectiveness of Chemotherapy

When metastatic lesions become widespread with involvement of the distant organs and most of the lymph nodes, chemotherapy is often the treatment of choice. The initial lymphangiogram is useful in demonstrating the extent of lymph node involvement. Follow-up lymphangiograms can evaluate the effectiveness of such therapy. Sequential examination of the contrast filled nodes may show a change in the size and configuration of the nodes. Any increase in the size or change in the architecture should be considered suspicious and indicates the ineffectiveness of such therapy. If there is inadequate residual contrast material remaining, a repeat lymphangiogram should be performed. Again, the same basic criteria exists as in the establishment of metastatic disease.

A Guide to Node Dissection

Prior to retroperitoneal lymphadenectomy, information concerning the extent of the metastatic lesion is desirable. Lymphangiography can demonstrate the location and extent of the metastases from testicular malignancies. Therefore, this procedure can be used as a guide to the surgeon in determining the advisability of nodal dissection (Fig. 6-25). Node dissections, regardless of the thoroughness or talents of the surgeon, are seldom complete. Roentgenograms of the abdomen obtained in the operating room during the surgical procedure must be undertaken to determine the completeness of dissection. Radioactive iodine and marker dyes such as chlorophyl in Ethiodol have been utilized in an attempt to achieve a more complete dissection. A cross-over of the lymph drainage between the two sides in the para-aortic region is a normal finding. Contralateral metastases of testicular carcinoma is not uncommon; consequently, bilateral nodal dissection is essential. The extent of the dissection should be determined by the lymphatic distribution. This depends, in part, on the level at which the testicular and lumbar lymphatic trunks empty into the thoracic duct. At times, this continues above the L-2 level to the T-10 or even higher (Fig. 6-26). Under such circumstances, it is somewhat difficult to surgically approach the complete lymphatic drainage from the testis.

Demonstration of Postlymphadenectomy Changes

Lymphatic alterations are encountered following pelvic retroperitoneal nodal dissection, i.e. lymphocysts (Fig. 6-8), lymphatic obstruc-

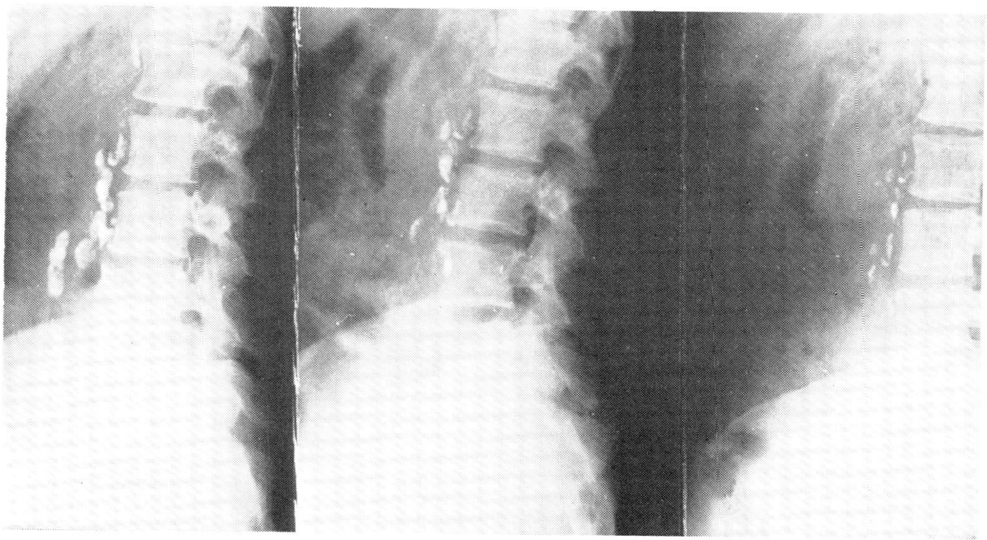

Fig. 6-23. Aid to therapy. The preoperative and postoperative examinations revealed residual nodes following the retroperitoneal dissection. Radiation therapy reduced the size of the residual nodes.

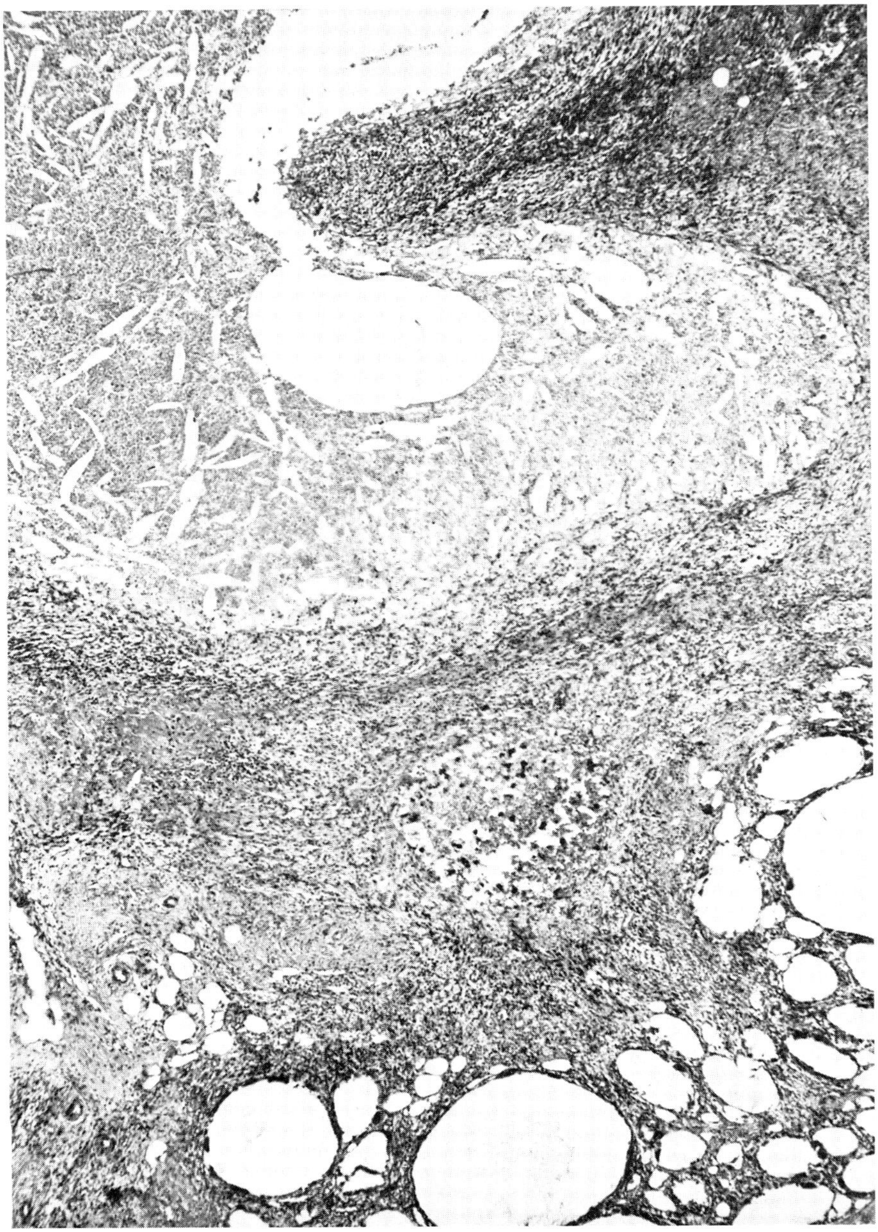

Fig. 6-24A. Excised lymph node showing reaction to lymphangiographic media in the lower half. In the upper portion is an irregular area of necrosis with multiple cholesterol-like spaces. H+E×20.

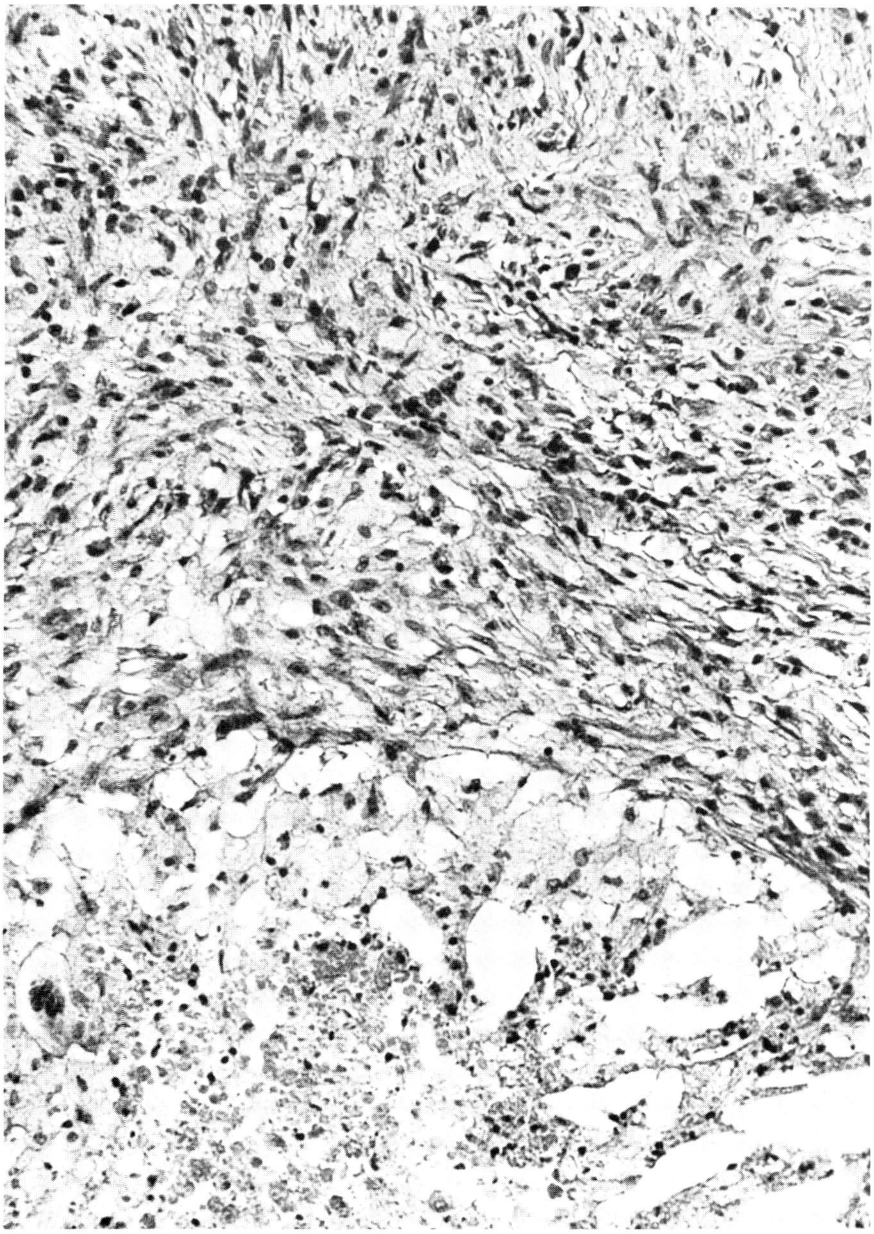

Fig. 6-24B. Higher magnification. Necrosis is present in the upper half. Foamy macrophages are in the periphery of the necrosis. In the lower half there is prominent fibrovascular proliferation. Tumor is not seen. H+E×100.

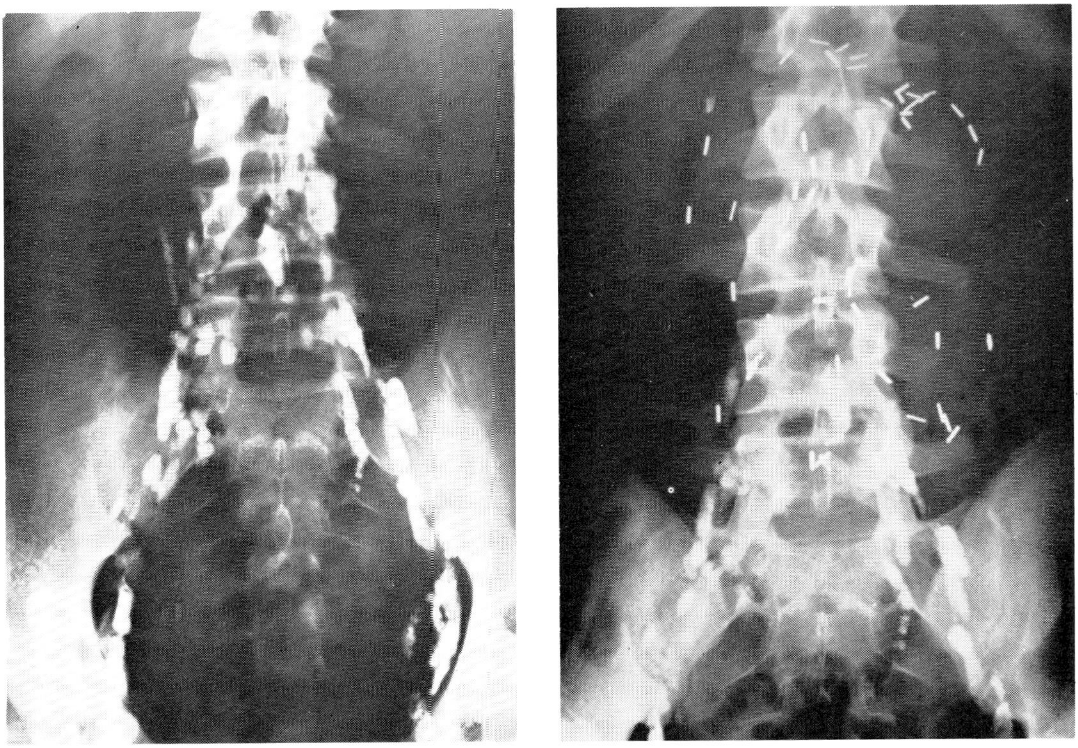

Fig. 6-25. Guide to node dissection. A, Preoperative. B, Postoperative.

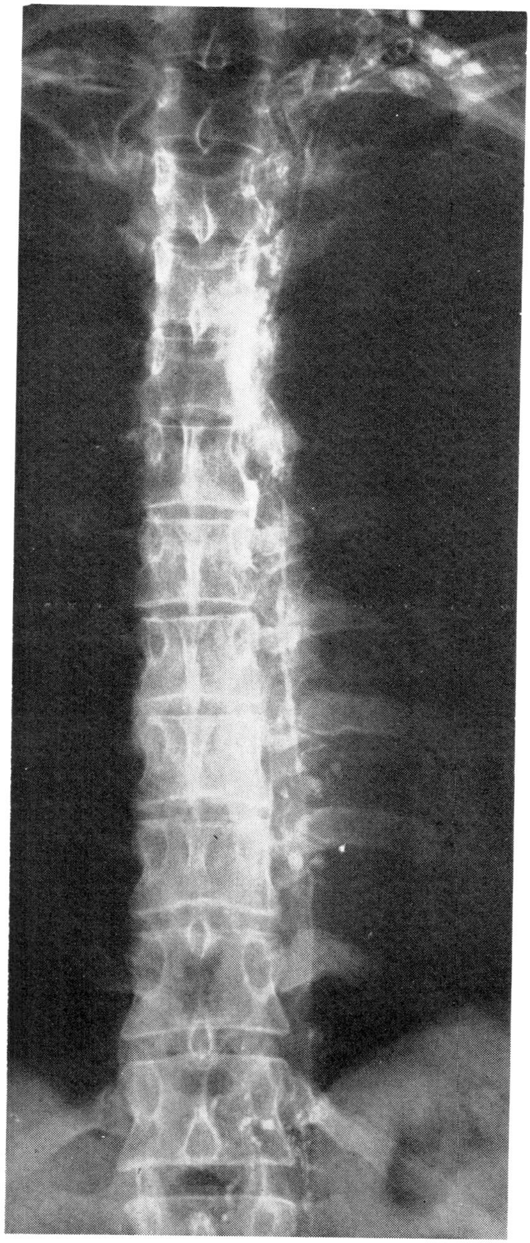

Fig. 6-26. Mediastinal nodes. Mediastinal and supraclavicular nodes opacify as a manifestation of variations in the normal distribution of the thoracic duct. A, Lymphatic phase.

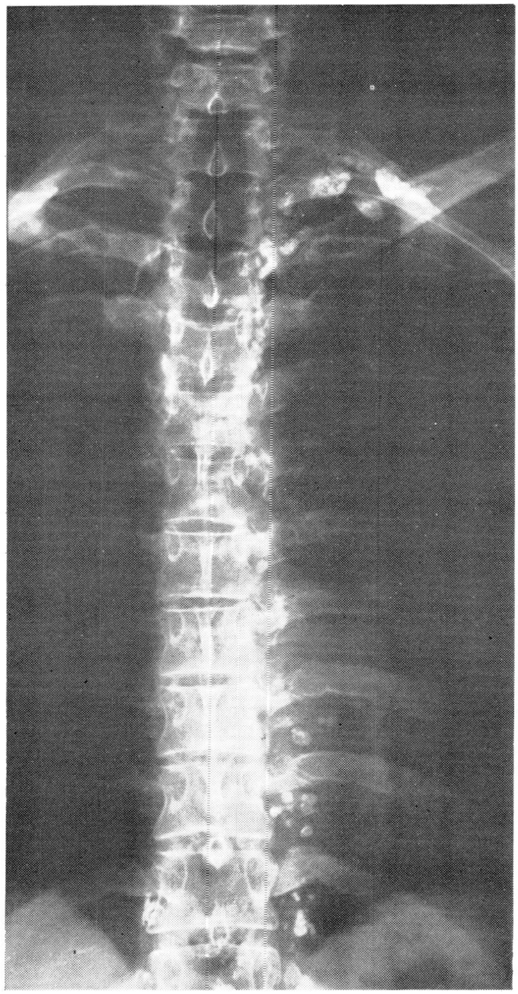

Fig. 6-26. Mediastinal nodes. B, Nodal phase.

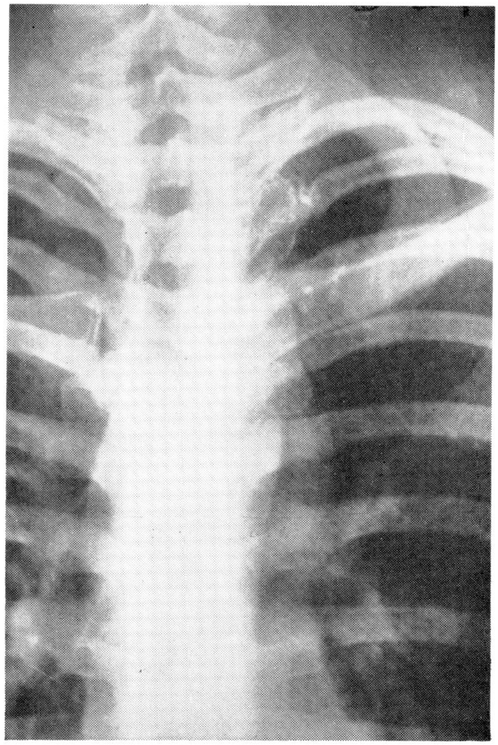

Fig. 6-26. Mediastinal nodes. Mediastinal nodal metastases in a patient with embryonal carcinoma of the testis.

tion or distortion (Fig. 6-7), and lymphatico-venous anastomoses (Fig. 6-11). Lymphocysts developing after nodal dissection may exert pressure effects on the urinary tract, gastrointestinal viscera and blood vessels. These effects may interfere with the function of the involved structures.

RESULTS AND SUMMARY

In evaluating the patient with testicular malignancy it is preferable to perform both testicular and pedal lymphangiography (Busch and Sayegh 1963; Arvay and Picard 1964; Cook et al. 1965; Chiappa et al. 1966; Sayegh et al. 1966; Wallace and Jing 1970). The lymphatic drainage is delineated more completely so that therapy may be tailored to the individual anatomic distribution. If the testicle has been removed pedal lymphangiography should be complemented by inferior vena cavography, bilateral renal venography, and follow-up pyelography. These studies provide maximum information as to the staging and extent of nodal metastases.

Our experience with 291 cases of testicular malignancies studied by pedal lymphangiography is described in Table XIV. Patients with seminoma of whom 25 per cent had abnormal findings by lymphangiography were treated by radiotherapy alone, making specific nodal correlation impossible. All other testicular malignancies were managed by a combination of surgery and radiotherapy, permitting closer scrutiny of the lymphangiographic findings. A normal lymphangiogram and normal findings at surgical exploration negate the necessity of any further treatment.

Surgical or autopsy findings, or both, were correlated with the lymphangiographic findings (Table XV). Retroperitoneal node dissections were

TABLE XIV

LYMPHANGIOGRAPHIC INTERPRETATION

(291 CASES)

	Positive	Negative
Seminoma	28	76
Carcinoma	76	105
Rhabdomyosarcoma	2	4
Totals	106	185

TABLE XV

LYMPHANGIOGRAPHIC - PATHOLOGIC CORRELATION

121 SURGICAL AND/OR AUTOPSY CASES

Positive	37	Carcinoma	117
False Positive	1	Rhabdomyosarcoma	4
Negative*	70		
False Negative**	13		
Totals	121		121

*For the purpose of correlation and patient management, all equivocal or suspicious readings are considered negative.

**1 case - 2 nodes positive in 11 central para-aortic group. 45 nodes in right and left para-aortic area all negative. The metastases were microscopic.

1 case - No evidence of metastasis on lymphangiogram. The metastasis was microscopic.

8 cases- Positive nodes in primary testicular lymphatics.

3 cases- Microscopic lesion, less than 3 mm.

performed at times following radiation therapy. Of the 50 dissections in which positive nodes were found, 37 patients (74 per cent) were diagnosed preoperatively by pedal lymphangiography. Positive roentgenographic interpretation had excellent correlation (96 per cent). Surgical exploration was not uniformly undertaken especially in patients with more advanced disease. If all cases of non-seminomatous malignancies of the testicle were included, 76 (85 per cent) of a total of 89 patients with retroperitoneal nodal metastasis were diagnosed by pedal lymphangiography. Eight of the 13 patients who exhibited false-negative findings were found to have metastases in nodes lateral to those usually opacified by pedal lymphangiography; these metastases may have been diagnosed by the testicular route.

In 7 patients, repeat lymphangiography was performed following retroperitoneal node dissection. Ligation of lymphatic channels resulted in the utilization of collateral pathways. These collateral pathways resulted in opacification of nodes beyond the usual drainage from the testicle. Any subsequent metastases might therefore occur along this new route of lymph flow. In another patient a postoperative lymphocyst displaced the ureter and kidney. Follow-up lymphangiography opacified the large cyst which was then treated surgically. Still another effect of para-aortic node lymphadenectomy was the utilization of lymphatico-venous anastomoses as a collateral pathway in the face of surgically produced lymphatic obstruction.

The importance in constant monitoring of the disease by lymphangiography is illustrated in a patient with a seminoma of the right testicle (Fig. 6-27). The right testicular lesion invaded the scrotum. The testicle as well as a portion of the scrotum were surgically removed and the right iliac and para-aortic areas were treated by radiation therapy. Follow-up evaluation demonstrated collateral pathways to the lymphatics and nodes in the inguinal and iliac areas. Metastases subsequently appeared in these nodes.

Lymphangiography should be utilized as a guide in the management of patients with testicular malignancy. In seminomas, when lymphangiography is positive, radiotherapy should be given to the ipsilateral iliac and bilateral retroperitoneal nodes to the diaphragm. The mediastinum and both supraclavicular areas are also treated. In the presence of a negative lymphangiogram, radiotherapy is given only to the level of the diaphragm.

In non-seminomatous malignancies, a patient with a positive lymphangiogram is treated by radiotherapy to a tumor dose of 2500 rads to the nodes up to the level of the diaphragm. A retroperitoneal node dissection is then undertaken to remove residual tumor tissue with additional radiotherapy following the retroperitoneal node dissection. In the presence of negative lymphangiographic findings, the retroperitoneal node dissection is undertaken initially. If the node dissection is negative, no further treatment is instituted.

Therefore, at M. D. Anderson Hospital and Tumor Institute lymphangiography has become an essential tool in the evaluation as well as the management of the patient with testicular malignant disease.

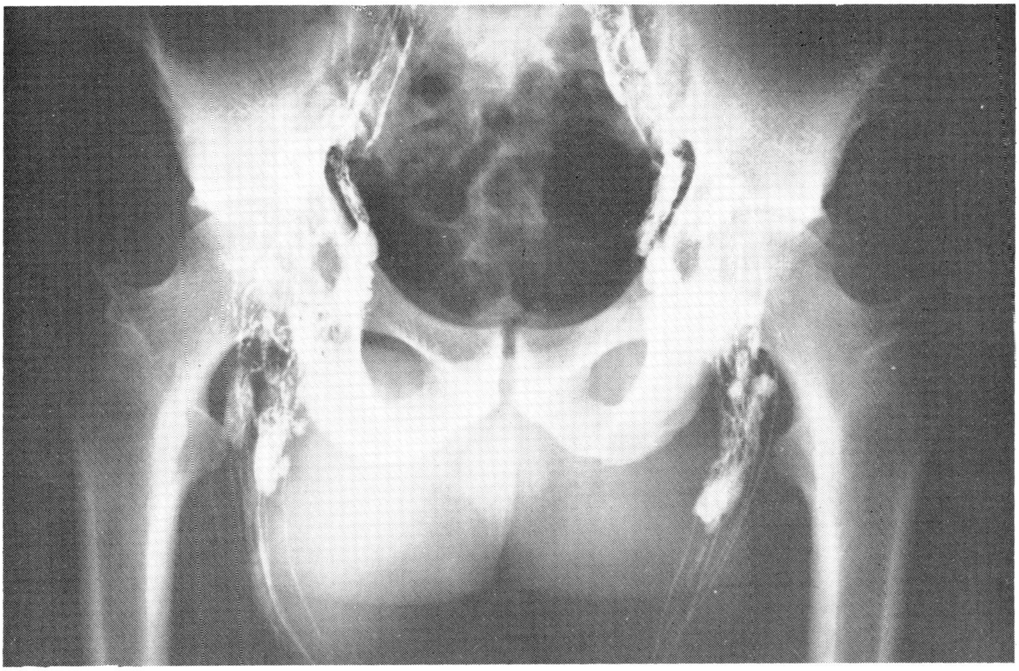

Fig. 6-27. Demonstration of the progress of disease. This patient was examined because of a seminoma of the right testis with scrotal involvement. A, Lymphatic phase prior to treatment.

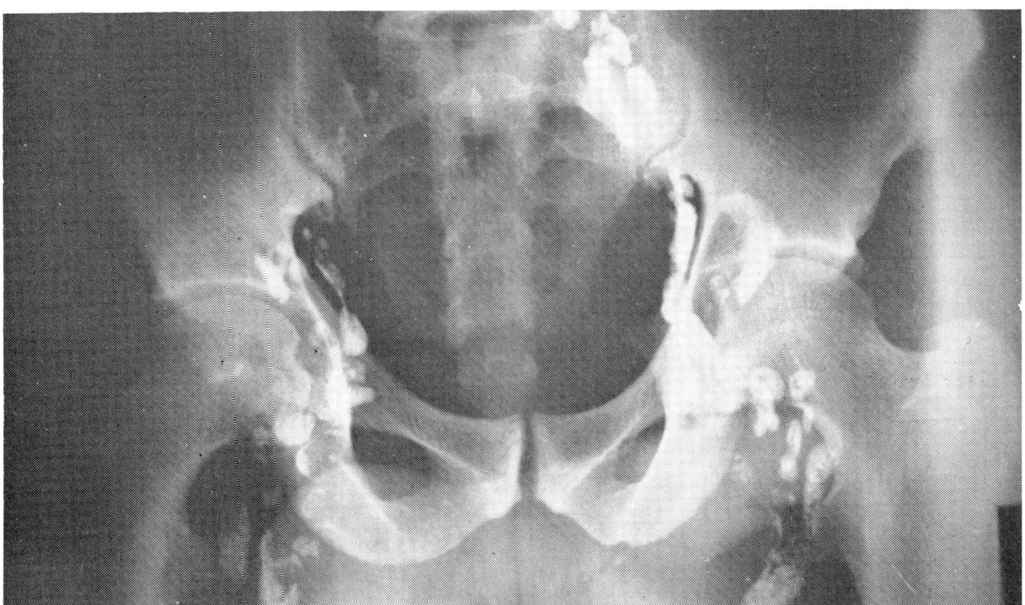

Fig. 6-27. Demonstration of the progress of disease. B, Nodal phase prior to treatment. One and one-half years later there was progression of the disease to involve the contralateral inguinal and iliac nodes.

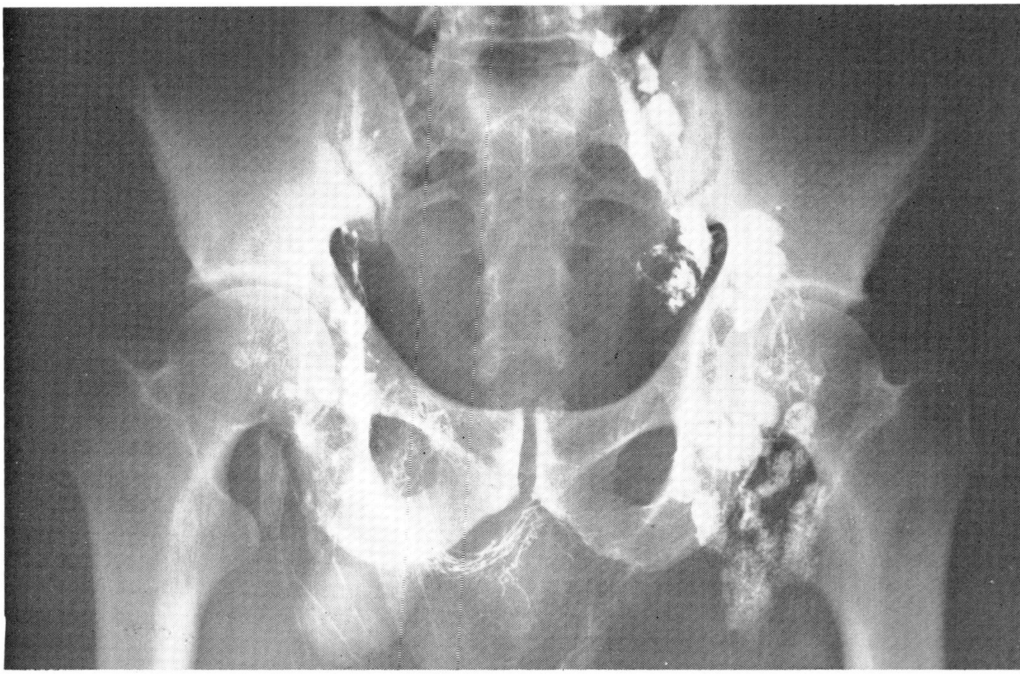

Fig. 6-27. Demonstration of the progress of disease. C, Lymphatic phase. Note the collateral pathways crossing over from right to left in the perineum.

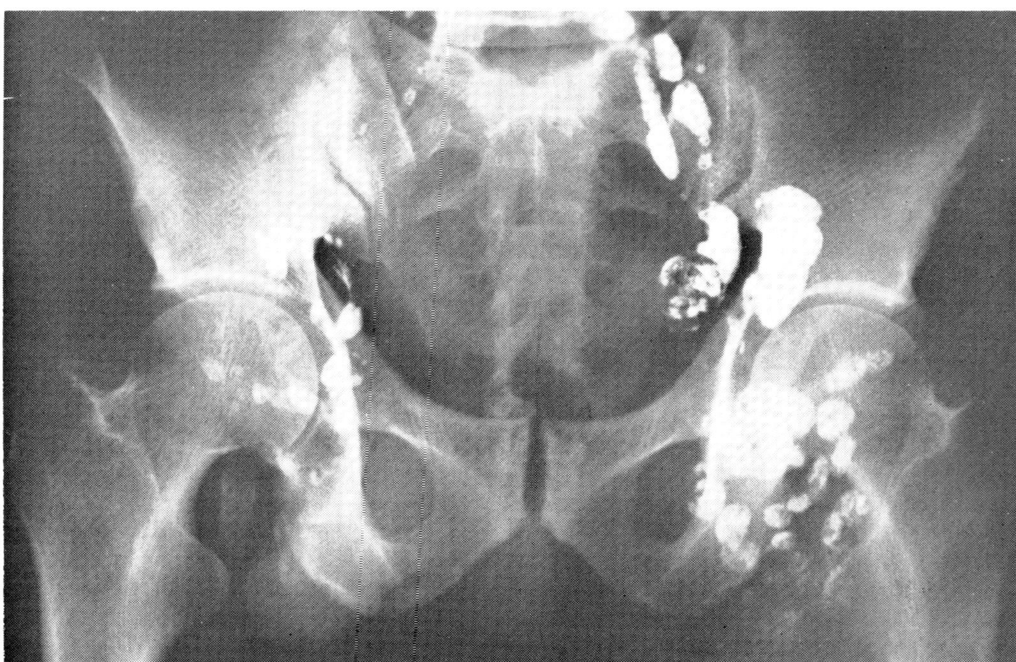

Fig. 6-27. Demonstration of the progress of disease. D, Nodal phase. The left inguinal and iliac nodes are now involved by metastatic seminoma.

CHAPTER 7

TREATMENT: SURGICAL MANAGEMENT

by

Gene A. Guinn

Radical orchiectomy with high ligation of the spermatic cord at the internal inguinal ring is the treatment of choice for every scrotal mass suspected of harboring malignant testicular disease (Figs. 7-1, 7-2, 7-3 and 7-4). This procedure facilitates removal of the primary tumor with the lowest incidence of local recurrence and provides the pathologist with the necessary tissue for accurately assessing the morphological features of the tumor and the extent of local invasion. In those cases exclusive of seminoma where a scrotal orchiectomy has inadvertently been used to excise a testicular tumor, removal of the remaining portion of the spermatic cord through an inguinal approach is mandatory. Occult metastases are occasionally present in the remaining portion of the cord and may be the cause of further spread of disease.

Significant improvement in survival rates for patients receiving surgical or irradiation therapy to the primary lymphatic drainage areas dictates the employment of additional treatment following orchiectomy. In the absence of figures from prospective studies demonstrating the superiority of either therapeutic modality, today's physician is often faced with the dilemma of choosing the appropriate form of treatment.

A systematic approach for staging the disease in patients with testicular tumors allows an orderly plan for therapy and evaluation of the end results of treatment. While it may appear redundant to mention the importance of a thorough physical examination, this is often one of the studies omitted in the evaluation of the patient. Asymptomatic abdominal masses, enlarged peripheral lymph nodes, and abnormalities in the remaining testis may be found. The presence or absence of demonstrable metastases in the lung can be discerned quite readily with a routine chest roentgenogram. Standard excretory urography is a useful method for detecting enlarged lymph nodes in the perirenal areas which may not be opacified by lymphangiography. The pedal lymphangiogram is invaluable in the staging of the tumor (Wallace and Jing 1970; Maier and Schamber 1972). Testicular lymphangiography has been of help in defining the normal testicular drainage, but is extremely time-consuming and has not proved useful in the routine evaluation of these patients. In selected cases, opacification of the inferior vena cava may aid in delineation of retroperitoneal masses.

The main controversy in the treatment of testicular tumors is concerned with the management of the lymph nodes in the primary and secondary lymphatic drainage areas. Few clinicians would argue that pure seminoma is best controlled by radical orchiectomy, followed by irradiation of

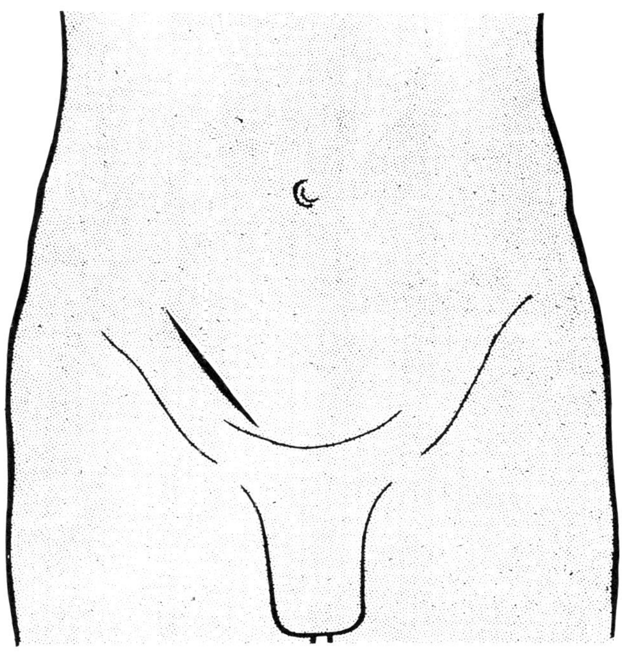

Fig. 7-1. The incision for an inguinal orchiectomy.

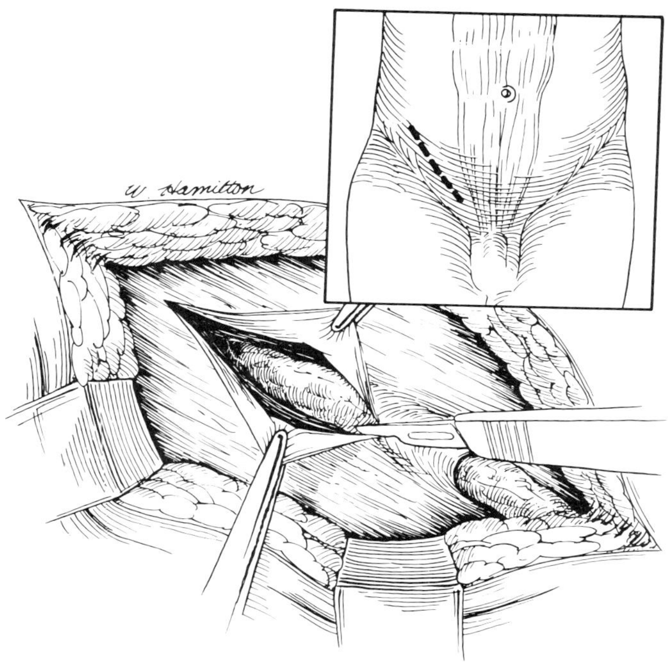

Fig. 7-2. After incising the skin and subcutaneous tissue, the external oblique aponeurosis is opened in the direction of its fibers.

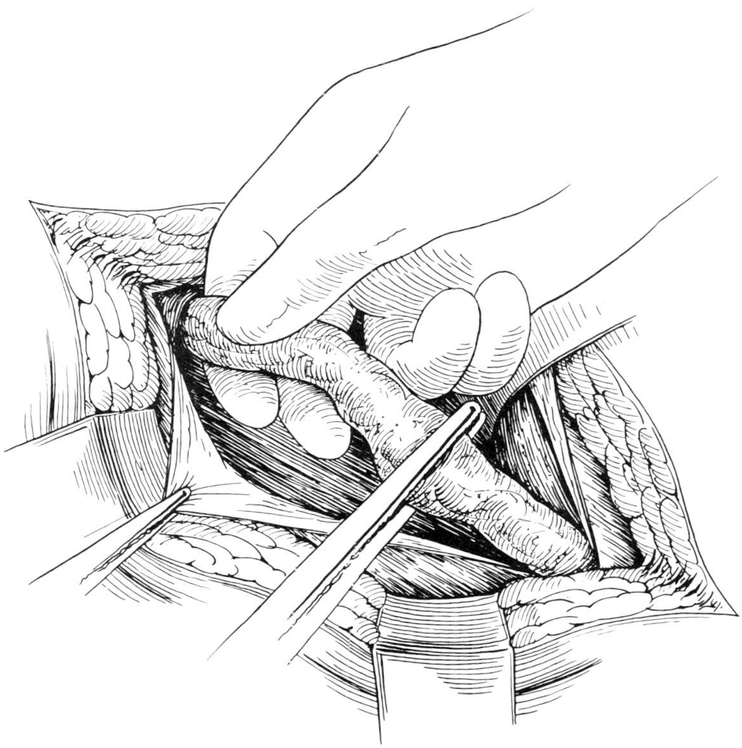

Fig. 7-3. The spermatic cord is isolated and a non-crushing clamp is applied to prevent escape of malignant cells during mobilization of the testis.

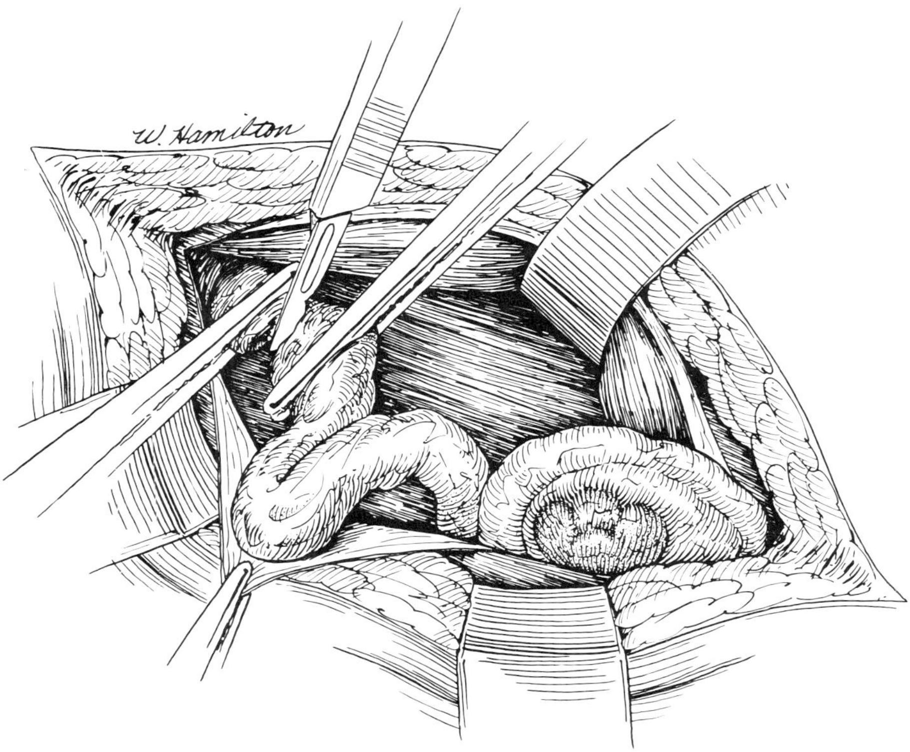

Fig. 7-4. Once the diagnosis is established, the spermatic cord is divided at the level of the internal inguinal ring and the cord is doubly ligated.

the ipsilateral groin area and retroperitoneal lymph nodes. The technique has yielded a 90 to 95 per cent five year survival rate. The addition of retroperitoneal lymph node dissection by Maier et al. (1968) in 39 patients with seminoma did not enhance their survival. The dilemma that exists today, therefore, arises in the management of patients with malignant testicular disease other than pure seminoma (Caldwell 1969; 1971). Retroperitoneal lymphadenectomy was added to the physicians' therapeutic armamentarium for testicular tumors by Roberts in 1902, and has been employed with varying degrees of thoroughness and enthusiasm. The major difficulty in evaluating this procedure has been that most reported patients with lymph nodes involved by metastatic disease have received supplemental postoperative irradiation. The only sizeable group of patients who have undergone retroperitoneal lymphadenectomy without postoperative irradiation, performed by one individual with the technique clearly stated, are those treated by Staubitz et al. (1969). He reports 22 of 26 patients with malignant testicular tumors, other than seminoma, alive at four years after operation. In this group, eight patients had lymph nodes with metastatic disease and seven of these were alive at the end of four years. Other authors have reported smaller groups of patients treated with only lymphadenectomy, but problems arise in evaluating their results as many of the excisions were unilateral and the degree of thoroughness with which the dissections were performed fluctuated among the various surgeons (Whitmore 1962).

Radiotherapy alone, after orchiectomy, has been used extensively by British and European physicians. Smithers and Wallace (1962), Cox (1954), Ekman et al. (1965), Blandy et al. (1970), Smithers (1972) and Earle et al. (1973) have discussed the radiotherapeutic approach and believe that the results from radiotherapy give comparable survival figures to those from lymphadenectomy. We believe that retroperitoneal lymphadenectomy allows a more accurate assessment of the stage of disease and, in patients with uninvolved lymph nodes, is a more benign procedure than is prophylactic irradiation. Radiotherapy, combined with lymphadenectomy, is reserved for cases of proved regional metastatic spread.

CHOICE OF INCISIONS

Surgical extirpation of the retroperitoneal lymph nodes can be performed through a variety of incisions (Fig. 7-5). Although the first recorded retroperitoneal lymph node dissection for a testicular tumor utilized a transperitoneal approach (Roberts 1902), the extraperitoneal route became almost exclusively employed until the modern era of antibiotics. Hinman (1914, 1919, 1923 and 1935) described several incisions but preferred one which paralleled the lower border of the twelfth rib and ran anteriorly and inferiorly to the region of the internal inguinal ring. The spacial limitations imposed by this incision influenced Cooper et al. (1950), and later Lewis et al. (1952), to extend the incision to form a combined thoracoabdominal approach.

The thoracoabdominal approach begins in the posterior axillary line over the tenth rib and runs anteriorly and inferiorly over this structure onto the lower abdominal quadrant to the region of the external inguinal ring. The incision provides superior exposure of the area above the renal vessels but usually limits the dissection to one side. It may be performed with or without entering the pleural cavity. However, the pleural cavity is usually entered, requiring a chest tube. Although it would appear that this approach would result in increased morbidity, Skinner and Leadbetter (1971) report minimal morbidity with patients leaving the

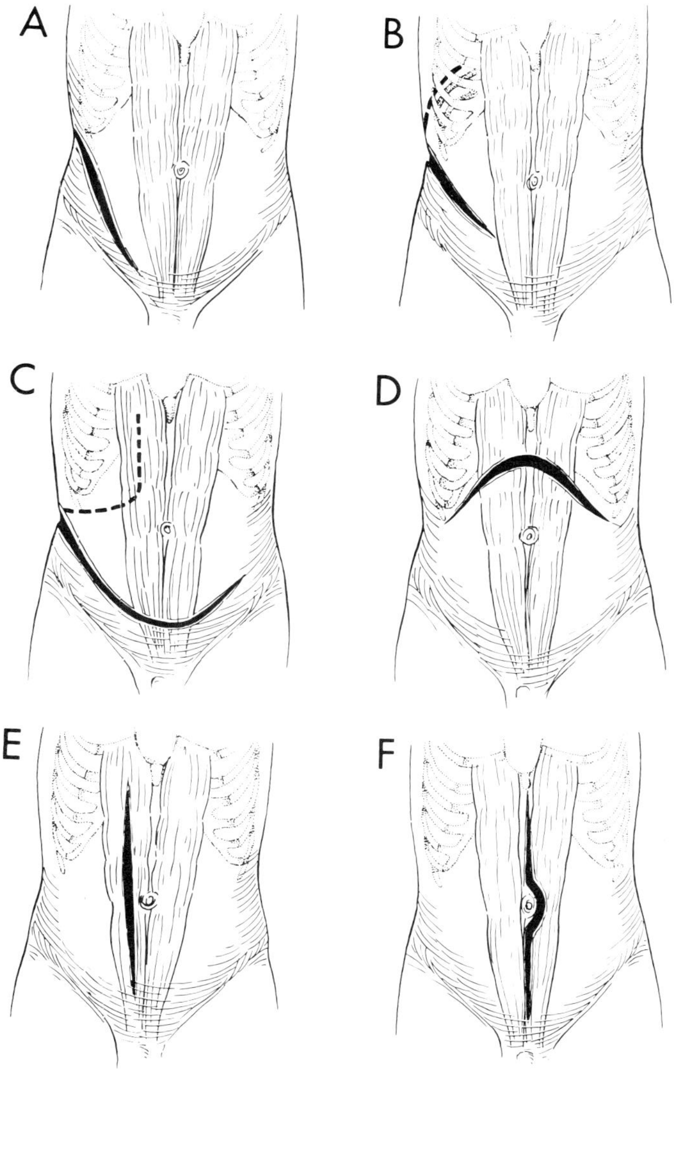

Fig. 7-5. Incisions for retroperitoneal lymphadenectomy. A. Hinman's incision. B, Thoraco-abdominal approach. C. Extrapleural, extraperitoneal incision of Nagamatsu. D. Chevron incision. E. Paramedian incision. F. Classical midline incision.

hospital in 7 to 10 days.

An extrapleural, extraperitoneal approach for simultaneous bilateral retroperitoneal lymph node dissection has been described by Nagamatsu (1963). It is a combination of his dorsolumbar incision with a Cherney incision. Recently, good results have been reported with the transverse upper abdominal Chevron incision (Chute et al. 1967). In addition, retroperitoneal lymphadenectomy may be performed through a transabdominal, transperitoneal approach utilizing either a vertical midline or a paramedian incision.

The relative merits of these approaches relate to the location of the primary testicular lymph drainage area, contralateral spread of tumor in the absence of ipsilateral node involvement, and the technical feasibility of completely excising the lymph nodes. Studies of the testicular lymphatics by Jamieson and Dobson (1910) and Most (1899) originally showed the primary testicular lymph drainage area to lie below the renal vessels. However, recent roentgenographic studies (Busch and Sayegh 1963; Cook et al. 1965) using testicular lymphangiography suggest that, in adults, the primary lymph drainage area of the testes may range from the level of L-4 to T-1. Nevertheless, most surgeons believe that removal of lymph nodes above the left renal pedicle is of little value. Contralateral spread of tumor occurs occasionally in the absence of ipsilateral involvement (Jamieson and Dobson 1910; Busch and Sayegh 1964; Cook et al. 1965) and, for that reason, we recommend bilateral lymphadenectomy.

The anterior transperitoneal approach allows for excellent exposure of the primary lymphatic drainage area, except for the lymph nodes located superior to the renal vessels and permits bilateral simultaneous dissection. This approach has been employed at the University of Texas System Cancer Center, M. D. Anderson Hospital and Tumor Institute at Houston for the last ten years with minimal postoperative morbidity and no deaths.

OPERATIVE TECHNIQUE TRANSABDOMINAL RETROPERITONEAL LYMPHANDENECTOMY

A midline vertical incision is made which should extend from the xiphoid to below the umbilicus (Fig. 7-6). It is imperative that the incision always extend superiorly to the xiphoid in order to obtain optimal exposure of the perirenal area. Whenever preoperative studies raise doubts as to operability, it is wise to make only the supraumbilical portion of the incision. If the operative findings suggest that lymphadenectomy is feasible the incision can then be completed.

Upon entering the abdomen exploration of the major structures is performed. This can be facilitated by thorough preoperative evacuation of the colon and by removal of the gastric contents through a nasogastric tube inserted shortly after endotracheal anesthesia has been achieved. Complete muscular relaxation of the patient is mandatory throughout the procedure. A self-retaining retractor is introduced, the transverse colon and greater omentum are exteriorized onto the anterior abdominal wall, and the small intestines are displaced to the right by appropriately placed retractors which will require readjustment as the dissection proceeds. The incision (Fig. 7-7) in the posterior parietal peritoneum is begun over the distal aorta. It should extend superiorly so that adequate exposure of the renal vessels is provided and inferiorly to adequately expose the proximal portion of each iliac artery. Care should be taken at this point to prevent incising the sigmoid mesocolon. To increase exposure, the inferior mesenteric vein can be divided without fear of adverse consequences. The anterior surface of the aorta is exposed by sharply incising the loose areolar tissue containing the lym-

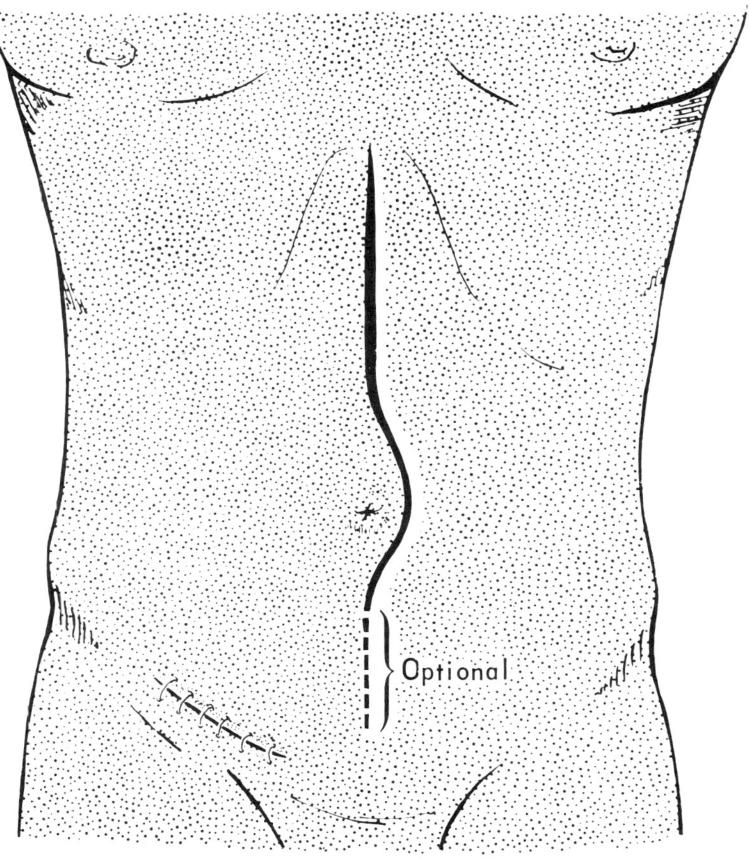

Fig. 7-6. Incision used for optimum exposure of the retroperitoneal area. The lower portion of the incision is frequently not necessary in thin individuals.

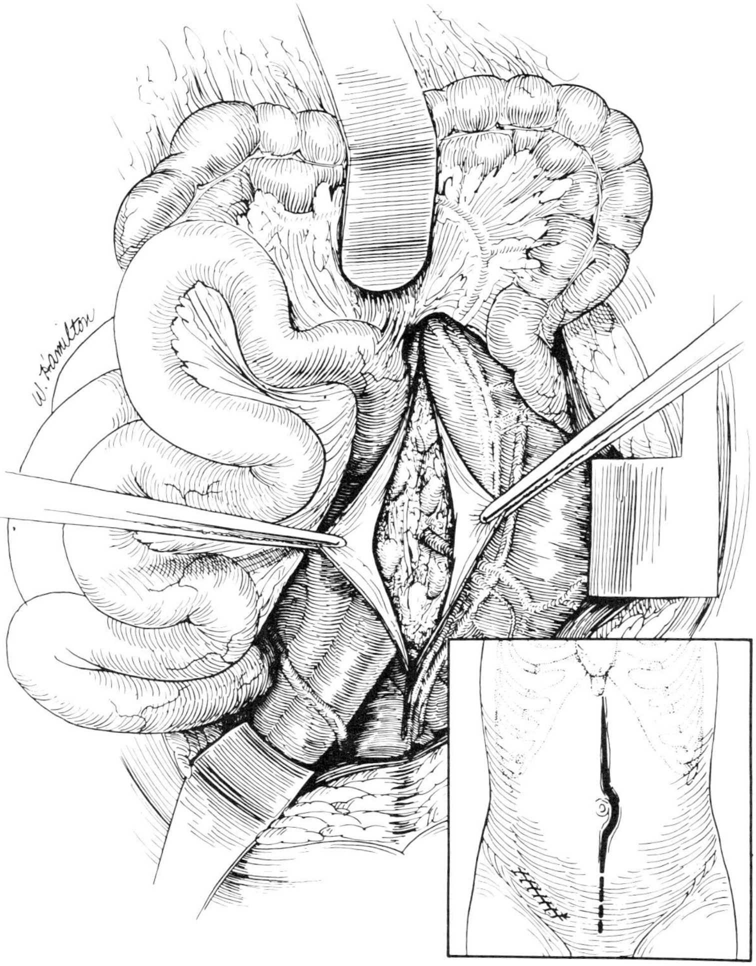

Fig. 7-7. Incision in the posterior parietal peritoneum over the aorta. The exposure superiorly can be increased by division of the inferior mesenteric vein.

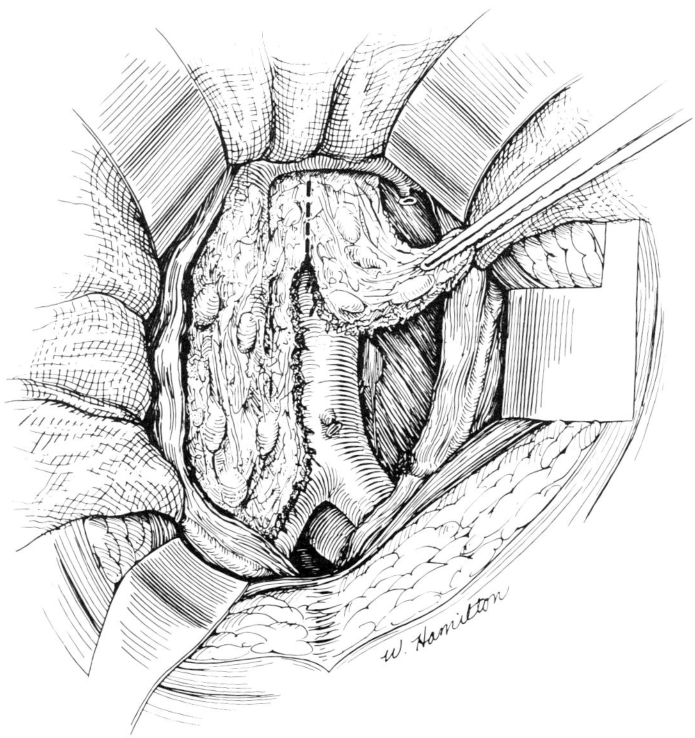

Fig. 7-8. Method of removal of retroperitoneal lymphatics on the left side of aorta. Note that division of the inferior mesenteric artery has allowed improved exposure. The sympathetic chain is left intact.

phatics and periaortic sympathetic nerve plexuses. Beginning with the lymphatics on the left side, the inferior mesenteric artery is ligated at its origin to expedite the procedure and to allow for a more complete removal. It is important that this artery be ligated before it divides, to assure the preservation of the collateral circulation of the sigmoid colon and rectum. Caution, however, is advised in the ligation of this artery when it appears large since enlargement suggests that it may supply a major portion of the intestinal blood supply. This is especially true in older individuals where atherosclerotic occlusion of other vessels is common. The left lateral aspect of the aorta (Fig. 7-8) is exposed from the renal vein to approximately three centimeters below the aortic bifurcation. A useful guide for determining the lateral boundary of the dissection is the angle formed by the joining of the spermatic and left renal veins. As the left posterior aspect of the aorta is exposed, the posterior layer of Gerota's fascia is encountered and must be sharply incised approximately three centimeters below the aortic bifurcation. A useful guide for determining the lateral boundary of the dissection is the angle formed by the joining of the spermatic and left renal veins. As the left posterior aspect of the aorta is exposed, the posterior layer of Gerota's fascia is encountered and must be sharply incised in order to expose the retroaortic lymph nodes. Tobin (1944) has described in detail the relation of this fascia to the aorta and vena cava. Anomalies of the venous return and arterial supply of the kidneys are common and can produce technical problems in the dissection. A venous collar caused by variation in the venous drainage of the left kidney is frequently seen around the aorta (Anson 1961; Thomas 1970). The posterior vein usually passes caudally, emptying into the vena cava several centimeters below the main renal vein.

The lymphatic chain may be removed in a caudad or cephalad direction. Generally, it is well defined inferiorly and the procedure can be initiated lateral to the iliac artery, excising the tissue in a cephalad manner. Meticulous hemostasis, using either silver clips or fine ligatures, is mandatory to ensure complete removal of the lymph nodes and to prevent excessive blood loss. It is important to remain constantly aware of the location of the ureter (the lateral limit of the dissection on the left), the stump of the inferior mesenteric artery, and the lumbar sympathetic chain.

When the dissection is terminated superiorly the transected lymphatic vessels should be ligated to prevent lymph accumulation in the retroperitoneal space. The inferior lymphatic chain should be ligated for the same reason. A warm sponge is placed in the dissected area and attention directed toward the removal of the tissue lying between the aorta and vena cava and lateral to the vena cava.

For proper exposure at this stage of the procedure, the posterior parietal attachment of the small bowel mesentery should be incised. It is usually unnecessary to mobilize the cecum. The key to adequate exposure and excision of the lymphatics around the vena cava is to work immediately adjacent to this vessel. A longitudinal incision is made through the areolar tissue to the anterior aspect of the vessel wall. As on the left, it is usually easier to remove the lymph nodes in a cephalad direction. Counter-traction of the vena cava by an assistant (Fig. 7-9) is necessary if the right primary lymphatic chain is to be adequately exposed and removed. Should hypotension result from obstruction of the venous return to the heart, the pressure on the vena cava must be removed temporarily. Ligation of the right spermatic vein will aid exposure and should be performed at a convenient

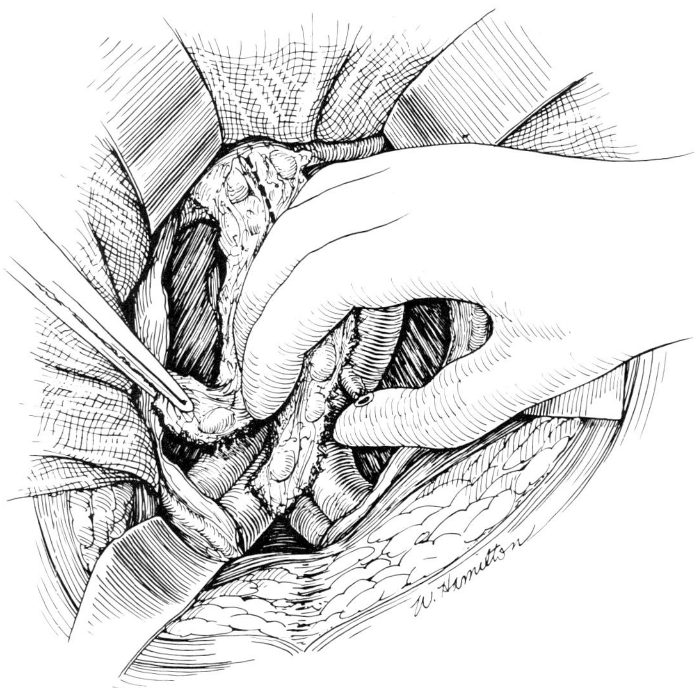

Fig. 7-9. Exposure of the right lymphatic chain by rotation of the inferior vena cava to the left side.

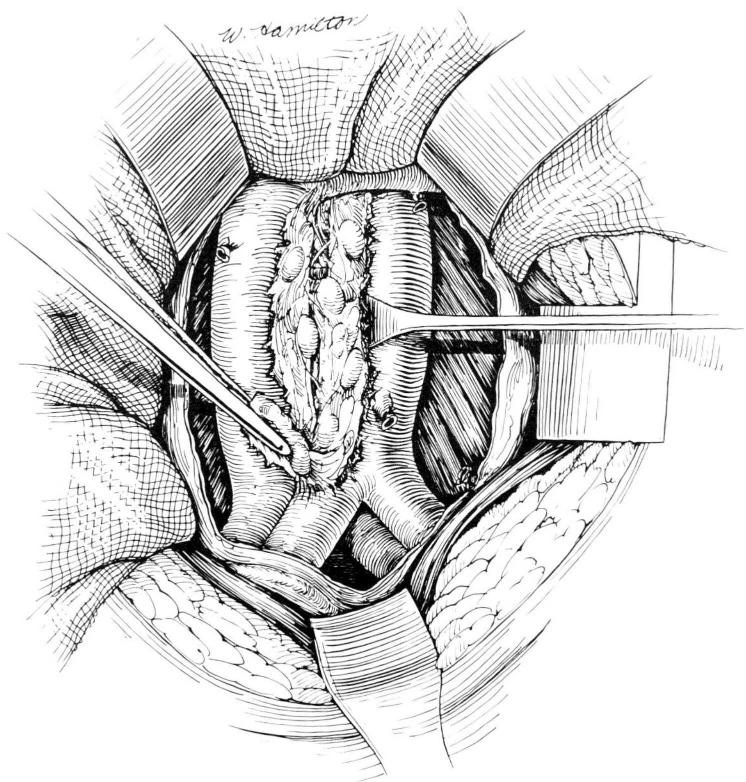

Fig. 7-10. Technique for exposure and removal of lymphatics between aorta and vena cava. Retraction of these vessels away from each other aids in exposure when the more superficial portion of the dissection is completed.

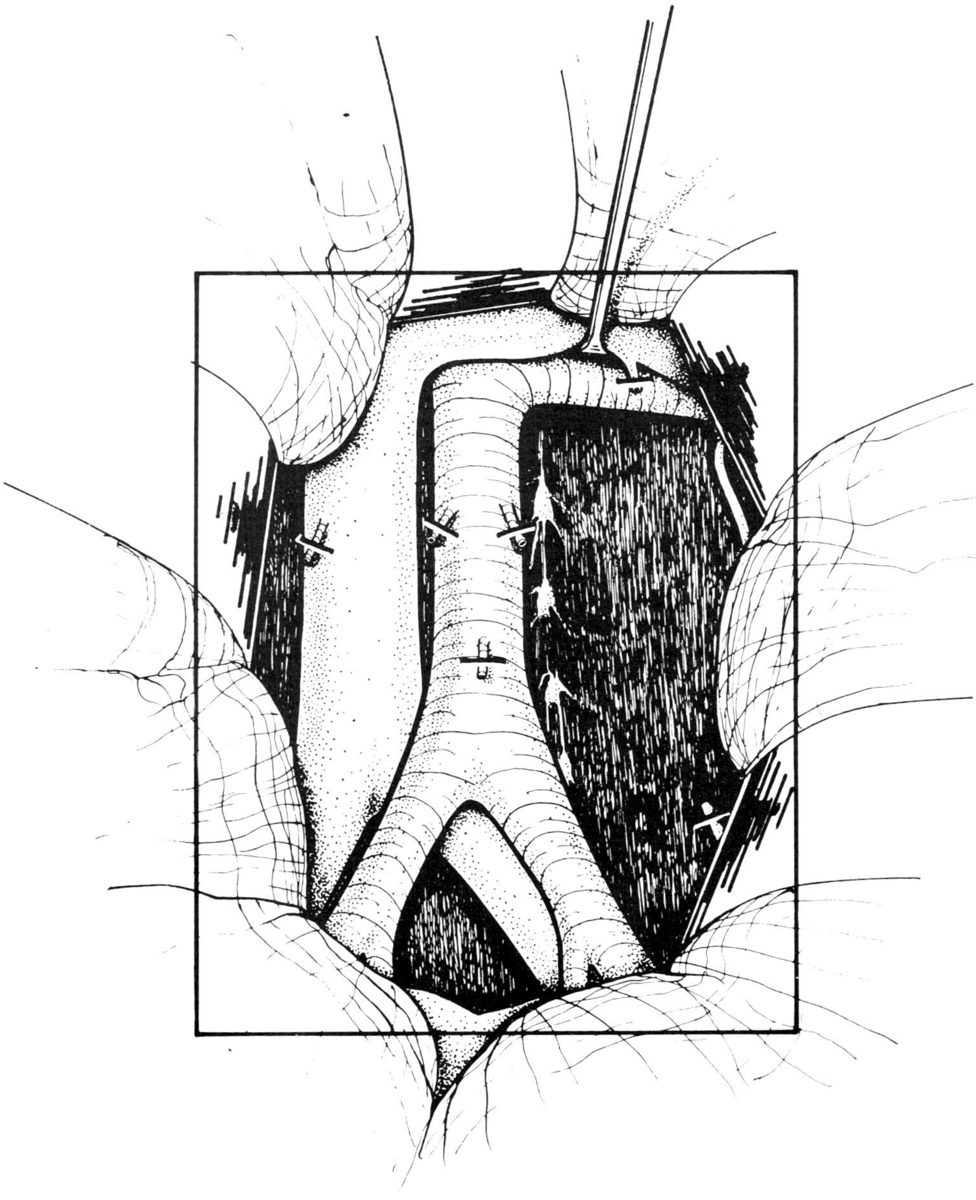

Fig. 7-11. The extent of the completed dissection is represented by the superimposed lines.

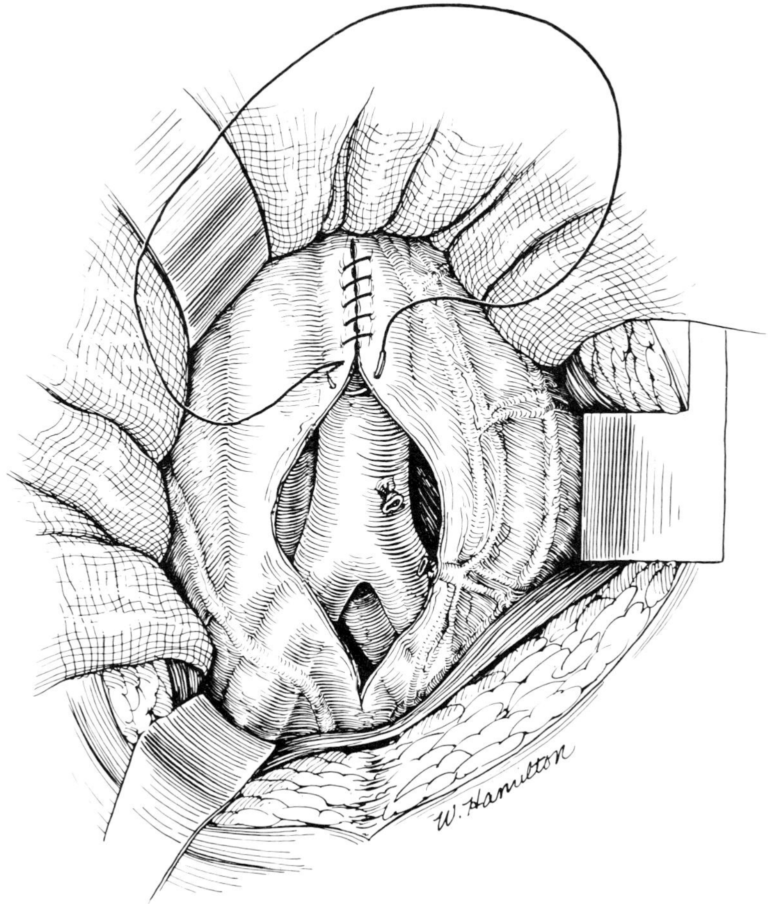

Fig. 7-12. Method of closure of retroperitoneal area.

time before being torn.

The central dissection is well delineated but often tedious because of the intimate relation of the aorta, vena cava, and lumbar vessels to the lymphatics (Fig. 7-10). It is important to remember that the lumbar arteries arise from the posterior aspect of the aorta. After passing over the vertebral bodies, they course posteriorly between the posas muscles and the vertebral bodies. Dissection in the central zone is terminated with exposure of the right renal artery at the inferior edge of the left renal vein. It is important that the dissection in this area be thorough since these lymph nodes may be involved with tumor and are easily overlooked.

Thorough inspection of the entire area with removal of residual lymph nodes is vital to ensure an adequately performed lymphadenectomy (Fig. 7-11). After adequate hemostasis is obtained, the posterior parietal peritoneum is closed with a continuous chromic catgut stitch (Fig. 7-12). Closure of the abdomen is done in a routine layered fashion with retention sutures having been unnecessary in our experience except for patients in a debilitated state or where wound sepsis is anticipated.

POSTOPERATIVE COMPLICATIONS

The occurrence of postoperative complications following retroperitoneal lymphadenectomy are similar to those following any intra-abdominal operative procedure. In addition, complications peculiar to retroperitoneal lymph node dissection have occasionally developed. Brief periods of partial intestinal obstruction have occurred but in all instances they have responded to nasogastric suction and intravenous fluid administration. In one of our patients, severe postoperative pancreatitis developed but subsided with supportive therapy. In another patient, postoperative recovery was prolonged by chylous ascites. This complication regressed on conservative therapy and did not require either drainage or surgical intervention.

The formation of a lymphocyst following pelvic lymphadenectomy occurs frequently (Rutledge et al. 1959). Griffith and Carlton (1970) reported a large pelvic lymphocyst developing after a gynecological surgical procedure which required surgical aspiration to relieve ureteral obstruction. A similar situation was encountered after retroperitoneal lymphadenectomy was performed for malignant testicular disease in one of our patients. The preoperative roentgenogram demonstrated a large mass displacing the left ureter anteriorly and laterally with moderate hydroureteronephrosis. A large, thick-walled cyst, adherent to the surrounding structures, was found at operation (Fig. 7-13). The roof of the cyst was excised and an omental flap was used to fill the evacuated space. The patient's postoperative course was uneventful. To our knowledge, this is the first report of a symptomatic lymphocyst following retroperitoneal lymphadenectomy.

Ejaculatory disturbances following bilateral retroperitoneal lymphadenectomy have been troublesome. Approximately 50 per cent of our patients have noted some loss of ejaculatory powers but, in most instances, this has been only temporary. Several men in our study have fathered children after bilateral lymphadenectomy, revealing that all patients do not experience this loss. An excellent discussion of the problem is provided by the report of Leiter and Brendler (1967).

RESULTS

The results reported in the literature on retroperitoneal lymphadenectomy are difficult to evaluate. Maier (1968) found no improvement in the survival of patients with seminoma who had undergone lymphadenectomy

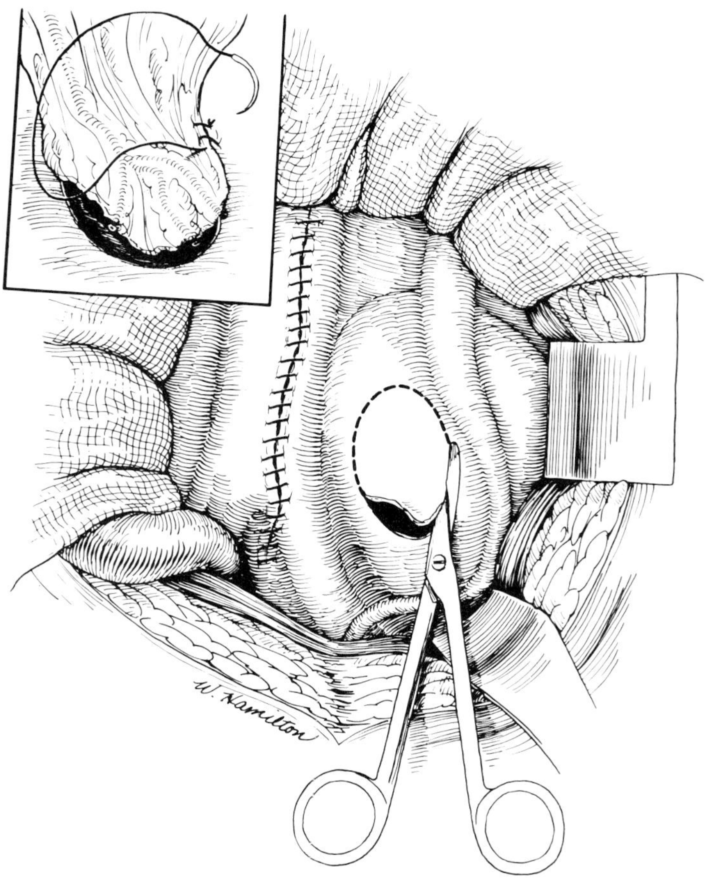

Fig. 7-13. Lymphocyst following lymphadenectomy causing displacement of aorta and ureter. The anterior wall has been excised and an omental flap was used to fill the cyst cavity (see insert).

and the procedure is no longer advocated for this type of tumor. For other types of testicular tumors, the value of lymphadenectomy has been more difficult to assess. Not only has the extent of the operative procedure varied among surgeons but the frequent use of postoperative irradiation in patients with metastatic lymph node disease has contributed to the lack of uniformity in reported series. The procedure often serves merely as a diagnostic tool for determining the advisability of employing immediate irradiation since the removal of all lymph nodes is unlikely (Thompson 1961). Currently, Staubitz et al. (1969) is the only author reporting routine lymphadenectomy without postoperative irradiation for patients found to have metastatic periaortic lymph node involvement.

Our own approach (Castro 1969) has been to treat those patients having a positive lymphangiogram with preoperative irradiation. After delivering 2,500 rads of Cobalt 60 irradiation to the retroperitoneal area in three weeks, a bilateral retroperitoneal lymphadenectomy is performed. An additional 2,500 rads of Cobalt 60 is given during the postoperative period if the removed lymph nodes are shown histologically to contain metastatic tumor. In those patients having a negative lymphangiogram, a bilateral retroperitoneal lymph node dissection is performed. In those instances where histologic examination reveals metastatic involvement, 5,000 rads of Cobalt 60 irradiation is given postoperatively over a five week period. This program evades the issue as to the value of lymphadenectomy. It is our belief, however, that lymphadenectomy is to be preferred to the routine use of proplylactic radiotherapy.

Special problems arise in the management of patients with testicular malignant disease who have undergone previous scrotal or inguinal surgical procedures. Alterations in the normal testicular lymphatic drainage may result from these operations and inguinal lymph node metastases may occur (Witus et al. 1959; Bowles 1962). Ilioinguinal lymphadenectomy combined with retroperitoneal lymph node dissection is recommended in these rare instances where non-seminomatous tumors are encountered (Herr et al. 1973).

Treatment of distant metastases usually requires irradiation, chemotherapy or a combination of these modalities. Occasionally, surgical extirpation of isolated lesions may be indicated. Resection of pulmonary metastases with prolonged survival has been reported (Thomford et al. 1965; Spratt and Yuen 1966; Woodhead et al. 1968; Thompson and Goldstein 1969; Rees and Cleland 1971). Cases considered for aggressive surgical management must be carefully selected. Patients having multiple or bilateral pulmonary nodules or those having other evidence of disease do not usually benefit from surgical excision of lung metastases.

CONCLUSIONS

1. Masses in the testicle should be excised through an inguinal approach with high ligation of the spermatic cord at the internal inguinal ring. If the patient is found to have a tumor following scrotal orchiectomy, the spermatic cord should be excised through a separate inguinal incision.

2. Proper staging of the disease in patients found to have a testicular tumor is necessary to ensure appropriate therapy and to evaluate the end results of treatment. A chest roentgenogram, excretory urogram, pedal lymphangiogram, and in selected instances, inferior cavogram are necessary for proper staging.

3. Seminomas of the testicle are managed by orchiectomy and irradiation to the ipsilateral groin and retroperitoneal area.

4. Germ cell tumors other than

seminoma should have retroperitoneal lymph node dissections initially when the lymphangiogram is negative or following preoperative irradiation when lymph node involvement is minimal to moderate.

5. When massive retroperitoneal nodal involvement is known, irradiation and chemotherapy are advised. Surgical excision in these instances is difficult, often incomplete, and rarely affects survival.

CHAPTER 8

TREATMENT: RADIATION THERAPY

by

David H. Hussey and John F. Doornbos

The management of malignant tumors of the testis at the University of Texas System Cancer Center, M. D. Anderson Hospital and Tumor Institute is by a team approach involving the pathologist, the urologist, the radiotherapist, and the chemotherapist. The treatment planning is influenced by the histopathological classification and the clinical stage of the disease.

HISTOPATHOLOGICAL CLASSIFICATION

Over 95 per cent of testicular tumors arise from the germinal cells. The other 3 to 5 per cent comprise a miscellaneous category including interstitial cell tumors, lymphosarcomas, reticulum cell sarcomas and rhabdomyosarcomas. Dixon and Moore (1952) have subdivided the germinal cell tumors into the following classification of prognostic importance:

Group I	Seminoma, pure
Group II	Embryonal carcinoma, pure or with seminoma
Group III	Teratoma, pure or with seminoma
Group V	Choriocarcinoma, pure or with either seminoma or embryonal carcinoma or both
Group IV	Teratoma, with either embryonal carcinoma, choriocarcinoma, or both, with or without seminoma

Table XVI shows the distribution of histological types and the influence of the initial histological diagnosis on prognosis in 377 patients treated in the Radiotherapy Department at M. D. Anderson Hospital between March 1944 and July 1971. Thirty-six months with no evidence of disease (3-year NED rate) is used as an indicator of cure since over 95 per cent of the treatment failures appeared within 36 months.

The data show that a diagnosis of pure seminoma carries the best prognosis and choriocarcinoma the worst. Embryonal carcinoma and choriocarcinoma alone do not have as good prognoses as when teratoma is also present.

For purposes of treatment planning, the germinal tumors may be divided into two categories: (1) pure seminoma, and (2) all other histological types (Groups II-V), hereafter referred to as "mixed tumors."

This investigation was supported in part by Public Health Service Research Grant CA-06294 and Training Grant CA-5099 from the National Cancer Institute.

TABLE XVI

DISTRIBUTION OF PATIENTS
AND
INFLUENCE OF INITIAL HISTOLOGY ON PROGNOSIS
(March 1944-July 1971)

	Number of Patients Treated	3-yr NED rate (all stages)
Seminoma, Pure	141 (37%)*	114/141 (81%)
Embryonal Carcinoma, pure or with seminoma	97 (26%)	45/97 (46%)
Teratoma, pure or with seminoma	33 (9%)	23/33 (70%)
Teratoma with embryonal carcinoma, choriocarcinoma, or seminoma	74 (20%)	44/74 (59%)
Choriocarcinoma, pure or with seminoma and/or embryonal carcinoma	19 (5%)	2/19
Miscellaneous	13 (3%)	7/13

* Includes seven patients initially diagnosed as having pure seminomas who were subsequently found to have mixed tumor metastases.

Radiosensitivity

Pure seminoma is a very radiosensitive tumor. Even huge masses are permanently eradicated with relatively low doses of irradiation. Mixed tumors have the same order of radiosensitivity as the epithelial tumors and higher doses are required than for pure seminomas. Bulky retroperitoneal metastases from mixed tumors are likely to persist after 5000 rads which is at the limit of normal tissue tolerance. Control in that area is improved by resection of the gross masses, leaving only microscopic disease to be eradicated by irradiation (Table XVII).

Routes of spread

Pure seminoma usually metastasizes in a stepwise fashion to retroperitoneal and then to mediastinal and supraclavicular lymph nodes. Early hematogenous spread is rare. With embryonal and teratocarcinoma, the initial metastasis is usually to retroperitoneal nodes but hematogenous spread is not uncommon. Hematogenous metastases occur early in the course of nearly all choriocarcinomas.

The testicular lymphatics usually drain into the ipsilateral periaortic nodes lying between the renal pedicles and the aortic bifurcation (Fig. 8-1). However, the network of collateral and retrograde lymphatics is extensive. Lymph nodes lying slightly lateral to the lumbar nodes at the level of the renal veins may not be visualized by pedal lymphangiography, but have been filled by testicular lymphangiography (Wallace and Jing 1970).

The iliac nodes may be involved primarily when the tumor has involved the epididymis or secondarily when there is periaortic disease. Inguinal metastases may occur when the tunica albuginea has been invaded. Although periaortic node involvement is frequently bilateral, iliac extension is usually unilateral. However, patients who have had a previous inguinal herniorrhaphy or orchiopexy, may develop contralateral inguinal metastases (Maier and Van Buskirk 1970). There were two such patients in the present series.

Mediastinal and/or supraclavicular metastases occur but are rare in the absence of clinical involvement of the periaortic area. Left supraclavicular nodes may be involved in the absence of mediastinal disease.

CLINICAL STAGING

The staging system used at M. D. Anderson is:

Stage I	Tumor clinically limited to the testis
Stage II_A	Clinical or radiographic evidence of tumor beyond the testicle but limited to the regional lymphatics below the diaphragm; excluding massive retroperitoneal disease
Stage II_B	Retroperitoneal lymphatic disease greater than 15 cm in diameter
Stage III_A	Extension beyond the diaphragm but still confined to the mediastinal or supraclavicular lymphatics
Stage III_B	Extranodal metastases

The staging work-up includes a complete history and physical examination, CBC, urinalysis, liver function tests, and BUN. Radiographic studies include a chest radiograph, intravenous pyelogram, lymphangiogram and, if indicated, an inferior vena cavagram. Surgical findings at lymphadenectomy do not alter the clinical staging.

TREATMENT PLANNING

Treatment for the primary tu-

TABLE XVII

MIXED TUMORS OF THE TESTIS

FAILURE IN POSITIVE PERIAORTIC NODES
March 1944 - July 1971
(Analysis July 1974)

	PERIAORTIC TREATMENT		
	Radiation Therapy Only	Node Dissection Only	Node Dissection + Radiation Therapy
Number with Positive Periaortic Nodes	8*	6**	27**
Number with Failure in Periaortic Nodes	4	3	1 (3.7%)

* Positive nodes on lymphangiogram and/or IVP
** Positive nodes at lymph node dissection

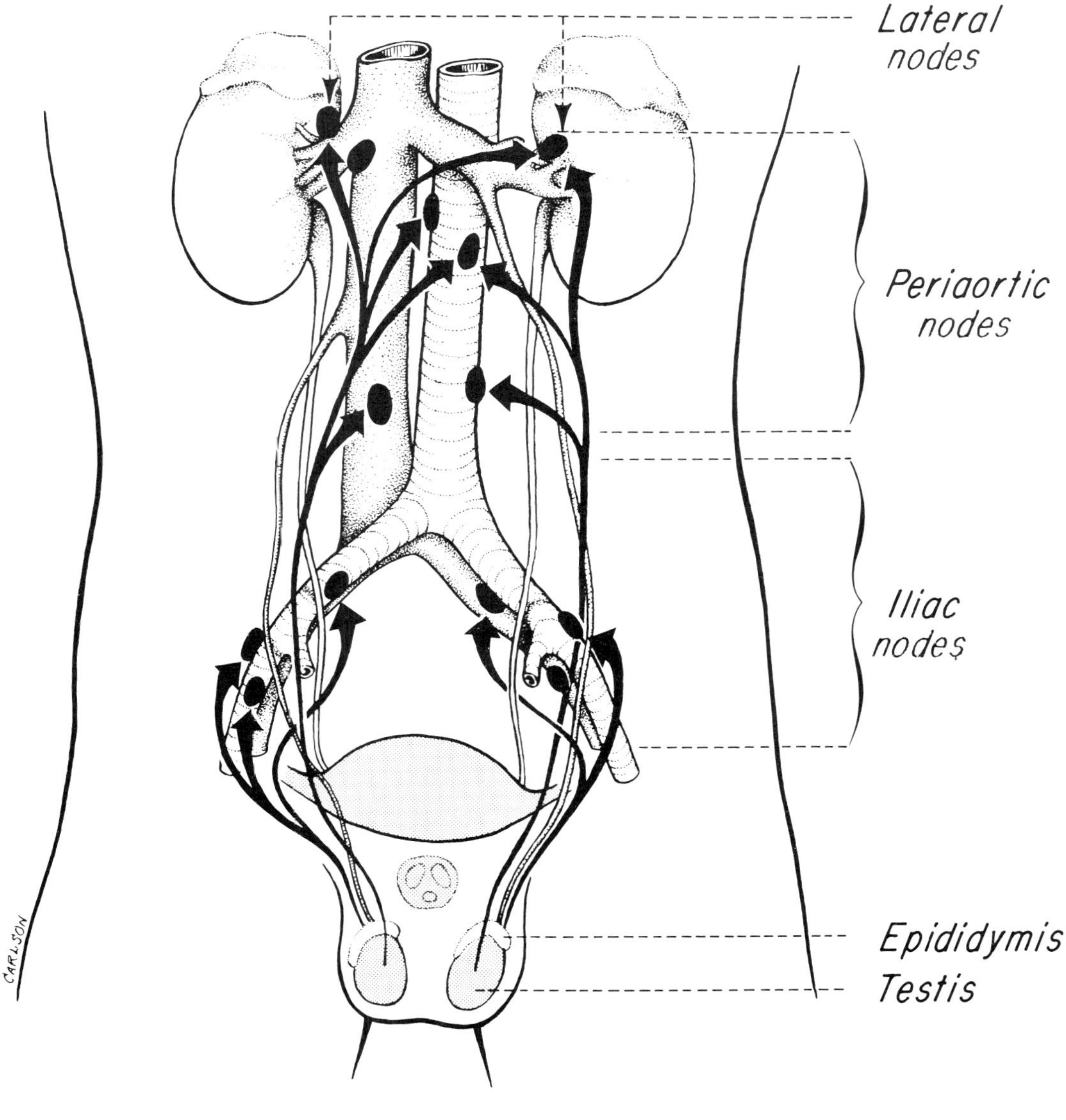

Fig. 8-1. Lymphatic drainage system from the testis and epididymis. The "laterial" nodes may not be filled by pedal lymphangiography.

mor, regardless of the histological type, is a radical orchiectomy through an inguinal incision with high ligation of the spermatic cord. If the patient has been referred after an incisional biopsy or scrotal orchiectomy, a radical orchiectomy or resection of the spermatic cord is performed before proceeding to further therapy. The exception is the case of pure seminoma where irradiation of the spermatic cord and scrotum may be substituted for further surgical intervention.

The lymphatics are treated by radiotherapy and/or lymphadenectomy. The treatment plan depends on the histopathological type and the stage.

Pure Seminoma

Pure seminoma is a radiosensitive neoplasm that has an orderly lymphatic spread. High cure rates are achieved with orchiectomy and radiotherapy (Table XVIII). The regional lymphatics are treated with radiotherapy. Lymphadenectomy is not indicated since even large masses are curable with relatively low doses of irradiation.

Stage I

The incidence of occult retroperitoneal node metastasis in Stage I pure seminoma is uncertain because, for at least three decades, patients have received elective regional lymphatic irradiation. Nevertheless, most authors accept a figure of 10 to 20 per cent (Notter and Ranudd 1964; Maier et al. 1968 and Castro 1973). This incidence justifies elective irradiation of the periaortic and iliac areas.

A tumor dose of 2500 rads in 3 weeks is delivered to the periaortic and ipsilateral iliac areas (Table XIX and Fig. 8-2). If there is a scrotal incision it is included in the treatment field together with the inguinal lymph nodes. The remaining testicle is shielded since the incidence of bilateral tumors is low (2/141 - 1.4 per cent).

In our experience, prophylactic irradiation of the mediastinum and supraclavicular areas is not indicated in Stage I. Of 62 patients electively treated only to the iliac and periaortic areas, only one developed subsequent metastatic disease in the mediastinal or supraclavicular areas (Table XVIII). The 3-year NED rate with irradiation to the iliac and periaortic lymphatics only (59/62 - 95.2 per cent) is equal to that achieved with additional treatment to the mediastinal and supraclavicular areas (20/22 - 90.9 per cent).

Stage II

In early Stage II disease (II_A), the ipsilateral iliac and periaortic areas are irradiated to a basic dose of 2500 rads in 3 weeks. An additional 1000-1500 rads may be given through reduced fields overlying the initially involved areas shown on the lymphangiogram.

With retroperitoneal masses greater than 15 cm in diameter (Stage II_B), a basic dose of 2000 rads is given to the whole abdomen in 3 weeks. This is followed by an additional 1000-2000 rads through reduced fields over the residual nodal masses. Care is taken to limit the dose to both kidneys to no more than 1500 rads.

Elective irradiation of the mediastinum and left supraclavicular area is indicated in Stage II, since two of ten patients treated to fields limited to below the diaphragm have developed disease in these areas at 5 and 81 months (Table XVIII). The prophylactic dose to the mediastinum and left supraclavicular area is 2500 rads in 3 weeks.

Stage III_A

In Stage III_A seminoma, aggressive treatment will still salvage many patients. The abdominal lym-

TABLE XVIII

PATIENTS INITIALLY DIAGNOSED AS HAVING PURE SEMINOMA:
NED at 36 months#
(March 1944 - July 1971)

Stage	AREAS TREATED: Iliac & Periaortic Only	AREAS TREATED: Iliac, Periaortic, Mediastinum, & Left SC	AREAS TREATED: Whole Abdomen, Mediastinum, & Left SC	NED @ 36 months
I	59/62 1- rec mediast + SC + ENM 1- met as embryonal Ca 1- 2nd primary (emb Ca opp testis)	20/22 2- acute leukemia		79/84 (94.0%)
II_A	5/9* 1- SC + ENM Δ 2- met as embryonal Ca 1- LTF	12/13 1- perforated gastric ulcer	8/9 1- marginal recurr mediastinum	25/31 (80.6%)
II_B	0/1 1- ENM**	1/3 1- marg rec abd + ENM 1- ENM	6/8 1- periaortic nodes + ENM 1- rad nephritis	7/12 (58.3%)
III_A		2/3 1- marginal recurr abdomen	1/2 1- met as embryonal Ca	3/5 (60.0%)
III_B	Nine patients irradiated palliatively with limited fields (includes three patients subsequently found to have choriocarcinoma or embryonal carcinoma)			0/9

\# Abbreviations: SC = supraclavicular area; ENM = extranodal metastases (lung, liver, bone, brain); LTF = lost to follow-up

Δ SC + ENM at 5 months; salvaged with additional radiotherapy

* One patient scored as NED at 36 months, developed metastases in mediastinal, supraclavicular, and axillary nodes at 81 months, but was salvaged with additional radiotherapy

** ENM at 28 months; salvaged with additional radiotherapy

TABLE XIX

PURE SEMINOMA: TREATMENT PLAN FOLLOWING RADICAL ORCHIECTOMY

Clinical Stage	TREATMENT AREAS		
	Whole Abdomen (Fields G&H)	Periaortic & Iliac (Fields A, B, & C)	Mediastinum & Left Supraclavicular (Fields D, E, & F)
I		2500 rads/3 wks Elective Irradiation	
II_A		2500 rads/3 wks Basic dose + 1000-1500 rads/1-1-1/2 wks Boost to initial nodal masses	2500 rads/3 wks Elective Irradiation
II_B	2000 rads/3 wks	1000-2000 rads Boost to residual disease	2500 rads/3 wks Elective Irradiation
III_A		2500 rads/3 wks Basic dose* + 1000-1500 rads/1-1-1/2 wks Boost to residual disease	2500 rads/3 wks Basic dose + 500-1000 rads/1/2 - 1 wk Boost to residual disease
III_B	Radiotherapy and/or chemotherapy on an individualized basis.		

* Patients with extensive retroperitoneal disease are treated initially with whole abdominal irradiation (see Stage II_B).

phatics are treated as outlined for Stage II. The mediastinum and left supraclavicular areas are treated to similar doses depending on the extent of the disease in these areas.

Stage III_B

Extranodal disease such as pulmonary or bony metastases is treated with local radiotherapy with or without chemotherapy. Long-term palliation and occasional cures are obtained.

Results

The 3-year NED rates for Stages I, II, and III_A pure seminoma are 94.2 per cent, 74.4 per cent, and 60.0 per cent respectively (Table XIX). Of 14 patients developing further disease (Stages I-III_A), only one developed recurrent pure seminoma in the treated area. Six patients developed lymphatic metastases of seminoma outside the treated area (with or without distant metastases), and two died of distant metastases only. Four patients developed metastases which were diagnosed as mixed tumors and one developed a second primary tumor (embryonal carcinoma) in the opposite testis.

MIXED TUMORS

Mixed tumors are considered as a single clinical entity for the purposes of treatment planning. Again, a radical orchiectomy with high spermatic cord ligation is the treatment for the primary tumor. The results are outlined in Tables XX and XXI.

Stage I

Patients with normal, or small abnormal, nodes seen on the lymphangiogram are treated initially with a transabdominal bilateral lymphadenectomy (Table XXII). Postoperative radiotherapy is, or is not, given depending on the findings in the surgical specimen:

Negative nodes - If the lymphadenectomy specimen is negative for tumor, no further treatment is given since only a rare patient (2/68 - 3 per cent) will develop recurrent cancer in the inguinal-iliac or periaortic areas (Table XX).

Positive nodes - If positive retroperitoneal disease is found, control in that area is improved with postoperative radiotherapy. Three of six patients treated with surgery alone for positive lymph nodes have developed a local recurrence; while only one of 27 recurred locally following a combination of surgery and irradiation (Table XVII). Since mixed tumors have the same order of radiosensitivity as do the epithelial tumors, 4500-5000 rads over a 4 to 6 week period are given.

Elective irradiation of the mediastinum and left supraclavicular area is not advocated for mixed tumors, since only three of 33 patients with positive lymphadenectomy specimens (Stages I and II), have developed disease in the mediastinal or supraclavicular areas. Two of these presented with concurrent extranodal metastases. Nine patients with positive periaortic nodes have developed extranodal metastases (Table XXI). Prophylactic chemotherapy is presently advised for this group, and the initial results have been promising. Irradiation to these areas would compromise subsequent chemotherapy.

Stage II

Retroperitoneal nodes which are interpreted as positive on lymphangiography receive 2500 rads in 3 weeks preoperatively. A bilateral lymphadenectomy is performed within 1 to 2

TABLE XX

PATIENTS WITH MIXED TUMORS (EXCLUDING CHORIOCARCINOMA):
NED at 36 months
(March 1944-July 1971)

Clinical Stage	Orch. Alone	Orch. + XRT	Orch. Node Dissection (-) nodes	Orch. Node Dissection (+) nodes	Orch. Node Dissection + XRT (-) nodes	Orch. Node Dissection + XRT (+) nodes	TOTAL
I	2/2	6/10	58/65* (89. 2%)	3/3	5/6**	7/9	81/95 (85. 3%)
II		0/8	2/3	0/3	9/9	11/18	22/41 (53. 7%)

* 1 - lost to follow-up
** 1 - dead, auto accident (18 months)

TABLE XXI

SITES OF FAILURE IN MIXED TUMORS
(March 1944-July 1971)

Clinical Stage	Orchiectomy + XRT	Orchiectomy + node dissection (-) nodes	Orchiectomy + node dissection (+) nodes	Orch. + node dissection + XRT (-) nodes	Orch. + node dissection + XRT (+) nodes
I	4/10 1- periaortic nodes + ENM 2- ENM only 1- bowel infarction	7/65 1- scrotal rec. * 1- periaortic nodes + ENM 4- ENM only 1- LTF	0/3	1/6 1- ID	2/9 1- medias. nodes + ENM 1- ENM only
II	8/8 4- periaortic nodes + ENM 2- ENM only 2- uncertain	1/3 1- medias. nodes + ENM	3/3 1- periaortic nodes only 2- periaortic & medias. nodes + ENM	0/9	7/18 1- periaortic nodes + ENM 1- marginal rec. abd. + ENM 4- ENM 1- bowel obstruc.

Abbreviations: SC = supraclavicular area; ENM = extranodal metastasis (lung, liver, bone, brain); LTF = lost to follow-up.

* Scrotal recurrence treated with surgery & chemotherapy - died of septicemia secondary to chemotherapy.

TABLE XXII

TREATMENT PLAN FOR MIXED TUMORS (GROUPS II-V)

Stage	Primary		Regional Lymphatics		Systemic
I	Radical Orchiectomy		Lymphadenectomy	Neg nodes: No further treatment Pos nodes: Post op XRT (4500 rads/5-5-1/2 wks)*	ChemoRx
II	Radical Orchiectomy	Preop XRT (2500 rads/3 wks)	Lymphadenectomy	Post op XRT (2500 rads/3 wks)*	ChemoRx
III	Radical Orchiectomy	Chemotherapy and/or radiotherapy on an individualized basis			

* The final 500-1000 rads is delivered through reduced fields to areas of known involvement marked by silver clips.

weeks. Following surgery, an additional 2500 rads in 3 weeks is given. The final 500-1000 rads is given through reduced portals to areas of known involvement marked with silver clips. The periaortic area is preferably treated with 25 MeV megavoltage x-rays. Because of the superficial location of the nodes, the inguinal-iliac fields are treated with ^{60}Co. The surgical morbidity has not been increased with this treatment regimen.

Stage III

The presence of mediastinal or supraclavicular lymphatic disease in patients with mixed tumors usually means extranodal metastases which will quickly become evident. Chemotherapy forms the basis for treatment in these cases and radiotherapy is reserved for the management of local problems.

Results

The results of treatment for mixed tumors are shown in Table XX. Choriocarcinoma has been excluded because of virtually complete failure (2/19 NED at 3 years). The 3-year NED rates for the other mixed tumors are 85. 3 per cent for Stage I and 53. 7 per cent for Stage II.

RADIOTHERAPY PORTALS

The treatment portals employed depend on the extent of disease and are similar for pure seminoma and mixed tumors (Figs. 8-2 through 8-4). Because of their anterior location, the inguinal and iliac nodes are ordinarily irradiated through a single anterior field (Field A). The tumor dose is assessed 3 cm anterior to midplane. The inguinal nodes are included in the inguinal-iliac field if the scrotum was involved with tumor. The opposite testis is shielded (Fig. 8-2). A portion of the scrotum may be included if the orchiectomy incision reaches the scrotum.

The periaortic nodes are treated through parallel opposed portals (Fields B & C) and the tumor dose is assessed at midplane. These fields are usually 0-11 cm wide, utilizing the lymphangiogram to insure proper coverage of the nodes. Care must be taken to include nodes at the renal hila, especially on the left where the spermatic vein enters the left renal vein. As was previously discussed, the lateral nodes draining the testis may not be filled by pedal lymphangiography. The kidneys are localized with intravenous pyelograms with the patient in a prone position. The lateral two-thirds of both kidneys is excluded whenever possible.

With massive abdominal disease, total abdominal portals (Fields G & H are used initially. The kidneys are shielded posteriorly with 2 HVL's of lead. When the tumor location requires inclusion of one kidney, the contralateral kidney is shielded anteriorly and posteriorly with 5 HVL.

Mediastinal and left supraclavicular fields (Fields D, E & F) are used in Stages II and III_A pure seminomas (Figs. 8-3 and 8-4). The mediastinal fields are 9-10 cm wide and the tumor dose is assessed at midplane. Since the supraclavicular nodes lie just beneath the skin, only an anterior field is employed.

TOLERANCE AND COMPLICATIONS

There are few complications with the doses customarily used for pure seminoma, provided renal shielding is employed to limit the dose to both kidneys to 1500 rads. Of 141 patients with pure seminoma, three patients developed complications related to radiotherapy. One patient died of radiation nephritis after irradiation of the whole abdomen with the ^{60}Co trunkbridge technique to an estimated dose of 3700 rads. A second patient developed acute sigmoiditis (4500 rads) re-

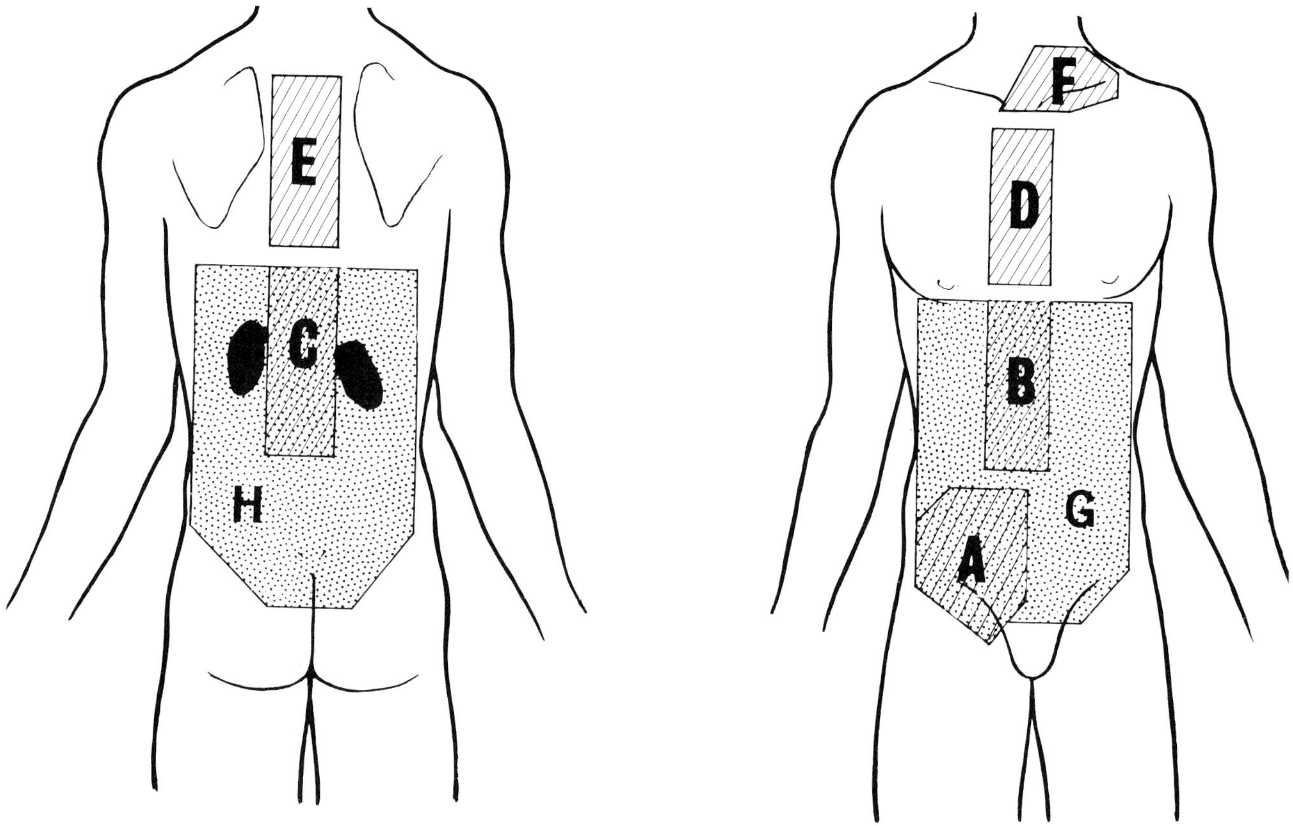

Fig. 8-2. Typical field arrangements for testicular tumors.
Stage I pure seminoma - Fields A, B, & C.
Stage II pure seminoma - Fields A, B, C, D, & E. With extensive retroperitoneal disease, a portion of the treatment is delivered through whole abdomen portals (Fields G & H).
For tumors other than pure seminoma, the mediastinal and supraclavicular areas are not irradiated.

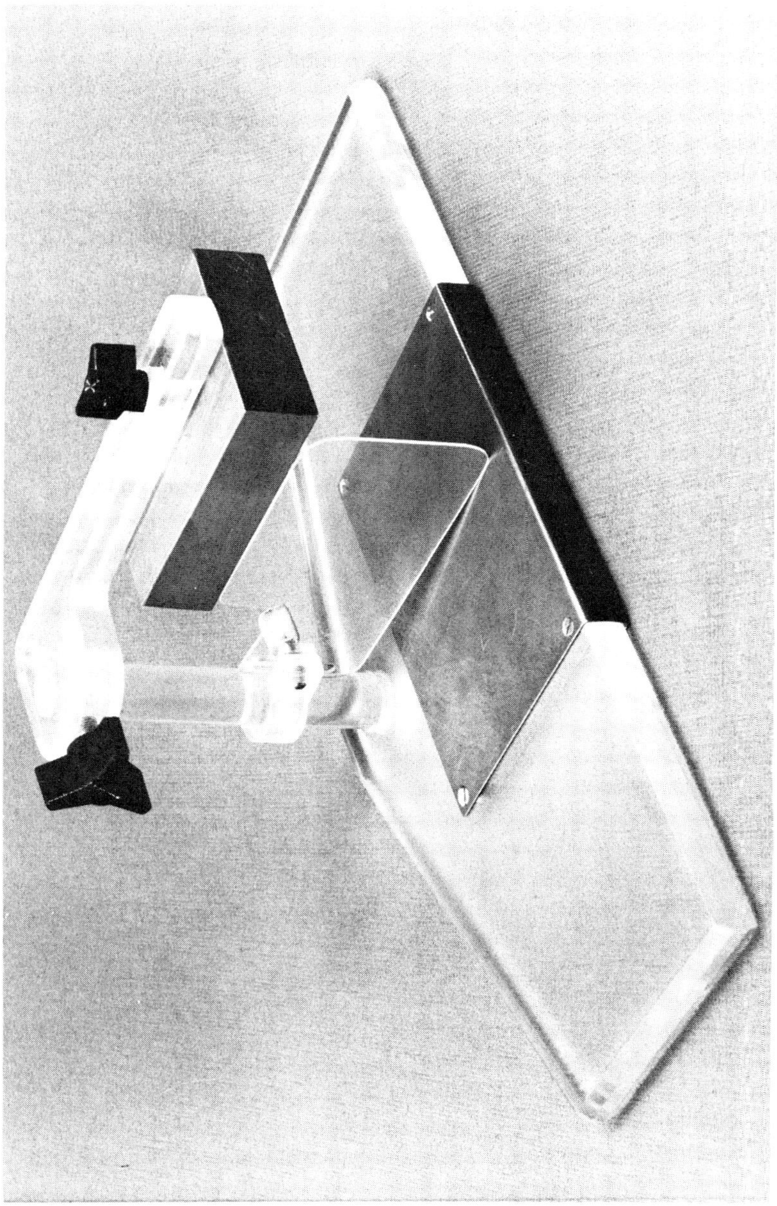

Fig. 8-3A. Device to shield the contralateral testis while irradiating a portion of the scrotum (Courtesy Harter, D., Delclos, L., and Hussey, D.).

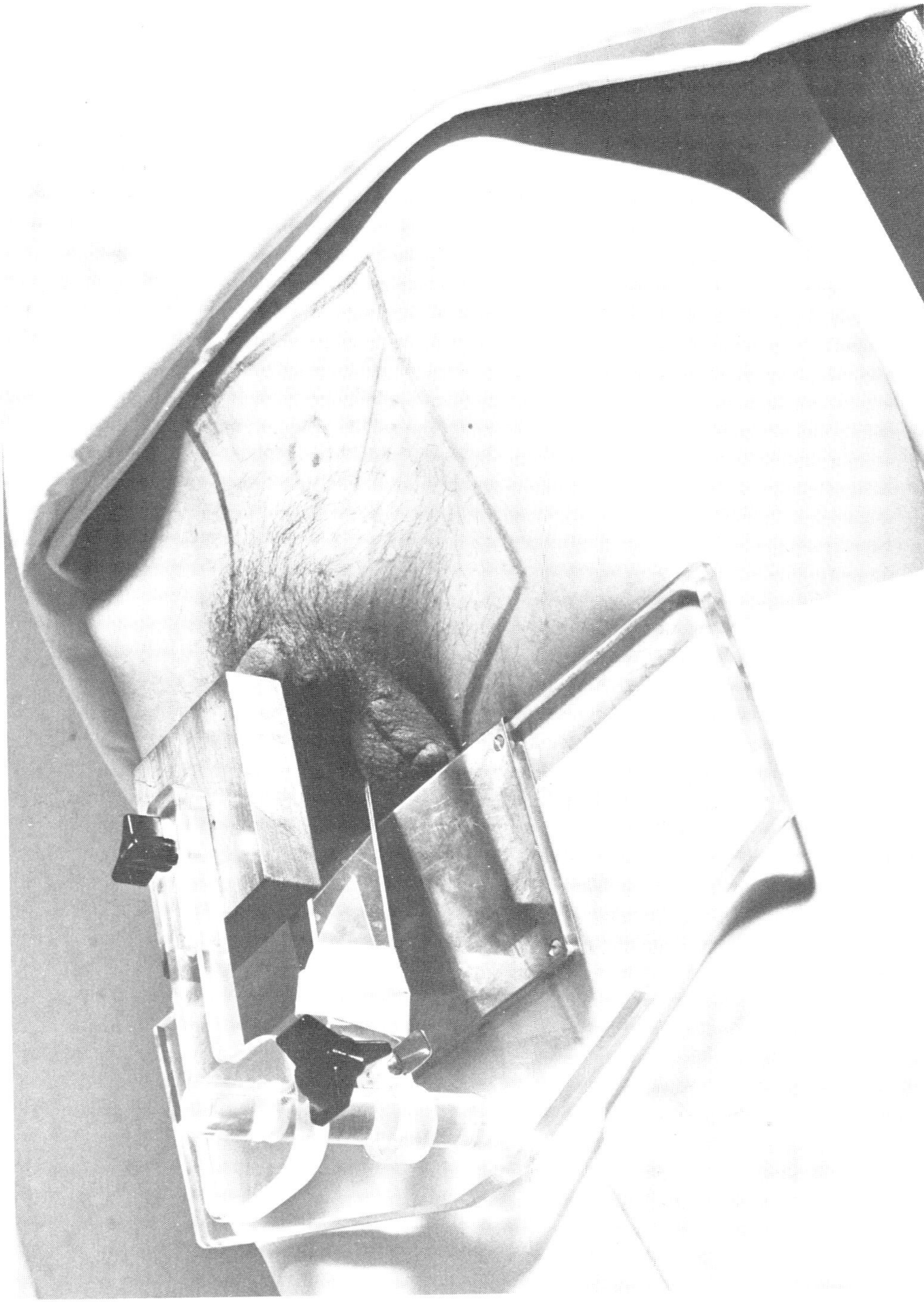

Fig. 8-3B. Device in position for patient receiving radiation to the left scrotum.

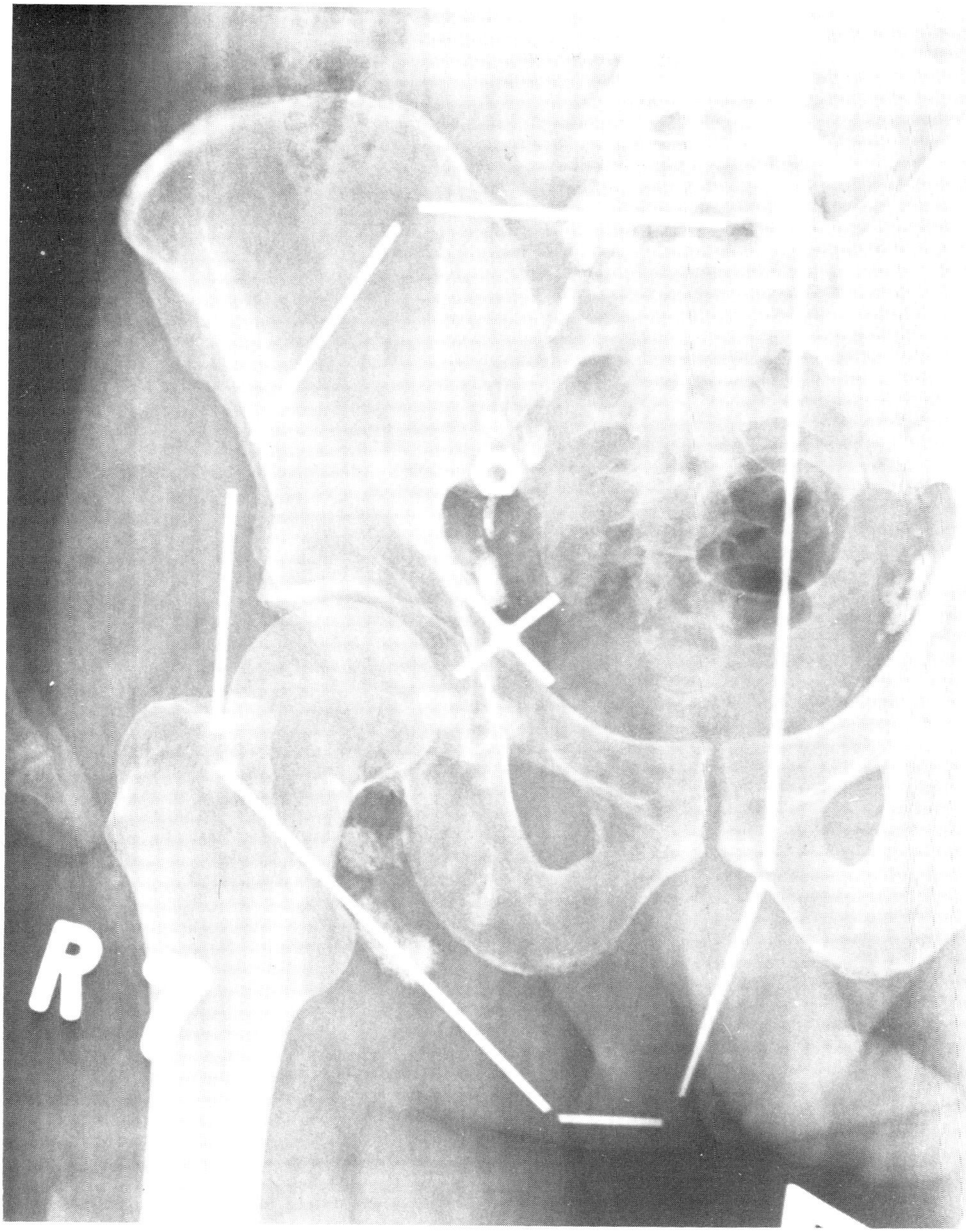

Fig. 8-4A. Portal film of the inguinal-iliac field A. Since the iliac and inguinal nodes lie anteriorly, only an anterior portal is used. The tumor dose is calculated 3 cm anterior to midplane. Only the ipsilateral nodes are included unless there has been a previous herniorrhaphy or orchiopexy. The superior margin is at the L_5S_1 level. The medial margin extends 1 cm across midplane on the skin.

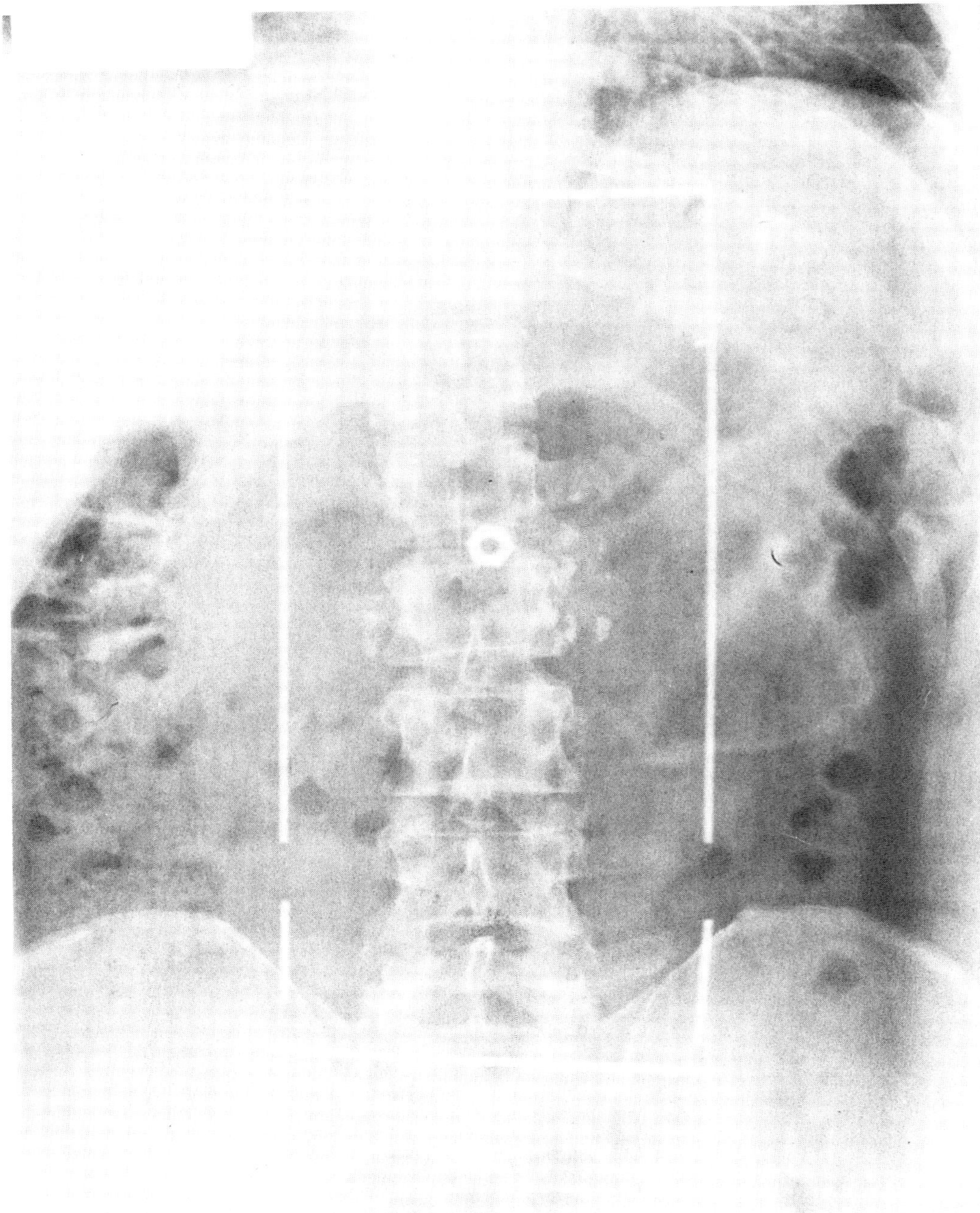

Fig. 8-4B. Anterior portal film of the periaortic field B. The fields are usually 10-11 cm wide. Care is taken to cover the "lateral" nodes at the renal hila which may not be filled by pedal lymph-angiography.

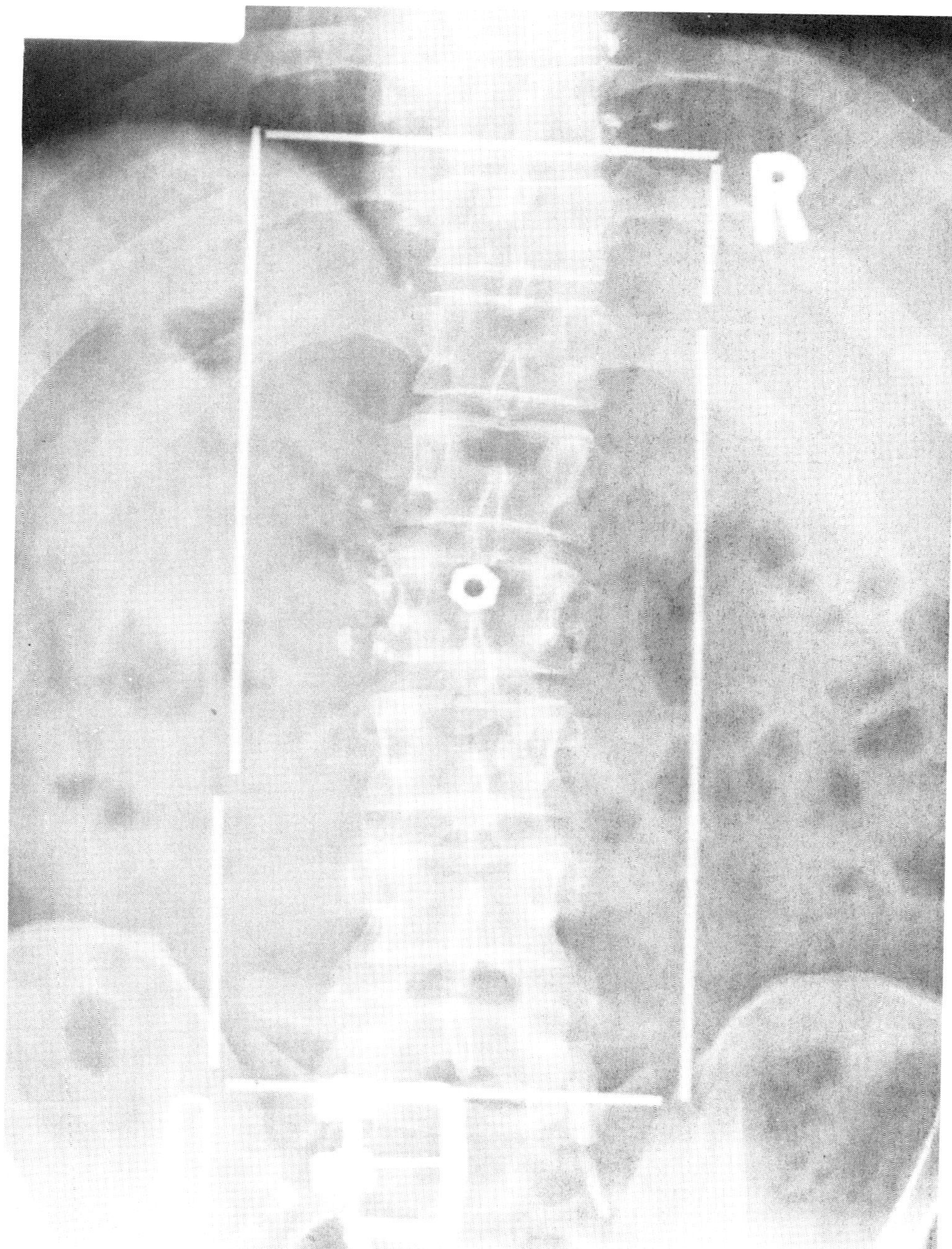

Fig. 8-4C. Posterior portal film of the periaortic field C.

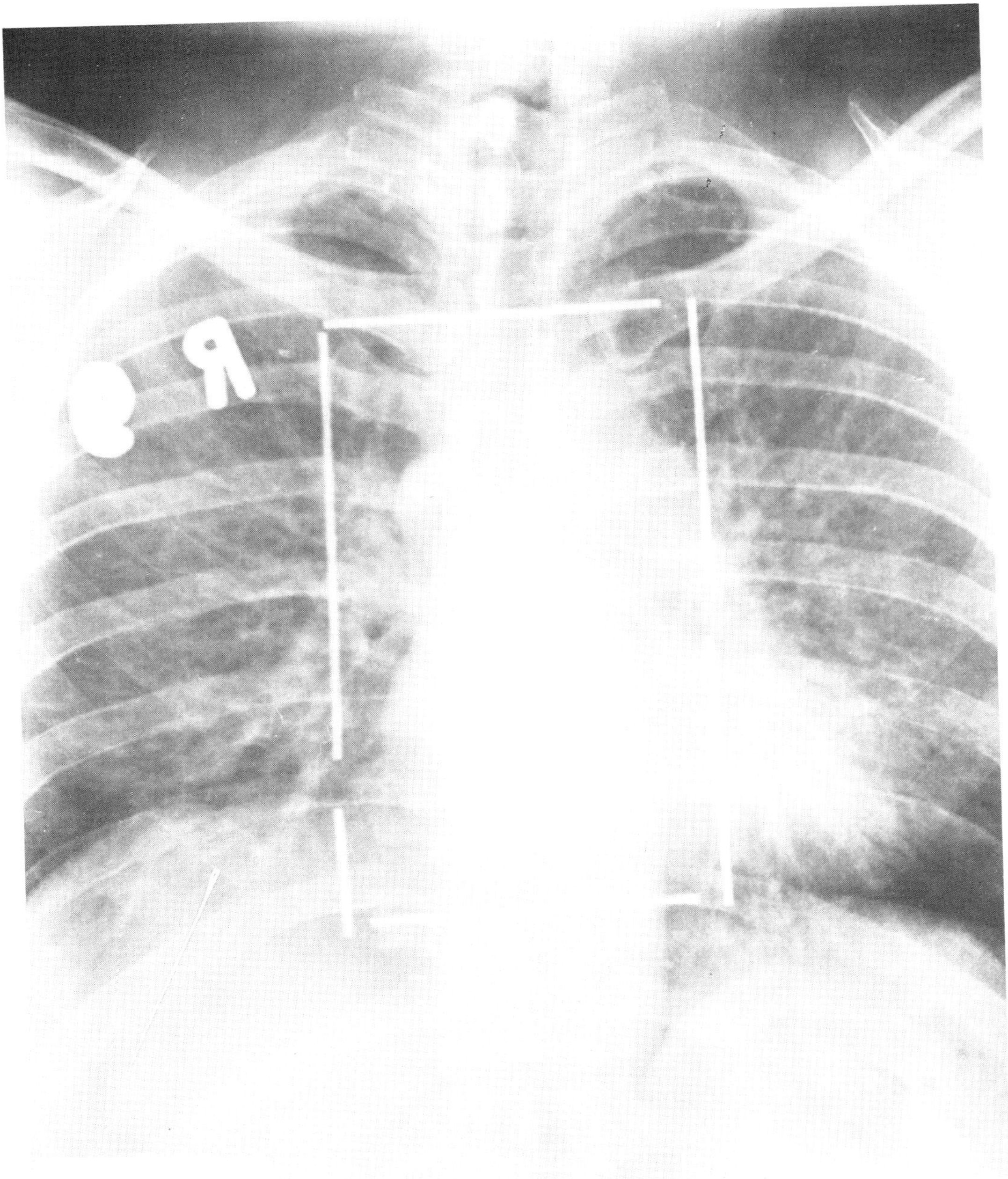

Fig. 8-4D. Anterior portal film of the mediastinal field D. Care is taken to avoid an overlap with the periaortic fields at the spinal cord.

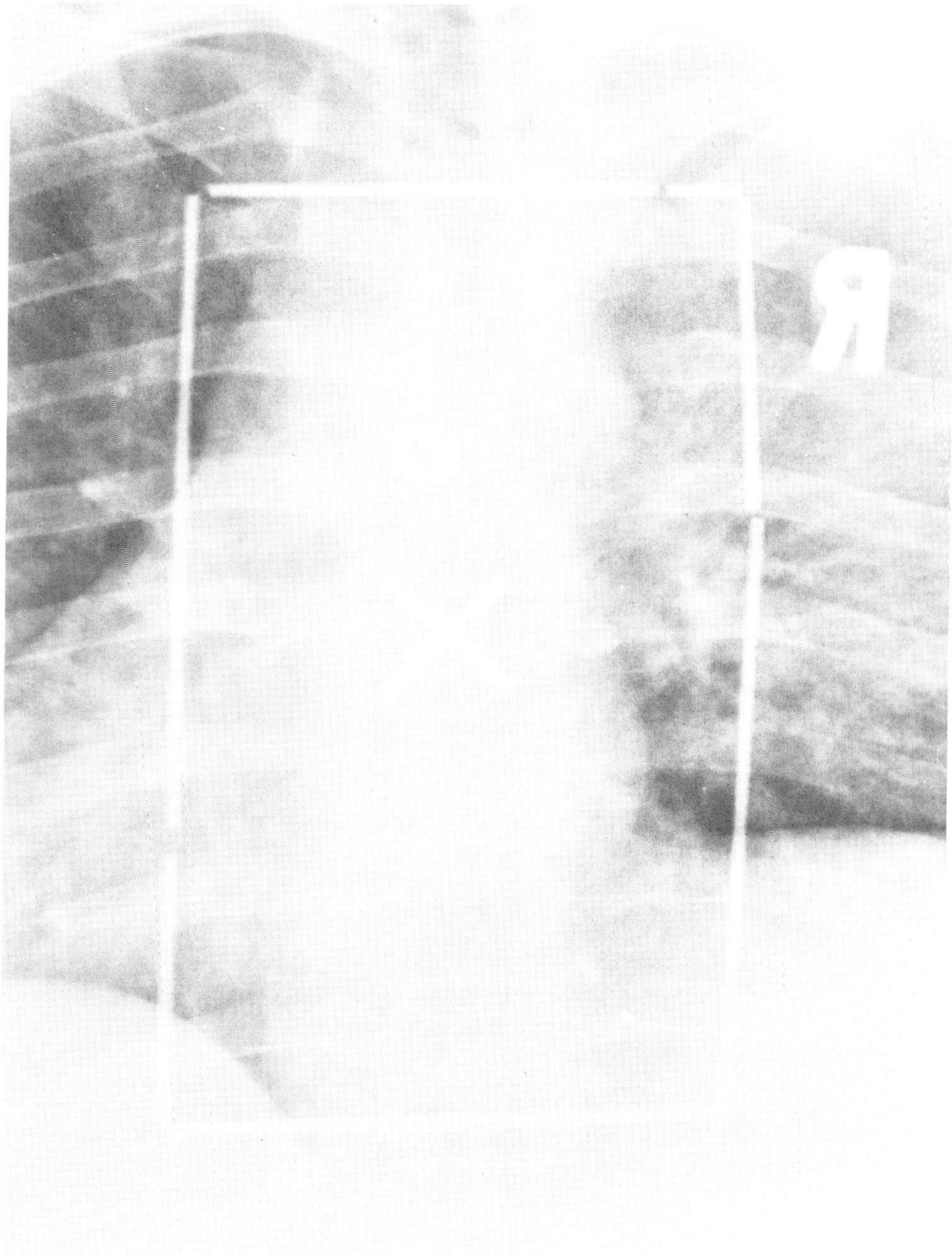

Fig. 8-4E. Posterior portal film of the mediastinal field E.

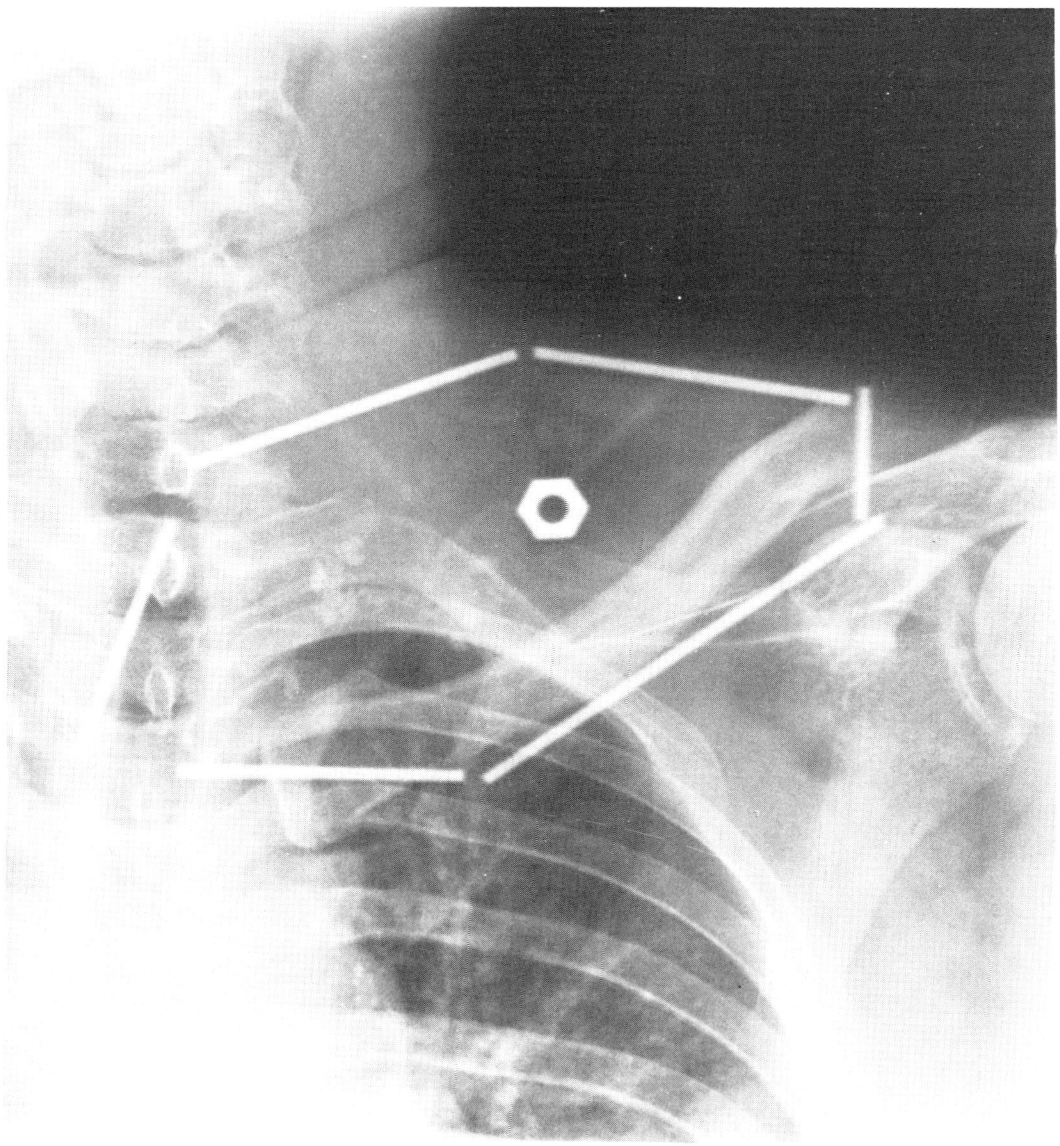

Fig. 8-4F. Portal film of the supraclavicular field F. Since the nodes lie just beneath the skin, the tumor dose is assessed as the given dose (0.5 cm).

quiring a partial colectomy. A third patient developed scrotal necrosis after 3750 rads.

Two patients died of acute myelogenous leukemia following 2500 rads to the inguinal-iliac, periaortic, mediastinal, and left supraclavicular lymphatics; and one patient died of a perforated gastric ulcer at the edge of a periaortic field treated to 2500 rads. Although these events may possibly be classified as complications of treatment, the relationship is not proven.

The mixed tumor groups require doses in the range of 4500-5000 rads in 4-1/2 to 6 weeks, and the risk of complications is greater. Doses at this level have been known to cause neurologic and bowel complications and should not be exceeded.

CHAPTER 9

TREATMENT: CHEMOTHERAPY

by

Melvin L. Samuels

INTRODUCTION AND REVIEW OF CHEMOTHERAPY

Germinal tumors of the testis are more responsive to chemotherapeutic attack than other malignancies of genitourinary tract origin. This is probably related to their very rapid growth rate since the mean volume doubling time of pulmonary metastasis has been found to be 27 days as compared to 28 days for malignant lymphoma (Charbit et al. 1971). Thus, agents which act predominantly during the mitotic cycle can be expected to be more active than in more common slower-growing solid tumors. As a corollary to this premise, untreated Stage 3 patients with widespread metastatic disease should have a short survival and indeed, it has been shown that 90 per cent of such patients will be dead within 1 year, and most within 6 months (Collins and Pugh 1964). The mechanism of death is usually pulmonary failure from massive lung metastases, but a small number of patients will die as the result of liver metastases, bilateral ureteral obstruction with uremia or rarely brain metastases. In these situations, palliation is difficult with radiotherapy alone and drug treatment must assume the primary role.

In 1958, Blokhin et al. reported the results of a 4 year clinical trial with sarcolysin (DL-p-di(2-chlorethyl) aminophenylalanine hydrochloride), an alkylating agent which was synthesized in 1953. Of 23 patients with seminoma, complete response was observed in 11 and considerable reduction of tumor size was noted in 8 patients. Prolonged control up to 2.5 years was obtained in 3 patients. There were no complete responses in 9 patients with nonseminomatous germinal tumors. This study represents the first in-depth trial of chemotherapy in testicular cancer and provided the stimulus for future trials. Subsequently, we confirmed the activity of alkylating agents in seminoma, but found virtually no activity in the nonseminomatous tumors. Cytoxan, thiotepa and melphalan appeared to be equally active against seminoma. Since the greater majority of seminoma patients are cured with radiotherapy and therefore do not present to the chemotherapist, interest in alkylating agents waned. Antimetabolites received a brief unsustained period of trial and it was demonstrated that methotrexate and 5-fluorouracil were active (Wyatt and McAninch 1967; Hyman et al. 1962; Wilson 1960; Allaire et al. 1961). However, Li et al. (1958) reported that while choriocarcinoma in the female is very responsive to parenteral methotrexate, choriocarcinoma in the male, either pure or mixed with embryonal carcinoma or teratocarcinoma, is refractory. Methotrexate produced minor fluctuations in gonadotropin titers with no significant change in tumor mass. Thus, further trials were abandoned in favor of a new class of compounds, the antitumor antibiotics. Actinomycin-D, a product of streptomyces parvullus fermentation, was introduced into testicular cancer protocols in 1955 by Li (1960). It has a highly selective mechanism of action resulting from binding to helical DNA. This results in inhibition of DNA-dependent RNA synthesis. However, actinomycin-D has many effects that are not related to inhibition of RNA synthesis. These include inhibition of protein and phospholipid synthesis, inhibition of replication of RNA viruses (polioviruses), inhibition of amino acid transport and stimulation of breakdown of messenger RNA (Pastan and Friedman 1968). Introduction into clinical trials preceded adequate pharmacology studies and trials were accelerated when activity was observed in Wilms' tumor. Very few studies have been reported with actinomycin-D used alone in testicular cancer, but results suggest that objective remission can be obtained in one-third to one-half of the patients with advanced disease when used as initial therapy. When used as secondary therapy in patients refractory to other chemotherapy programs, responses are few, and almost never complete. Mithramycin (Pitts 1970), another antibiotic belonging to the genus streptomyces, has received extensive clinical trial with 305 evaluable patients reported. There were 113 responses of which 33 (28 per cent) were complete but only 12 patients survived beyond 1 year in complete remission. Serious liver, kidney and marrow toxicity in the face of poor salvage has resulted in virtual abandonment of further trials.

The periwinkle alkaloid, Velban and Oncovin, have been proven to be important drugs with significant activity in Hodgkin's disease and non-Hodgkin's lymphoma. We initiated a study in 1962 (Samuels and Howe 1970) using large dose Velban in Stage 3 disease and found striking objective regressions in 50 per cent with one-third of the responses being complete. Of 40 patients studied, only 2 survived beyond 4 years in complete remission, again emphasizing poor salvage with single drugs.

Combination chemotherapy was introduced by Li (1960) in an attempt to improve the remission rate and duration of response. Three drugs, each from a different class, were combined in an intensive 25 day regime. Chlorambucil, an alkylating agent, was given in a dose of 10 mg orally per day and methotrexate, an antimetabolite, 5 mg orally for 16 to 25 days as toxicity permitted. Actinomycin-D, 0.5 mg intravenously was started on day 3 and given for 5 consecutive days. A second 5 day course was started on the 12th day and a third 5 day course on the 21st day. Enhancement of drug toxicity is to be expected when such combinations are used and severe stomatitis, diarrhea and myelosuppression may prove life-threatening. Of 23 patients initially reported by Li, there were 12 responses with 7 complete or near complete. In a subsequent report from the same hospital, MacKenzie (1966) described 90 trials with a 50 per cent response rate. However, there were only 10 complete responses with 3 long term survivors. Ansfield et al. (1969) obtained a 50 per cent response rate with the Li regime but noted that reactivation usually occurred within 3 months. Jacobs (1970) reported on the combination of actinomycin-D, vincristine, and cyclophosphamide and found no improvement over the Li regime. Mendelson and Serpick (1970) reported a 4 drug combination of cyclophosphamide, vincristine, methotrexate and 5-fluorouracil, all given by rapid intravenous administration in 5 day courses. Cyclophosphamide and methotrexate were given on days 1 and 4 in a dose of 7.5 mg/kg body weight and 0.75 mg/kg respectively, vincristine on day 1 and 4 in a dose of 0.25 mg/kg and 5-fluorouracil 7.5 mg/kg/day daily for 5 days with repeat courses given as toxicity permitted. Five of 17 patients achieved a complete response with the median duration of remission only 9 months. Thus, it is quite clear that combination chemotherapy trials have not improved the salvage over single active drugs given to maximum toxicity.

BLEOMYCIN

In 1970, the Clinical Screening Cooperative Group of the European Organization for Research on the Treatment of Cancer (1970) reported objective regressions in 4 of 6 patients with advanced testicular cancer treated with a new antitumor antibiotic, bleomycin. There were two complete responses, both in patients with choriocarcinoma. Bleomycin, a product of fermentation of streptomyces verticullus, a soil actinomycote found in Japan, is a mixture of 14 high molecular weight glycoproteins. The bleomycins can be separated by paper chromatography into 2 fractions, bleomycin A and bleomycin B. Further separation by sephadex chromatography results in the following separation: A_1 through A_6, B_1 through B_6, A_2'-a and A_2'-b (Umezawa et al. 1966; Umezawa 1971). The major component of the commercial preparation is bleomycin A_2 comprising about 50 per cent. Bleomycin is especially attractive for combination chemotherapy since it does not usually produce significant myelosuppression. The dose-limiting toxicity is interstitial fibrosis of the lung.

The mechanism of action of bleomycin is not completely understood. Suzuki et al. (1968, 1969) has hypothesized that bleomycin binds to DNA and causes strand scission. The points of breakage of DNA are randomly distributed along the DNA molecule (Haidle 1971) with many sites probably adjacent to one another. There is also inhibition of thymidine incorporation into DNA with impaired DNA synthesis. Bleomycin effects cells in all phases of the mitotic cycle, but certain phases are more sensitive. Thus, Chinese hamster ovary cells are more effectively destroyed in M and G_2 (Barranco and Humphrey 1971). However, Hela cells appear to be more sensitive in S phase. Umizawa et al. (1972) has demonstrated greater concentration of bleomycin in squamous carcinoma of the skin of the mouse as compared to methylcholanthrene-induced sarcoma. In this regard, clinical activity has been demonstrated in squamous carcinoma of the skin of the head and neck, and penis, as well as in malignant lymphoma (Clinical Screening Cooperative Group of the European Organization for Research on the Treatment of Cancer 1970; Katsuyuki et al. 1970; Blum et al. 1973).

THE M. D. ANDERSON HOSPITAL PROGRAM

In formulating drug combination programs one seeks to combine proven active agents with qualitatively different toxicities so that they can be administered together in full dosage. The antitumor effect should be at least additive and hopefully, synergistic. The combination of Velban and bleomycin seemed particularly attractive. Both showed impressive clinical activity and had different mechanisms of action. Their toxic manifestations were completely different. The dose-limiting toxicity of Velban is myelosuppression while it is interstitial fibrosis of the lung and occasionally, severe stomatitis or severe skin reactions for bleomycin. Hence, full dosage of each could be expected to be tolerated.

Seventy patients with Stage 3 testicular cancer were studied between

August 1, 1970 and January 1, 1974. In addition, 7 patients with extragonadal primary tumors and 13 patients with non-measurable disease (9 Stage 2, 4 post-surgical resection for isolated metastases) are also included in the evaluation. The criteria of Dixon and Moore (1958) were used for histological classification. Special criteria were used to stratify patients according to presentation (Table XXIII).

The initial treatment procedure for hospitalized patients termed the VB-1 program consisted of Velban 0.4 to 0.6 mg/kg body weight in 2 fractions given by IV push day 1 and day 2 and bleomycin 30 units IM twice weekly for a loading dose of 300 mg (10 doses). For patients of small stature with a body surface area less than $1.6M^2$, the dose of bleomycin was reduced to 15 units twice weekly for 10 doses. For outpatients, or for debilitated patients with borderline blood counts (usually from prior radiotherapy), Velban 10 mg IV push was given on day 1 and thereafter 5 mg increments every 7 days until significant myelosuppression was noted. The bleomycin dosage remained unchanged. Therapy was repeated at 4 to 6 week intervals for a total of 4 to 6 courses, provided toxicity permitted. A five drug program, bleomycin plus cyclophosphamide, vincristine, methotrexate and 5-fluorouracil (bleoCOMF) was initiated for Velban-bleomycin failures. Bleomycin was administered in a dose of 30 units IM twice weekly for 4 doses, cyclophosphamide 200 mg/M^2 p.o. daily x 14, vincristine 2.0 mg IV push day 1 and 7, methotrexate 15 mg/M^2 IV twice weekly x 4 and 5-fluorouracil, 400 mg/M^2 IV daily x 5 doses. Therapy was carried to 14 days provided the leukocyte level remained above $2500/MM^3$ and platelets above $100,000/MM^3$. Finally, a small group of patients were treated with continuous bleomycin infusion, termed VB-3 program. Thirty units of bleomycin in 1000 cc 5 per cent glucose/distilled water was administered over a 24 hour period for 5 days, following Velban administration in the initial program.

RESPONSE

Objective response to VB-1 was observed in 53 of the 70 Stage 3 patients giving a response rate of 75 per cent. These included 22 complete responses in which all evidence of tumor disappeared and 31 partial responses in which there was a reduction of at least 50 per cent of the maximum diameter of all tumor masses. Response by histological classification is given in Table XXIV. Note that all 5 Dixon and Moore groups showed significant response, but that complete response was more frequent in Class I and Class IV. Response and prior therapy is given in Table XXV. Note that 30 of 34 patients who had received no prior therapy showed response while only 7 of 14 patients receiving prior chemotherapy and/or radiotherapy were responders. The number of complete responders diminished significantly in the previously treated groups.

The significance of tumor presentation is shown in Table XXVI. Ten of 17 patients with minimal pulmonary disease achieved a complete response while only 4 of 21 with advanced pulmonary presentations were complete responders. Patients with hormonal presentations included gynecomastia, with or without elevated H. C. G. titers, but negative clinical or roentgenological evidence of measurable tumor. Three of 4 such patients achieved rapid complete response. The extragonadal primary patients are detailed in Table XXVII. An excellent partial response was obtained in 1 patient (J. R. see Fig. 9-1) and a brief partial response was obtained in a second patient. There were no complete responses in spite of aggressive therapy with Velban-bleomycin and bleoCOMF.

TABLE XXIII

DEFINITIONS OF PRESENTATIONS

1. Minimal pulmonary disease – no more than 5 metastases per each lung field – each no larger than 2.0 cm.
2. Advanced pulmonary disease – any mediastinal mass, hilar mass, pleural effusion or intrapulmonary mass > 2.0 cm in diameter.
3. Minimal abdominal disease – positive lymphangiogram with no ureteral displacement or pressure on inferior vena cava, plus minimal pulmonary disease.
4. Advanced abdominal disease – palpable mass, enlarged liver with metastases, ureteral displacement ± obstructive uropathy, inferior vena cava distortion, inguinal adenopathy.
5. Hormonal alone – gynecomastia either unilateral or bilateral ± elevated HCG titers.
6. Extragonadal primary – retroperitoneal or anterior mediastinum.

TABLE XXIV

RESPONSE AND TUMOR TYPE

	Dixon and Moore Classification					
	I	II	III	IV	V	Totals
Complete Response	4	7	1	9	1	22
Partial Response	2	19	3	4	3	31
No Response	1	6	3	7	0	17
Totals	7	32	7	20	4	70

TABLE XXV

RESPONSE AND PRIOR THERAPY

	No Prior Therapy	Prior XRT	Prior Chemotherapy and/or XRT	Total
Complete Response	15	6	1	22
Partial Response	15	10	6	31
No Response	4	6	7	17
Total	34	22	14	70

TABLE XXVI

RESPONSE AND PRESENTATION

	Complete Response	Partial Response	No Response
I. PULMONARY – 38			
Minimal – 17	10	5	2
Advanced – 21	4	13	4
II. ABDOMINAL – 28			
Minimal – 3	2	1	–
Advanced – 25	3	12	10
III. HORMONAL – 4	3	–	1
IV. EXTRAGONADAL – 7 PRIMARY	–	3	4

TABLE XXVII

PATIENTS PRESENTING WITH EXTRAGONADAL PRIMARY TUMORS
THERAPY AND RESPONSE

Patient	Primary Site	Histology	Therapy	Response	Survival
1. J. R.	Mediastinum	Teratoma & Embryonal	B. COMF	P. R.*	12 weeks – Alive
2. R. G.	Retroperitoneum	Embryonal	VB_1	P. R.	19 weeks – Dead
3. R. S.	Mediastinum	Seminoma	B. COMF	< 50%	20 weeks – Dead
4. S. M.	Mediastinum	Embryonal	B. COMF	< 50%	4 weeks – Alive
5. J. C.	Mediastinum	Chorio-carcinoma	VB_1	None	10 weeks – Dead
6. L. E.	Mediastinum	Teratoma & Embryonal	1) B. COMF 2) XRT for S.V.C. 3) VB_3	None N. E.	14 weeks – Alive (progressive disease)
7. R. K.	Retroperitoneum	Teratoma	VB_3	< 50%	4 weeks – Alive

* – Striking partial regression to 2 courses of B. COMF

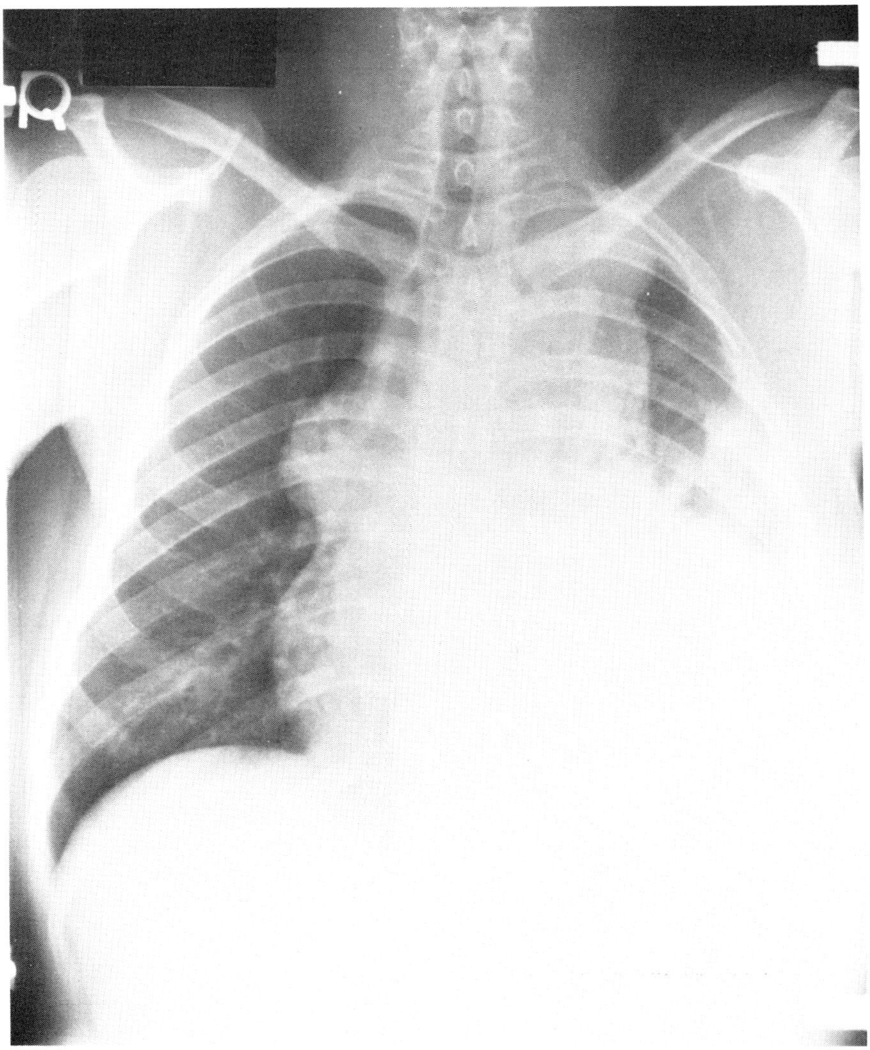

Fig. 9-1A. Extragonadal primary of anterior mediastinum.

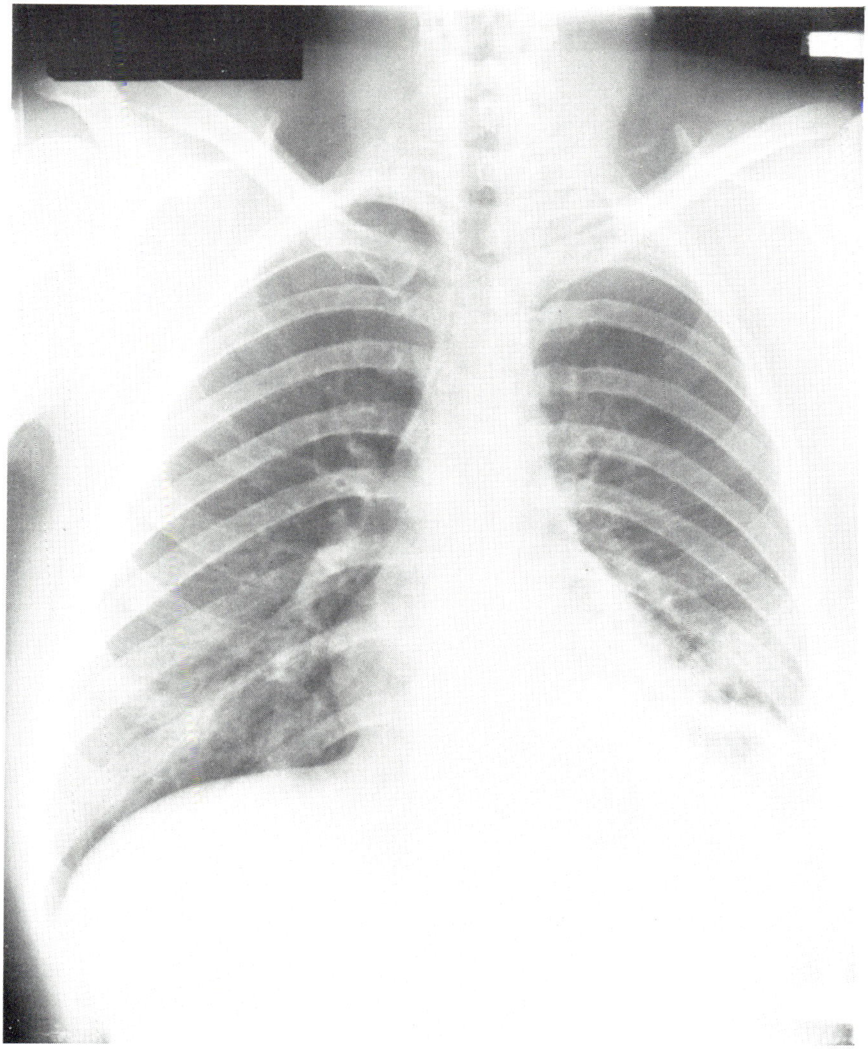

Fig. 9-1B. Extragonadal primary of anterior mediastinum following two courses of bleomycin-"COMF" chemotherapy.

As expected, patients with choriocarcinoma pure or mixed with embryonal carcinoma (Dixon and Moore Class V) proved quite responsive. Figure 9-2 shows such a response. We were also impressed with teratocarcinoma responses. Figure 9-3 shows a typical chest x-ray response to VB-1. Prior experience has shown that patients with metastatic liver disease are generally not responsive to chemotherapy. Figure 9-4 shows the liver scan of a patient with embryonal carcinoma, metastatic to liver. Following two courses of VB-1, there is a near complete response. In addition, 4 of 5 patients presenting with unilateral obstructive uropathy responded to the bleomycin program with complete relief of hydronephrosis.

The Stage 2 and Stage 3 post-surgical resection patients are summarized in Table XXVIII. In these situations chemotherapy was used "prophylactically" since there was no measurable disease, but a high likelihood of eventual failure. The numbers are small and survival extends only to 36 months post-orchiectomy. We are encouraged with 9 of 13 patients living and well in apparent complete remission. It is apparent that further trials will be necessary before any conclusions are justified.

As previously stated the bleo-COMF program was initially designated as a backup protocol for VB-1 failures. Of 24 such patients treated, remission was reinduced in 15 patients. Most of these responses were partial, but produced significant palliation. Eleven new untreated patients were subsequently entered in this program with impressive results. There were 4 complete and 3 partial responses.

The survival time and the duration of response are important parameters in judging the effectiveness of a drug program. Of the 22 complete responses, 3 have died and 4 have developed new metastatic disease. Two of the latter patients were reinduced to complete remission. The mean survival of this group is in excess of 2 years with the longest now at 4 years. Five of these patients with positive lymphangiograms prior to chemotherapy, had retroperitoneal lymphadenectomy after 4 courses of treatment in order to check the effectiveness of the therapy. Residual tumor, consisting of mature teratoid elements was found in only 1 patient. Figure 9-5 shows survival curves, plotted by the life table method, for complete, partial, and non-responders. There is a highly significant difference between complete responders versus the partial and non-responders.

TOXICITY

Severe leukopenia was the rule with the Velban-bleomycin programs but recovery was prompt. Thrombopenia was noted in only one-third of the trials, but was seldom severe and platelet transfusions were not required. Repeat courses did not result in cumulative hematological toxicity. Septicemia, usually due to pseudomonas, was encountered in 11 patients. Nine of this group had advanced abdominal disease with large masses, bowel invasion, or metastatic liver disease and 6 had received prior major radiotherapy to the abdomen or para-aortic nodes. There were 2 deaths, both occurring during the third course of chemotherapy.

Gastrointestinal side effects were common and consisted of glossitis, stomatitis, and vomiting with paralytic ileus. Figure 9-6 shows the peculiar form of glossitis commonly seen with the VB-1 program. The tongue becomes swollen and whitish-coated, with marginal dental impressions. Ulcerations along the lateral tongue border may be seen (Fig. 9-7) but healed promptly. Skin hyperpigmentation was universal in all patients receiving more than 3 courses. Tem-

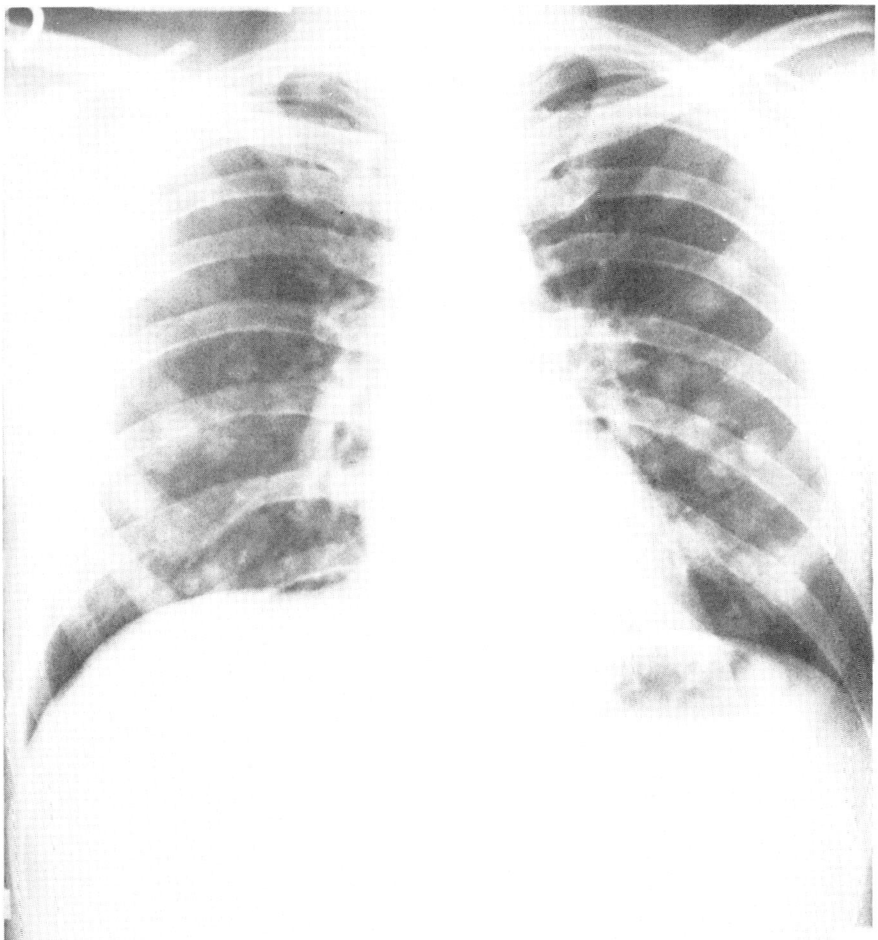

Fig. 9-2A. Metastatic choriocarcinoma rapidly appearing following orchiectomy.

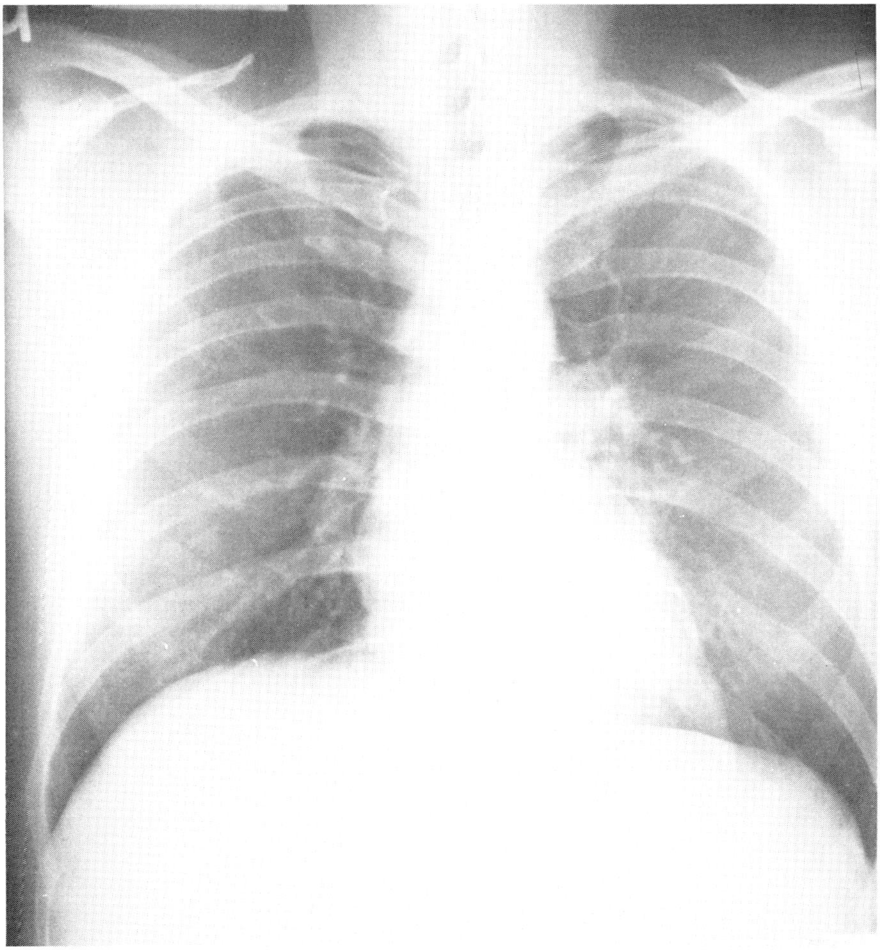

Fig. 9-2B. Metastatic choriocarcinoma rapidly appearing following orchiectomy after two courses of Velban-bleomycin.

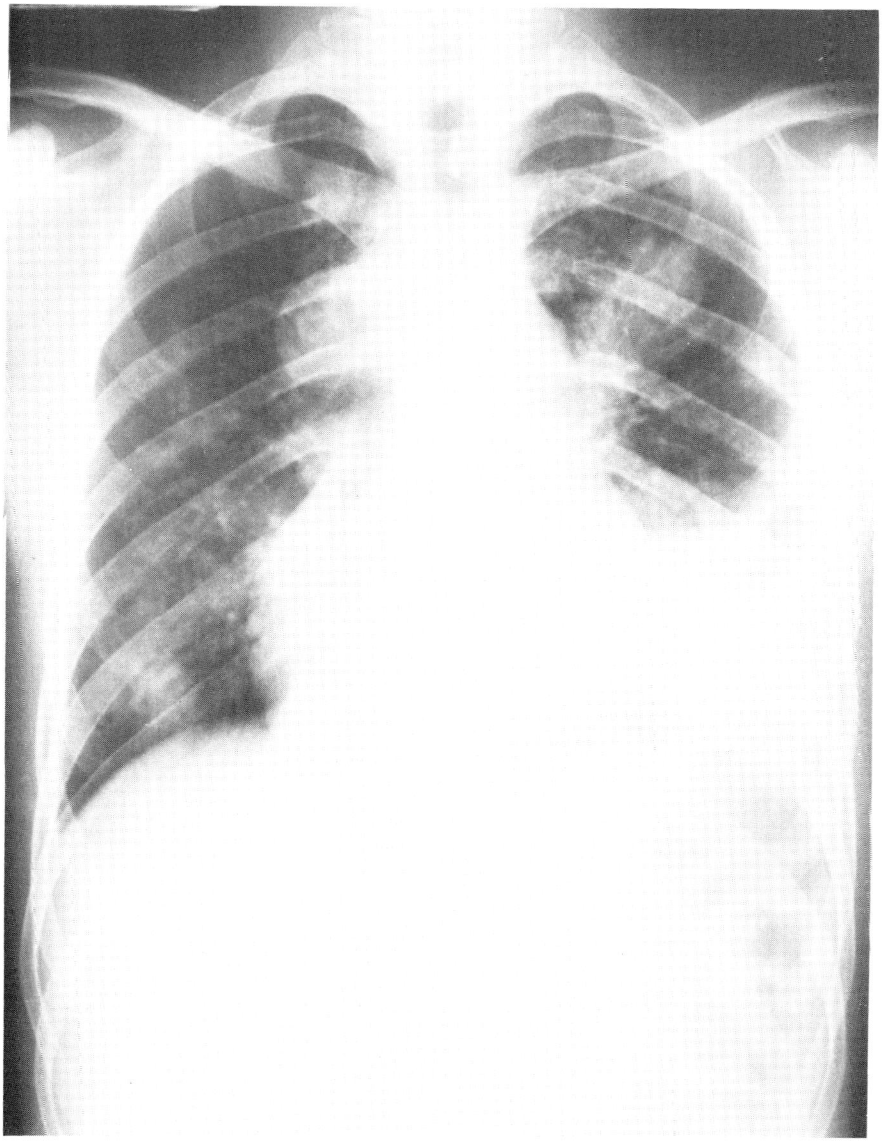

Fig. 9-3A. Metastatic teratocarcinoma and embryonal carcinoma unresponsive to Li regime.

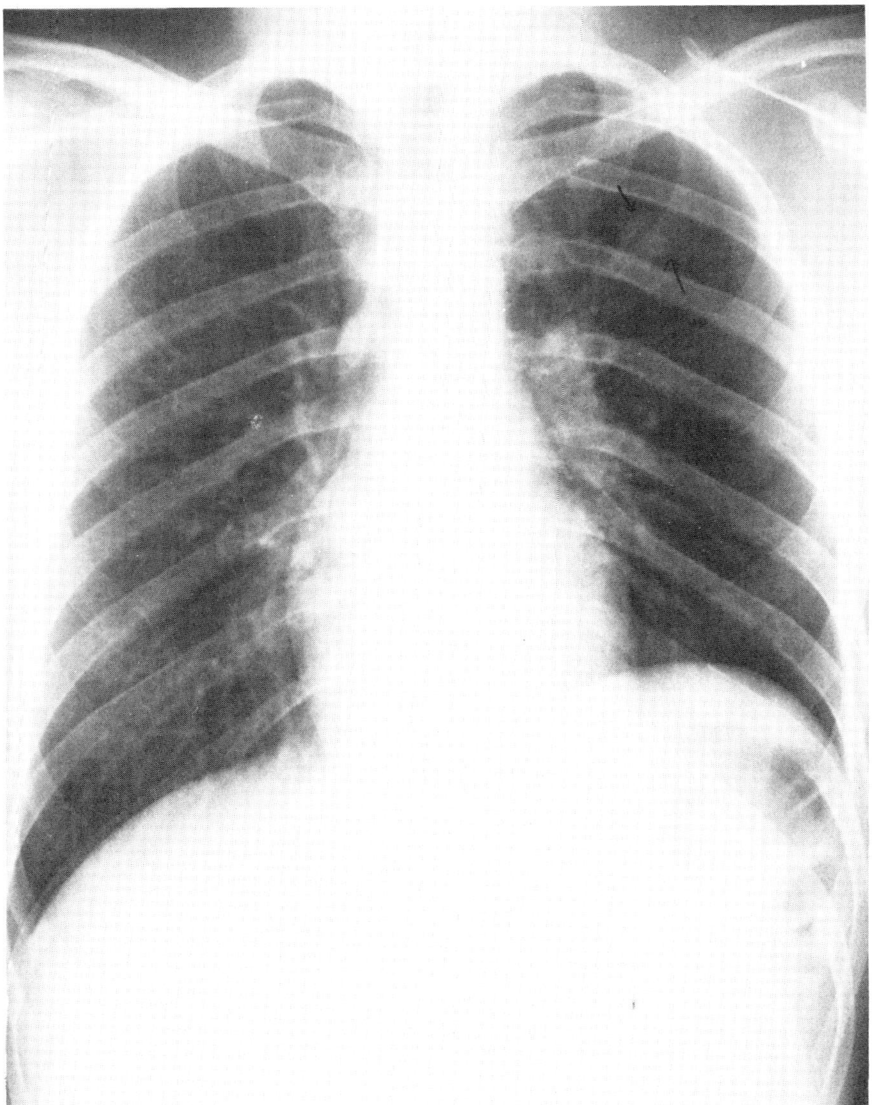

Fig. 9-3B. Metastatic teratocarcinoma and embryonal carcinoma unresponsive to Li regime following one course of Velban-bleomycin.

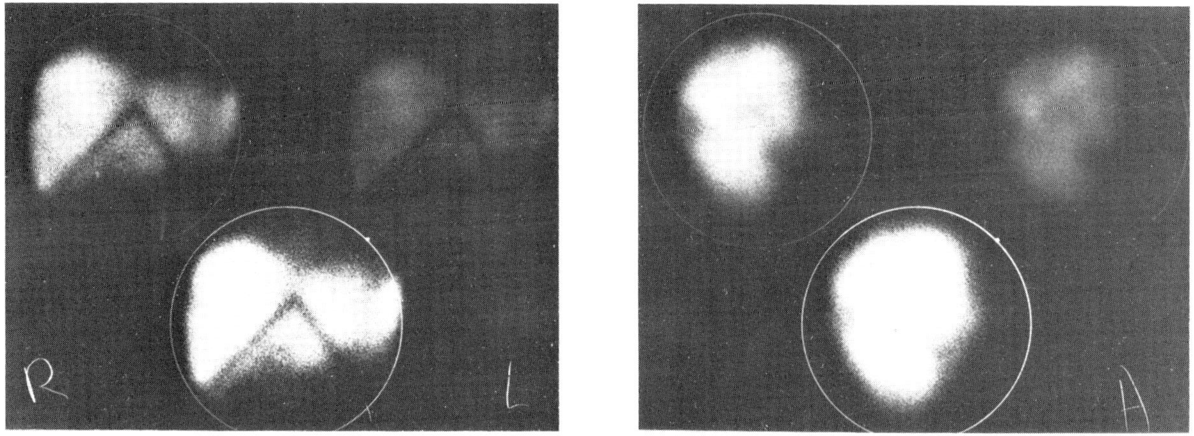

Fig. 9-4A. Liver scan with Technetium 99^{M} colloid showing metastasis from embryonal carcinoma.

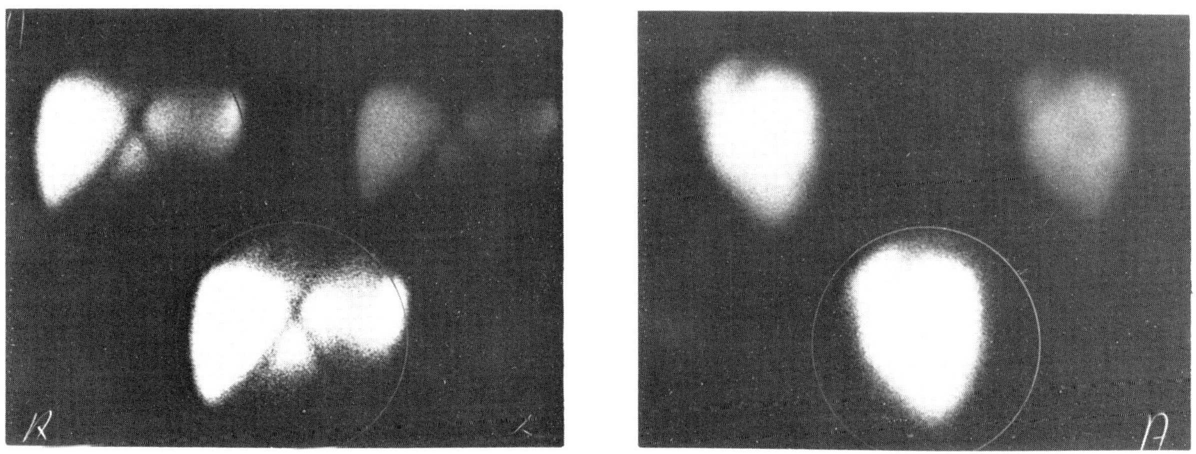

Fig. 9-4B. Liver scan with Technetium 99^{M} colloid showing metastasis from embryonal carcinoma following chemotherapy with V-B_1 program.

TABLE XXVIII

RESULTS OF PROPHYLACTIC BLEOMYCIN COMBINATION CHEMOTHERAPY IN PATIENTS AT GREAT RISK TO DEVELOP GENERALIZED METASTASES

	Patient Status				Median Survival (Months)	
	Number Patients	N.E.D.	Dead	Recurrent Disease	From Orchidectomy	Chemotherapy
Stage II post-X.R.T. or vascular invasion of primary tumor*	9	6	2	1[a]	23 (10 - 44)	14 (8 - 36)
Stage III post-surgical resection of isolated metastases**	4	3	1[b]	–	36 (12 - 60)	25 (5 - 28)
Total	13	9	3	1		

* 6 patients, Stage II, 2 patients with vascular invasion of primary

** Metastasis observed 5 - 8 months after orchidectomy except for 1 patient at 40 months

(a) At 5 months following 2 courses of Velban – Bleomycin

(b) Drug death – 3rd course of Velban – Bleomycin, post-mortem – no tumor

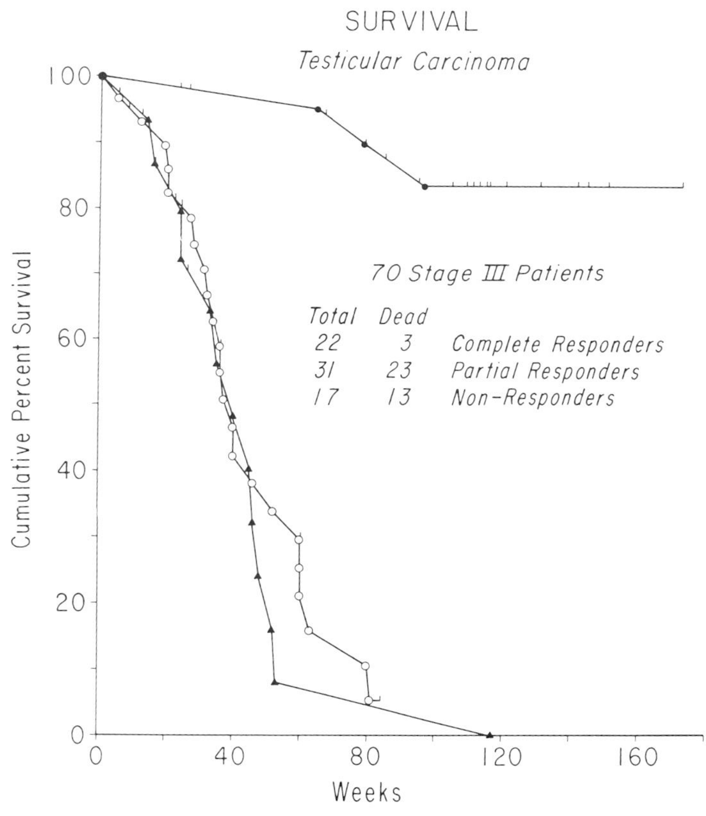

Fig. 9-5. Survival curves of complete, partial and nonresponders, Stage III. There is a highly significant difference between complete responders versus the partial and non responders. ($P < 0.01$).

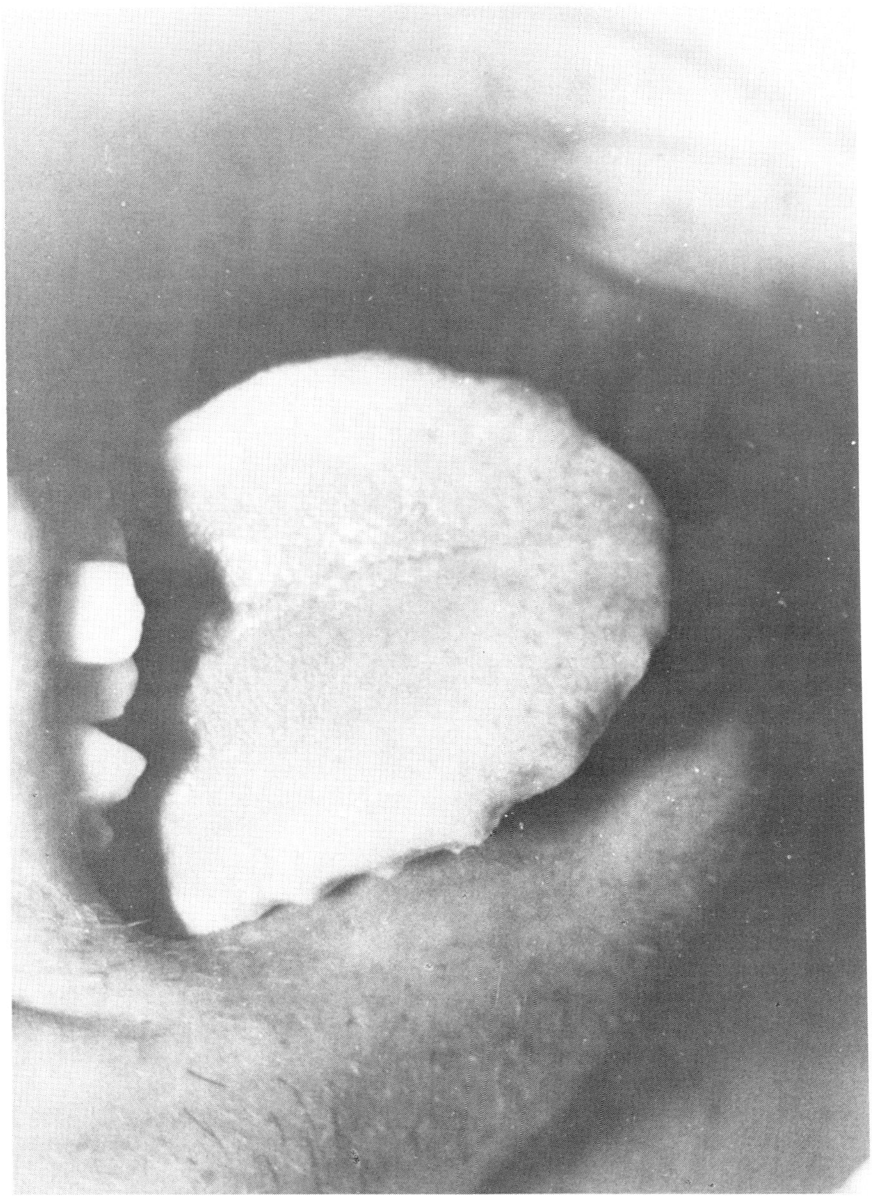

Fig. 9-6. Swollen white discolored tongue seen as early toxic manifestation of Velban-bleomycin.

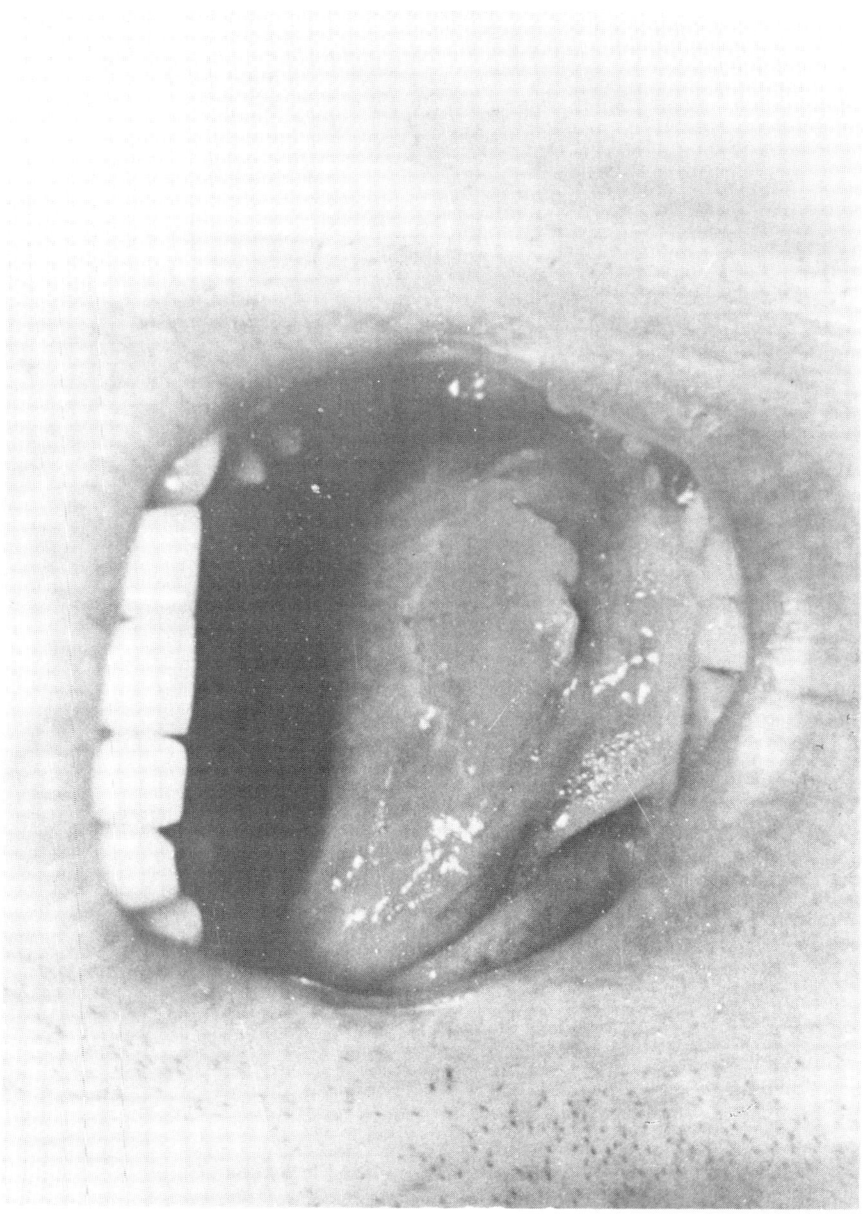

Fig. 9-7. Severe ulcerated tongue seen very occasionally with Velban-bleomycin programs.

porary alopecia was also quite common. Swelling of the hands and fingers with focal skin thickening at pressure points was noted in approximately 25 per cent of patients, but rapidly subsided after the completion of bleomycin.

Interstitial pneumonitis secondary to bleomycin was encountered in 5 patients. There were 2 deaths from pulmonary insufficiency. These patients presented with dyspnea at rest which rapidly worsened. Examination showed the characteristic fine dry "cellophane" rales in a scattered distribution and arterial blood gases revealed anoxemia with normal Ph and low partial pressure of carbon dioxide. Large dose corticosteroids were given to all 5 patients with doubtful effect. Table XXIX shows the mean spirometry values of the 5 pneumonitis patients in contrast to 12 normal patients. The pneumonitis group shows a drop of one-third of the forced vital capacity over 4 months while the normals show a lesser drop of 20 per cent over a longer period (almost 8 months). Thus, a steep rate of fall of the forced vital capacity should signal the discontinuation of bleomycin until pneumonitis can be excluded.

PRESENT STATUS

Although the bleomycin combination drug programs are very aggressive and produce significant morbidity with a mortality of 4 of 90 (4.4 per cent), the results in terms of the rate of remission induction and the duration of survival are superior to other programs. The median survival for the entire group is approximately one year while 35 per cent survive 2 years. More important, over half of the complete responders are beyond 2 years free of gross metastatic disease and represent potential cures. It is also apparent that previously untreated patients presenting with minimal disease are the most favorable and every effort should be made to produce complete remission. The aim is to produce cure. Patients presenting with large bulky abdominal masses are prone to develop septicemia, especially if previously irradiated and usually will not achieve complete remission. In this group, drug dosage can be decreased since the realistic aim is to produce palliation.

TABLE XXIX

SPIROMETRY AND BLEOMYCIN PNEUMONITIS

		Forced Vital Capacity					
	No. Patients	Initial (Liters)	Nadir (Liters)	% Fall	Time Nadir (Months)	F. E. V.* at nadir (1)	% F. E. V.
Pneumonitis	5	3.92	2.62	34.2	4.4	1.96	78
No Pneumonitis	12	4.88	3.77	22.8	7.2	2.31	81

* Forced expiratory volume at one second

All determinations are mean values.

CHAPTER 10

TESTICULAR TUMORS IN CHILDREN

by

Douglas E. Johnson

INCIDENCE

Testicular tumors can occur at any age, but they are rare under the age of 15 years. They rank seventh among malignancies seen in the pediatric age group, being exceeded in scarcity only by tumors of the intestine, tongue and ovary (Rusche 1952). In reviewing 244 necropsy cases of childhood malignancies at the University of Michigan, Hendrix (1956) could not find a single case of testicular malignant disease. Silvert (1957) states genital tumors account for less than one per cent of all childhood malignancy.

The incidence of testis tumors occurring prior to the age of 15 years is 0.5 to 2.0 per 100,000 males, with over one-half of these occurring before the age of five (Podis 1966). In most series of testicular tumors, the frequency of occurrence in children under the age of 15 years has ranged from 1.5 to 3.0 per cent (Pack and Le Fevere 1930; Scully and Parham 1948; Collins and Pugh 1964). Only Agarwal et al. (1967) and Bhargava and Reddy (1966) from India and Tsuji et al. (1973) from Japan, have reported significantly higher incidences, but their series are small. At the University of Texas System Cancer Center, M. D. Anderson Hospital and Tumor Institute, Houston, Texas from 1944-70, 13 cases of testicular tumors have been documented in children under the age of 15 years, within a group of 501 testis tumors, an incidence of 2.6 per cent.

AGE

The vast majority of testicular tumors occurring in children are diagnosed prior to the third year of life (Gross 1953; Doyle 1955; Collins and Pugh 1964; Li and Fraumeni 1972). In a collective review of 137 cases developing in children, Julien (1925) reported 20 tumors present from birth and 27 which appeared during the first year of life. Rusche (1952) reported 4 of 12 cases which appeared at birth with 75 per cent of the lesions present prior to age three. In a review of 73 cases of children with embryonal carcinoma of the testicle collected from the literature, Ravich et al. (1966) found 48 incidences in which the age of occurrence was noted. In only 11 of these 48 cases had the tumor occurred later than three years of age. At Anderson Hospital, 8 of 12 cases in which the age is known have occurred prior to age three (75 per cent).

CLINICAL FINDINGS

There are no pathognomonic symptoms of a testicular tumor in children. The usual clinical feature is a painless enlargement of the affected testis, which has been present for a varying period of time. The history of a bruise to the scrotum a few days prior to the examination is not uncommon (Anderson and Huston 1958). Occasionally, the tumor may arise in an undescended testis and present as an abdominal mass (Hansen 1967).

On physical examination a firm, symmetrically enlarged testis which fails to transilluminate is most frequently encountered. In cases with teratomatous elements, the lesion may be irregular and transillumination of cystic areas can mask the diagnosis. A delay in treatment occurs frequently due to a mistaken diagnosis of hydrocele. An associated hydrocele is present in 15 to 25 per cent of the cases occurring during childhood (Boehme et al. 1951; Abell and Holtz 1963) and may conceal the underlying lesion. In addition to hydrocele (Wakeley 1938; Paul 1952; Beard and Cooner 1966; Fraley and Ketcham 1968), testicular tumors in children have been mistaken for hematocele (Allen and Skaist 1961), inguinal hernia (Bormel and Mays 1961) and torsion (Batsakis 1961).

It cannot be overemphasized, irrespective of the patient's age, that a differential diagnosis of every testicular enlargement should include tumor until proven otherwise. Diagnosis will frequently necessitate exploration which should always be performed through an inguinal incision with cross clamping of the spermatic cord prior to delivery of the testis for examination. In the rare instance where visual and palpatory examinations fail to substantiate a diagnosis, biopsy with frozen histological evaluation may be indicated. It is usually preferable, however, in doubtful cases to proceed with orchiectomy and high ligation of the spermatic cord. Percutaneous needling of a scrotal mass in infants and children is to be condemned since tumor, hernia, torsion or hydrocele all require surgical intervention.

HISTOLOGIC TYPE

Similar morphological features have been described for testicular tumors developing during infancy and childhood, as have been noted for their counterparts in adults. Primary germinal tumors contribute to the majority of the cases, but non-germinal tumors are reported with higher frequency rates than in adults. Embryonal carcinoma, adult teratoma and teratocarcinoma comprise the germinal group. Seminomas as well as choriocarcinomas have not been documented in infancy or prepubertal adolescents (Melicow 1955; Phelan et al. 1957; Perskey 1969).

A lack of uniformity in nomenclature has arisen due to the rarity of germinal tumors occurring in children. Embryonal carcinoma is the most frequently occurring germinal tumor in childhood. Many authors (Magner and Bryant 1951; Darbari and Saxena 1960; Dutta and Mahanta 1968; Teoh et al. 1960; Deshmukh et al. 1967), however, have preferred to distinguish in infants an adenocarcinoma with clear cells (orchioblastoma) as a separate and distinct entity from other cases of embryonal carcinoma. Some authors continue to use the term "yolk sac" carcinoma (Ross and Morrow 1972) or "endodermal sinus tumor" (Klugo et al. 1972). Other investigators (Abell and Holtz 1963; Weitzner 1964; Ravich et al. 1966) believe such a distinction is arbitrary and prefer to group all such tumors as embryonal carcinomas with varying degrees of anaplasia.

The histologic adult teratoma is second in frequency of occurrence. Teratomas in adults are considered potentially malignant since metastases have developed in tumors thought to be histologically benign (Gray et al. 1950; Dixon and Moore 1952), but available data suggests that these lesions are invariably benign in the pediatric age group (Thompson 1955; Beard and Cooner 1966; Fraley and Ketcham 1968). Teratocarcinomas are the least common reported germinal tumor in infants, but in the Anderson Series comprised 25 per cent of the testicular tumors seen within the pediatric age group.

Non-germinal tumors occurring in children include: 1) Leydig (interstitial) cell; 2) Sertoli cell (Androblastoma); 3) Gonadoblastoma; 4) carcinoma of the rete testis; and 5) embryonal rhabdomyosarcoma. A more detailed discussion of these tumors is given in Chapter 1 and Chapter 11.

TREATMENT AND PROGNOSIS

The initial treatment for testicular malignancy, regardless of the patient's age, is radical orchiectomy with high ligation of the spermatic cord at the internal inguinal ring. Thereafter, careful and complete evaluation of the patient is necessary before planning further therapy. In addition to the routine clinical evaluation, a chest X-ray with both posteroanterior and lateral views, an excretory urogram and a lymphangiogram should be performed in order to adequately stage the disease. Infancy in itself does not preclude lymphangiography and studies have been performed safely in patients under five months of age.

Until recently neither radiotherapy nor retroperitoneal lymphadenectomy had been employed in a sufficient number of children with malignant testicular disease to warrant their conclusions as aids in improving survival. In the absence of disseminated disease physicians have often been reluctant to use either modality of treatment for purely prophylactic measures. The possibilities of delayed growth, bone marrow arrest, radiation nephritis and enterocolitis, as well as the sterilization of the other testis, frequently has limited the use of radiotherapy to those cases in which known disease existed. The fear of increased morbidity and mortality rates following retroperitoneal lymph node dissections in infants and children caused many investigators to decry the procedure as unnecessary. The fact remains, however, that embryonal carcinoma in children is characterized by a high degree of malignancy and a poor prognosis. Abell and Holtz (1963) reported that 7 of 12 children (58 per cent) with embryonal carcinoma of the testis died of metastatic disease within one-year of diagnosis. Phelan and associates (1957) at the Mayo Clinic treated four children with orchiectomy and all died within 13 months. Other series (Ravich 1966; Gangai 1968) suggest that a 50 per cent one year survival rate can be expected following orchiectomy for embryonal carcinoma in children. Too few patients with teratocarcinoma have been reported to conclude meaningful survival rates. Teratoma is the only germinal tumor in children with a favorable prognosis. Only one well documented case has been reported in which distant metastases have developed (Gordon-Taylor 1957).

In order to improve survival rates in children with malignant germinal tumors, either radiation therapy or lymphadenectomy is currently being recommended. Matsumoto et al. (1970) have treated 19 children with embryonal carcinoma ranging in age from 4 to 26 months with combination therapy consisting of simple orchiectomy and irradiation of the entire retroperitoneal lymph node chain. A daily dose of 100 rads given over a four to seven week period for a total dosage of 2000 to 3000 rads was administered with a linear accelerator. All patients were reported alive after more than 12 months without clinical evidence of recurrent disease or complications from the irradiation. Nine children were treated with only orchiectomy and four died within 15 months.

Other investigators (Staubitz et al. 1965; Gangai 1968; Johnson et al. 1970; McCullough et al. 1971; Boatman et al. 1973) have been equally encouraged by the results of retroperitoneal lymphadenectomy. The operation is no more difficult in the infant or young child than in the adult. Gangai (1968) collected 11 cases of embryonal carcinoma under the age of two from the literature and added a personal case which had been treated by retroperitoneal lymph node dissections. All patients survived from three months to 23 years with no reported complications developing from the surgical procedure.

Anderson Series

The experience at M. D. Anderson Hospital with 12 children with testicular tumors is given in Table XXX. The initial treatment for the six children with embryonal carcinoma was radical orchiectomy performed by their referring physician. Disseminated disease was present in two patients at the time of their referral, 13 and 16 months respectively after orchiectomy. In each instance chemotherapy was instituted without success, the patients succumbing to their disease within several months. The four remaining patients, seen within three weeks after their initial treatment, showed no evidence of metastatic disease. Three patients underwent bilateral retroperitoneal lymphadenectomy and are alive five months to three years later. One child underwent an ipsilateral retroperitoneal lymph node dissection followed by the administration of Cytoxan for ten days and was alive without disease six years later when he was lost to follow-up.

Three patients in this series had teratoma with an embryonal carcinoma component. These patients were evaluated at M. D. Anderson within three weeks following the diagnosis. Two were infants, ages 12 and 18 months respectively, and their evaluation revealed no evidence of metastatic disease. After receiving preoperative Cytoxan chemotherapy, they underwent ipsilateral retroperitoneal lymph node dissections followed by a short course of Cytoxan chemotherapy during the postoperative period. They are both alive without disease three years later. The third patient, age 14 years was found to have large retroperitoneal lymph nodes on lymphangiogram and he received 2000 rads irradiation therapy preoperatively. At the time of exploratory laparotomy, the lymph nodes were inoperable and he received an additional 2000 rads of irradiation to the retroperitoneal lymph nodes postoperatively. He has been maintained on Cytoxan chemotherapy, but a year later there is evidence of wide spread metastatic disease.

One child, age seven months, was evaluated after orchiectomy had been performed by his referring physician and a diagnosis of pure teratoma established. Although this lesion was thought to represent a benign disease, he underwent an ipsilateral retroperitoneal lymph node dissection and is alive without demonstrable disease seven years later.

Two additional children have been treated for testicular rhabdomyosarcoma. In the first child, age four years, the diagnosis was established by a needle biopsy performed by his local physician. On referral to Anderson Hospital he received Vincristine, Cytoxan and Actinomycin-D preoperatively and underwent a radical orchiectomy and an ipsilateral retroperitoneal lymph node dissection. A nephrectomy was also performed at that time due to severe retroperitoneal involvement by metastatic disease. He received chemotherapy postoperatively as well as 4000 rads irradiation therapy to the retroperitoneal and scrotal areas. At present, he is alive four years later without demonstrable residual disease. The second child, age four years, was seen shortly after an inguinal orchiectomy, performed by his referring physician, had substantiated the diagnosis of rhabdomyosarcoma. He was treated initially with Vincristine, and soon thereafter underwent an ipsilateral

TABLE XXX

SUMMARY OF CLINICAL FINDINGS

Age	Side with Tumor	Stage of Disease When seen at MDAH	Type of Tumor	Initial Treatment	Subsequent Treatment	Survival After Diagnosis	
						Alive	Dead
4 mos.	Rt.	I	Embryonal	Radical Orchiectomy	Bil. lymph node dissection	3 yrs. *	
16 mos.	Rt.	I	Embryonal	Radical Orchiectomy	Bil. lymph node dissection	2-1/2 yrs. +	
2 yrs.	Lt.	III	Embryonal	Radical Orchiectomy	Vincristine, cytoxan, hydroxurea		18 mos.
2 yrs.	Lt.	III	Embryonal	Radical Orchiectomy	Exploratory laparotomy, actinomycin-D, nitrogen mustard		16 mos.
2 yrs.	Rt.	I	Embryonal	Radical Orchiectomy	Ipsilateral node dissection, cytoxan X 10 days	6 yrs. +	
3 yrs.	Lt.	I	Embryonal	Radical Orchiectomy	Bil. lymph node dissection	5 mos.	
14 yrs.	Rt.	II	Terato-carcinoma	Radical Orchiectomy	Radiotherapy-4000 rads	1-1/2 yrs. *	
18 mos.	Rt.	I	Terato-carcinoma	Radical Orchiectomy	Ipsilateral node dissection	3 yrs.	
12 mos.	Rt.	I	Terato-carcinoma	Radical Orchiectomy	Ipsilateral node dissection	3 yrs.	
7 mos.	Lt.	I	Teratoma	Radical Orchiectomy	Ipsilateral node dissection	7 yrs.	
4 yrs.	Rt.	I	Rhabdomyo-sarcoma	Radical Orchiectomy	Vincristine, ipsilateral node dissection	4 yrs.	
4 yrs.	Lt.	III	Rhabdomyo-sarcoma	Needle Biopsy	1) Vincristine, cytoxan, actinomycin-D (preop. & postop.) 2) Radical orchiectomy with ipsilateral node dissection and nephrectomy 3) Radiotherapy-4000 rads to scrotal area 4) Cytoxan	4 yrs.	

*Alive with metastases
+Patient lost to follow-up

retroperitoneal lymph node dissection. He is alive four years later without evidence of residual disease.

The results from lymph node dissections in cases of embryonal carcinoma and teratocarcinoma have been encouraging. However, the failure to demonstrate metastatic disease in the removed lymph nodes in all the cases reviewed by Gangai (1968) and Young et al. (1970), as well as in our own, has caused some concern in recommending the routine employment of lymphadenectomy. It is possible that microscopic foci of neoplastic cells were present in the lymph nodes, but not identified at the time of histologic examination. In addition, lymphadenectomy allows for a more accurate staging of the disease and has prevented the unnecessary usage of radiotherapy with its inherent risks in this age group.

Considerable controversy surrounds the efficacy of unilateral as opposed to bilateral lymphadenectomy. The classic work of Jamieson and Dobson (1910), demonstrating cross communications of the lymphatic systems of the testes, has given support in the past to performing bilateral retroperitoneal lymph node dissections (See Chapter 6). However, Maier et al. (1969) at Walter Reed Army Hospital, in a review of 213 retroperitoneal node dissections performed for testicular tumors exclusive of seminoma were unable to demonstrate improved survival rates when comparing ipsilateral to bilateral node dissections. Although only two of the eight patients in the Anderson Hospital Series undergoing lymphadenectomy had bilateral lymph node dissections, we would presently recommend bilateral dissections when lymphadenectomy is indicated. We feel that lymphadenectomy can be performed without mortality and with minimal morbidity, but a larger number of cases so treated will be necessary before definite conclusions can be reached. In addition, a randomized series comparing lymphadenectomy to radiotherapy remains necessary before the superiority of either treatment modality can be established.

The prognosis for cases of testicular rhabdomyosarcoma has reportedly been hopeless (Kohler and Murphy 1959; Davis 1962; Arean and Kreager 1965). Our experience with two children has been most gratifying. Retroperitoneal lymphadenectomy combined with chemotherapy and/or irradiation appears to be of definite value in a planned therapeutic program for this malignancy.

CONCLUSIONS

Testicular tumors are infrequently encountered in infants and children and account for only two to three per cent of all testicular tumors. Their clinical presentation is similar to that seen in adults and the lesion is most frequently confused with hydrocele, hematocele, hernia and torsion. The evaluation of testicular malignant disease in children should parallel that which has been recommended for adults.

The treatment for teratoma in children is radical orchiectomy and careful periodic, postoperative follow-up examinations. For cases of embryonal carcinoma, teratocarcinoma and rhabdomyosarcoma, radical orchiectomy followed by bilateral transabdominal retroperitoneal lymphadenectomy is our procedure of choice. Radiation therapy is proving to be of equal benefit and may eventually eliminate the need for surgery.

CHAPTER 11

NON-GERMINAL TUMORS: INTERSTITIAL CELL TUMORS AND TUMORS OF SPECIALIZED GONADAL STROMAL ORIGIN

by

William D. Davis

INTERSTITIAL-CELL TUMOR

Sacchi in 1895 reported the first case of an interstitial (Leydig) cell tumor and in the ensuing 80 years over 170 cases have been reported (Gerwig) et al. 1964; Schoonees 1968; Hopkins 1970; Selvaggi et al. 1973). These tumors characteristically are composed of interstitial cells derived from primordial mesenchyme lying within the testicular interstitial tissue (Blundon et al. 1953). Tumor growth is a result of both the development of new Leydig cells from the indifferent cells of the interstitium and mitotic proliferation of neoplastic cells (Collins and Cameron 1964). These tumors, however, have been frequently confused with hyperplasia due to the absence of established criteria for differentiating them from interstitial-cell hyperplasia.

Hyperplasia versus Neoplasia

Interstitial cells are found in abundance during fetal life due to the influence of maternal hormones, but they rapidly disappear after birth. The cells remain inconspicuous during childhood but increase appreciably in number at puberty. Thereafter, the number of interstitial cells appears to correspond inversely with changes in spermatogenesis.

Interstitial-cell hyperplasia may be found in any condition in which spermatogenesis is decreased (Jemine 1937; Mayers 1952; Pomer et al. 1954) and has been reported in association with chronic disease such as tuberculosis, cirrhosis, pernicious anemia, syphilis or cancer, injury, cryptorchidism, radiation, environmental changes, drug administration, senility and following vasectomy. A diagnosis of hyperplasia is dependent upon finding an increase in interstitial cells between the tubules without destruction or displacement of the tubules beyond the limits of the growth (Warren and Olshausen 1943). A neoplasm, conversely, should be encapsulated or at least demarcated from the surrounding normal tissue with displacement of the testicular tissue and absence of seminiferous tubules throughout the lesion. Some investigators (Collins and Cameron 1964; Blandy et al. 1970) have suggested simplifying this distinction by designating all palpable tumor-like nodules in the testis which have been detected either by the patient or by the physician as neoplasms.

Incidence

Interstitial-cell tumors of the testis are uncommon although they are the most frequently encountered non-germinal testicular tumor. Dalgaard and Hesselberg (1957) collected 94 cases from the literature with many additional cases having been subsequently described. Dixon and Moore (1952) encountered 12 cases (1.2 per cent) among 1000 testicular neoplasms on file at the Armed Forces Institute of Pathology. In reviewing 104 cases of testicular tumors treated at the Atlanta Veterans Hospital, Ward et al. (1960) found two cases of interstitial-cell tumors, an incidence of less than two per cent. Among 995 tumors received by the British Testicular Tumor Panel and Registry, Collins and Pugh (1964) reported 14 cases of interstitial-cell tumors (1.4 per cent). In the Anderson Hospital Series of 652 testicular tumors, only three cases of interstitial-cell tumors have been reported.

Age Distribution

Analysis of the age incidence has revealed two distinct age maxima (5-10 and 30-35) and the one minimum (15-20) (Dalgaard and Hesselberg 1957). The youngest reported patient with an interstitial-cell tumor was two years and four months of age at the time of diagnosis (Newns 1952) and the oldest was 82 years (Nation et al. 1944). Excellent review articles detailing cases occurring in prepubertal children have been published (Bishop et al. 1960; Camin et al. 1960; Johnstone 1967).

Clinical Findings

Children: Interstitial-cell tumors in children produce a characteristic picture of sexual precocity which can be indistinguishable from virilizing adrenal hyperplasia (Allibone et al. 1969). The child typically undergoes rapid somatic growth, most marked in muscle development and enlargement of the penis. Pubic hair becomes well developed although axillary, facial and body hair may not be noticeable (Bishop et al. 1960). The voice becomes deeper and acne may appear. Gynecomastia is rarely present, but has been reported on five occasions (Huffman 1941; Tavares 1952; Jolly 1955; Jungck et al. 1957; Johnstone 1967). Psychosexual precocity has been noted in about one-half of the cases (Bishop et al. 1960) and occasionally abnormal behavior has preceded the physical changes (James and Shupe 1950; Jungck et al. 1957).

Radiological examinations demonstrate a marked increase in the bone age, but dental age is usually only slightly altered. Urinary 17-ketosteroid levels are elevated with the degree of elevation varying markedly among reported cases. Detailed hormonal studies have only occasionally been reported (Bishop et al. 1960; Martin et al. 1962; Richards and Neville 1973; Yuval et al. 1974).

Adults: In adults, endocrine manifestations are variable and may be completely absent. The most common presenting symptom reported by Collins and Cameron (1964) was gynecomastia, present in 6 of their 14 patients. A decrease in the libido or overt impotence is usually associated with the development of gynecomastia. Other findings of feminization (hyperpigmentation of the areolae, testicular and prostatic atrophy and loss of body hair) may be noted. Several investigators (Herrmann et al. 1958; Philip 1960), have found endocrine disturbances present in a minority of their cases. In patients who have no feminizing symptoms, testicular enlargement has been the prominent presenting complaint. The tumor is usually slow growing or stationary, circumscribed, firm and non-tender (Dalgaard and Hesselberg 1957). An occasional case with bilateral tumors has been reported (Kaufman 1907; Garvey and Daniel 1951; Flynn and Severance 1951; Staubitz et al. 1953; Rezek and Hardin 1955). Pain is a rare finding, although an interstitial-cell tumor presenting with an acute epididymo-orchitis has been described (Schoonees 1968). Leydig cell tumors have been associated in isolated instances with Klinefelter's syndrome (Arduino and Glucksman 1963) and insulin-resistant diabetes (Lopis et al. 1952). Occasionally, the tumor may be discovered during a routine physical examination, as was the finding in two of our cases.

Case 1 (83287): A 41 year-old Caucasian was noted to have a left testicular mass during the course of a routine physical examination. He admitted to its presence and gradual increase in size over the last three years. Twenty years previously, he had undergone surgical correction for bilateral cryptorchidism. A left inguinal orchiectomy was performed and he was referred to Anderson Hospital where a diagnosis of an interstitial-cell tumor was substantiated. Physical examination revealed no evidence of metastatic disease. Routine laboratory studies, as well as chest roentgenograms and an excretory urogram were within normal limits. A lymphangiogram could not be obtained because of his moderately severe emphysema. In the absence of metastatic disease, additional therapy was not believed warranted. He has been followed for five years without evidence of metastatic disease.

Case 2 (57327): A 22 year-old Caucasian was found to have a right testicular enlargement at the time of an employment physical examination. The lesion had been present for eight years with slow progression in size. On referral to Anderson Hospital, physical examination revealed a hard, non-tender right testis. The left testis was atrophic. Routine laboratory studies as well as chest roentgenograms and an excretory urogram were within normal limits. An inguinal orchiectomy was performed and examination of the excised tissue revealed an interstitial-cell tumor. He has been followed for ten years without evidence of metastatic disease.

Treatment and Prognosis

Initial treatment for an interstitial-cell tumor is identical to that for other testicular neoplasms - inguinal orchiectomy with high ligation of the spermatic cord at the internal inguinal ring. Partial or complete regression of secondary sexual characteristics as well as improvement in behavioral problems is to be expected in children following surgical removal of the lesion. In adults, regression and disappearance of gynecomastia frequently occurs and potency invariably returns. Body hair, however, may remain sparse.

Definite histologic criteria are lacking for determining malignancy, except for the presence of metastases. Approximately 15 cases of malignant interstitial-cell tumors are documented in the literature (Short and Coe 1963; Silverberg et al. 1966; Livesay et al. 1972; Mahon et al. 1973), and in no instance has metastatic disease developed in a child. Malignant tumors tend to occur in the older age group (average age - 51.6 years), without endocrine complaints and have usually shown presumptive pathologic evidence of malignancy (local invasion) or definite evidence (metastases) at the time of diagnosis (Silverberg et al. 1966). Survival has ranged from 45 days to 17 years, with only two patients living longer than five years (Masson 1943; Parker 1958). The regional lymph nodes, lungs, liver and bone are the most common sites of metastases (Mahon et al. 1973).

In view of the few documented cases with malignant disease, additional therapy following inguinal orchiectomy is unwarranted. Thorough evaluation at periodic intervals should be performed and appropriate therapy instituted at the time metastatic disease is demonstrated.

TUMORS OF SPECIALIZED GONADAL STROMA

A small number of testicular tumors believed to arise from primitive gonadal mesenchyme and capable of reproducing all the features of the supporting tissues of the gonads of both sexes have been reported. The lack of agreement with regards to their histogenesis and the paucity of cases have contributed to a marked confusion in the nomenclature of these lesions. Reports have appeared in the literature under a variety of names including Sertoli-cell tumor (Jones and Friedman 1950; Collins and Symington 1964), gonadoblastoma (Scully 1970), gonocytoma (Teter 1960), androblastoma (Teilum 1958), granulosa-cell tumor (Laskowski 1942), adrenocortical tumor (Ostergaard 1947) and tumors of specialized gonadal stroma (Mostofi et al. 1959). Although some investigators argue that the term "specialized gonadal stromal tumor" is imprecise (Collins and Symington 1964; Blandy et al. 1970), it appears preferable until a more complete understanding of their histogenesis has been substantiated. The danger lies not with differences in nomenclature, but with attaching too much importance to specific terminology. The morphological features of these tumors are described in Chapter 1.

Incidence

Tumors of specialized gonadal stroma comprise approximately 0.4 per cent of testicular neoplasms (Dixon and Moore 1953; Hope-Stone et al. 1963). Collins and Symington (1964) found 6 of 995 testicular tumors fulfilling their rigid criteria for Sertoli-cell origin (0.6 per cent). The majority of the tumors have been diagnosed in adults, but reports in the literature have described their occurrence in the newborn (Culp et al. 1956) to as late as the eighty-third year (Mostofi et al. 1959). In children, they account for as much as 9.5 per cent of all testicular tumors (Houser et al. 1965).

Clinical Features

The presenting symptom in the majority of the patients has been a slowly enlarging testicular mass, occasionally associated with pain. Gynecomastia has been documented in 10 of 38 patients (Mostofi et al. 1959) and has generally occurred as a late symptom after a period of increased tumor growth (Hopkins and Parry 1969). Sexual precocity has been reported on one occasion in a seven month-old infant (Gonder and Fadell 1960).

Hormonal investigations have resulted in conflicting data. Urinary excretion of androgens (Fuglsang and Ohlsen 1957; Gonder and Fadell 1960), estrogens (Ostergaard 1947; Gonder and Fadell 1960), pregnanediol (Fuglsang and Ohlsen 1957) and gonadotropins (Collins and Symington 1964) have been elevated in some cases, but normal levels of androgens and estrogens have also been reported (Lewis and Stockard 1950; Perch and Kirshman 1967).

Treatment and Prognosis

The preferred treatment is an inguinal orchiectomy with high ligation of the spermatic cord at the internal inguinal ring. Thereafter, laboratory and radiologic investigation should be undertaken as described in Chapter 5 for germinal tumors. Although histologic criteria for malignancy in these tumors has not been defined, prominent mitotic activity within the lesion is suggestive of a malignant potential (Hopkins and Parry 1969).

In the absence of metastatic disease, careful and prolonged observation is suggested. Gynecomastia has regressed following orchiectomy in the majority of the cases. If metastatic disease is demonstrated or subsequently develops, the patient should be managed along the outlines suggested for radio-resistant germinal tumors. To date, eleven cases with distant metastases have been reported (Talerman 1971; Koppikar and Sirsat 1973). Four patients died five months after orchiectomy (Mostofi et al. 1959; Pugh 1962; Collins and Symington 1964; Talerman 1971), one died four years following orchiectomy and prophylactic irradiation (Hopkins and Parry 1969), four are alive with clinical evidence of metastases (Pugh 1962; Koppikar and Sirsat 1973), one patient is alive and well 8 months after orchiectomy and retroperitoneal radiation (Talerman 1971) and one patient is alive free of disease two years after orchiectomy and retroperitoneal lymphadenectomy (Rosvoll and Woodard 1968).

CHAPTER 12

MALIGNANT LYMPHOMA OF THE TESTIS

by

Douglas E. Johnson and James J. Butler

Malignant lymphoma masquerading as a primary testicular tumor is rare. Malassez was the first to describe the condition in 1877, but in the ensuing 87 years less than 120 cases were recorded in the literature of Great Britain and America (Varney 1955; Gowing 1964). Sporadic cases have continued to be reported (Luedtke 1964; Westcott 1966; Ram and Burn 1969; Osman and Morrow 1969; Shivde and Junnarkar 1970; Kiely et al. 1970; Tanenbaum et al. 1972; Hamlin et al. 1972; Naranjo et al. 1974; Macnicol et al. 1974), but the cumulative number remains relatively small. In most series the incidence of malignant lymphomas of the testis has ranged from one to seven per cent of all malignant testicular tumors (Dockerty and Priestley 1942; Cohen et al. 1955; Eckert and Smith 1963; Gowing 1964). Diffuse histiocytic lymphoma presenting as a testicular tumor has been documented in 19 patients in a series of over 700 malignant testicular tumors evaluated at M. D. Anderson Hospital and Tumor Institute, Houston, from March 1944 to December 1974.

NOMENCLATURE

The term "malignant lymphoma" has been used by most authors to include all types of malignant lymphoreticular disease. Gowing (1964), in reviewing the pathological material from 63 patients with this disease, felt that the expression "malignant lymphoma," "poorly differentiated" best designated almost all the testicular neoplasms belonging to this group. In our previous material all the tumors had been designated as histiocytic reticulum cell sarcomas (Rappaport 1966; Butler 1970) but currently we prefer the term "diffuse histiocytic lymphoma."

ANDERSON HOSPITAL SERIES MARCH 1944 - DECEMBER 1974

The experience at the University of Texas Cancer System Center, M. D. Anderson Hospital and Tumor Institute at Houston with 19 patients with malignant lymphoma initially presenting as a testicular tumor is reviewed in the following case reports. In all cases the testicular lesion was the initial manifestation of the disease. Other cases in which secondary testicular tumor deposits were found during the course of the disease or at necropsy have been excluded from this series.

Case 1 (17250): This 54 year-old Caucasian man underwent a right orchiectomy on 7 September 1955 following a seven-month history of testicular enlargement. The initial pathologic diagnosis was seminocarcinoma and he was seen at M. D. Anderson Hospital on 30 September 1955. Physical examination, as well as a chest X-ray and an excretory urogram, were within normal limits. He underwent an exploratory laparotomy on 27 October 1955, for the purpose of having a bilateral retroperitoneal lymph node dissection performed. However, multiple enlarged lymph nodes were present in the periaortic region and an incomplete dissection was done. The histologic diagnosis revealed diffuse histiocytic lymphoma. A review of the testicular lesion demonstrated a similar pathologic process. He was treated with 3,000 rads total tumor dose to the right groin and periaortic regions over a six-week period. However, his course was one of progressive deterioration, and he died on 18 March 1956.

Case 2 (49164): The first symptom noted by this 64 year-old Caucasian man was hematuria. At the time of transurethral resection for grade II transitional cell carcinoma performed 10 July 1963, an enlarged right testicle was discovered and removed. The initial histologic diagnosis was granulomatous orchitis, although the pathologist suspected a lymphoma. He was seen three weeks later at Anderson Hospital and careful evaluation failed to reveal any evidence of metastatic disease. He returned to Anderson Hospital thirteen months later for evaluation of a five centimeter mass involving the bulk of the hard palate on the left (Fig. 12-1). Sinus X-rays revealed a tumor mass in the left maxillary antrum which had destroyed a portion of the floor and medial wall. This mass was biopsied and diagnosed as diffuse histiocytic lymphoma. A review of the original testicular lesion confirmed the presence of diffuse histiocytic lymphoma in that organ. He was treated initially with Cytoxan 100 mg per kg I. V. daily, and within seven days demonstrated a dramatic response. He was then maintained on oral Cytoxan 100 mg daily until November 1965. At that time, repeat sinus X-rays were interpreted as within normal limits with no evidence of malignancy. He was followed carefully and again placed on oral Cytoxan 100 mg daily in March 1966. However, because of progressive enlargement of the left testicle, he underwent an orchiectomy in September 1969 which revealed diffuse histiocytic lymphoma. All medications were withdrawn because of the recurrence of disease while receiving chemotherapy. He expired in March 1972 with recurrent disease.

Case 3 (51441): This 63 year-old Caucasian man underwent a left orchiectomy on 28 January 1964 after a two-day history of testicular swelling. He was seen at Anderson Hospital on 10 February 1964 and a review of the pathologic tissue was interpreted as granulomatous orchitis, although suspicion was raised concerning the possibility of lymphoma. Physical examination revealed no evidence of metastatic disease. While chest X-rays were normal, an excretory urogram suggested retroperitoneal adenopathy on the left. A bilateral pedal lymphangiogram was equivocal and suggested either an inflammatory reaction or lymphoma. Therefore, the patient underwent a right inguinal lymph node biopsy. The biopsy demonstrated reactive hyperplasia and no further therapy was instituted. However, within six weeks, skin lesions appeared and a biopsy demonstrated evidence of diffuse histiocytic lymphoma. The pathologic sections of the testicular lesion were reviewed and believed to represent the same tumor present in the skin. He was started on Cytoxan chemotherapy in April 1964, and continued on that drug until 26 May 1964. However, his condition was one of progressive deterioration and in June 1964 was started on Velban. He continued to deteriorate and died 15 July 1964.

Case 4 (51832): This 73 year-old Latin American man underwent a right orchiectomy for unknown reasons in December 1963 and a diagnosis of lymphoma was established. Approximately two months later, he developed subcutaneous lesions over the back and a biopsy again demonstrated poorly differentiated lymphoma. He was seen initially at Anderson Hospital on 11 March 1964 with a five-week history of progressive swelling and pain in the left eye. Physical examination revealed a hard nodule present in the left nostril, generalized lymphadenopathy, multiple subcutaneous nodules over the back and an enlarged, hard, firm left testis. Chest X-ray was interpreted as normal. Sinus X-rays revealed a destructive and infiltrative lesion involving the left maxillary, ethmoid and frontal sinuses with destruction of the superior medial left orbital margin. A review of the sections from both the testis and skin revealed diffuse histiocytic lymphoma. He was begun on chemotherapy with cyclophosphamide and received 2,000 rads tumor dose radiotherapy to the left orbit. There was initial marked improvement for several months, but he was re-admitted to the hospital in June 1964 with nausea, vomiting and weight loss. Chemotherapy with Velban was instituted but his course was one of progressive deterioration, and he died on 11 July 1964.

Case 5 (52116): This 72 year-old Caucasian man underwent a bilateral inguinal orchiectomy on 13 March 1964 after a two-month history of testicular enlargement. A diagnosis of diffuse histiocytic lymphoma was established and he was referred to M. D. Anderson Hospital. Physical examination was within normal limits and X-ray studies, including an excretory urogram and chest X-ray revealed no evidence of disease. He returned to Anderson Hospital in June 1964, at which time a large epigastric mass, as well as an enlarged right supraclavicular lymph node, were demonstrated. A biopsy of the supraclavicular lymph node again demonstrated diffuse histiocytic lymphoma. No therapy was instituted as his condition rapidly deteriorated and he expired on 22 June 1964.

Case 6 (52594): This 67 year-old Caucasian man underwent a right orchiectomy on 28 April 1964 following a one-month history of progressive pain and enlargement of that organ. Physical examination was within normal limits except for an enlarged left testis and a chest X-ray revealed old tuberculous lesions present in both lungs but no evidence of lymphomatous disease was demonstrated. A lymphangiogram was within normal limits. On review, the material from the right testis was interpreted as showing diffuse histiocytic lymphoma. He was treated with 3,000 rads total tumor dose to the periaortic and the right inguinal areas over a three-week period. In August 1964, at the time of surgery for a hiatal hernia, careful abdominal exploration revealed no evidence of metastatic disease. In November 1965, multiple subcutaneous nodules developed over the abdominal wall and he was started on oral cyclophosphamide, 150 mg daily. However, the disease progressed and the patient died on 20 November 1966.

Case 7 (57707): This 52 year-old Caucasian man noted progressive enlargement of the right testis for three months prior to its removal in July 1965. A pathologic diagnosis of seminoma was made and he was seen at Anderson Hospital on 28 July 1965. Physical examination at that time was within normal limits and an excretory urogram and chest X-ray were also normal. The testicular tumor was reviewed and interpreted as seminoma. A bilateral pedal lymphangiogram revealed right periaortic lymph node disease and he was, therefore, treated with 4,000 rads tumor dose to the periaortic lymph nodes and 2,500 rads to the right inguinal area. He returned one month later for prophylactic radiotherapy to the supraclavicular and mediastinal areas but at that time a right posterior cervical mass was noted. A biopsy was performed, demonstrating diffuse histiocytic lymphoma. Following the biopsy, the testicular tumor was again reviewed; the diagnosis was diffuse histiocytic lymphoma. He subsequently received 2,500 rads tumor dose to the right supraclavicular mass. The enlarged lymph nodes disappeared following therapy but in January 1966 he returned with nausea, vomiting, weight loss and axillary lymphadenopathy. In addition, an upper GI series demonstrated a lymphomatous lesion in the distal ileum as well as anterior displacement of the stomach. Gastroscopy revealed obstruction of the stomach at the pylorus with a submucosal tumor nodule present at the junction of the lesser curvature and posterior wall of the body of the stomach at the level of the fundus. He underwent a gastrojejunostomy and was then treated with two five-day courses of cyclophosphamide I. V., Vincristine, and Prednisone. This produced a marked regression in the size of the lymphadenopathy and abdominal mass, but within four weeks there was progressive deterioration and he died on 22 April 1966.

Case 8 (64538): This 62 year-old Caucasian man noted progressive enlargement of both testes for four weeks at which time he consulted his physician and underwent a left orchiectomy on 16 December 1966. A diagnosis of reticulum cell sarcoma was established and he was referred to Anderson Hospital for radiotherapy. The testicular tumor was interpreted as diffuse histiocytic lymphoma at this hospital. Physical examination, as well as a chest X-ray were within normal limits. However, an excretory urogram as well as a bilateral pedal lymphangiogram revealed evidence of retroperitoneal disease. He received 3,000 rads tumor dose to the abdomen with an additional 1,500 rads delivered to the right testis and 1,000 rads to the area of nodal involvement. He has subsequently been lost to follow-up.

Case 9 (66544): This 72 year-old Caucasian man was found to have an enlarged right testis at the time of a routine physical examination performed in April 1966. He underwent a right orchiectomy and a seminoma was diagnosed. He was treated with 3,000 rads to the right inguinal and periaortic lymph node areas. Twelve months later, a biopsy of an enlarged right cervical lymph node revealed the diagnosis of diffuse histiocytic lymphoma. He was seen at Anderson Hospital on 29 May 1967 and a review of the pathologic material demonstrated diffuse histiocytic lymphoma both in the lymph node and in the testis. He received radiotherapy with 3,000 rads delivered to both sides of the neck and an additional boost of 1,000 rads to the anterior aspect of the right neck. Eleven months later, in May 1968, he was found to have a right axillary mass and a chest X-ray revealed nodular metastases in the lung parenchyma as well as bilateral hilar lymphadenopathy. A biopsy of the right axillary mass revealed histiocytic reticulum cell sarcoma and he was started on chemotherapy with cyclophosphamide. Within two weeks there was marked regression in the palpable tumor mass in the right axillary area, as well as regression of the pulmonary nodules. A chest X-ray obtained eight weeks later was interpreted as within normal limits with no evidence of metastatic disease. Although there had been immediate regression in the size of the right axillary and intraclavicular masses, their failure to completely disappear necessitated institution of radiotherapy in August 1968. He received 3,000 rads tumor dose to those areas. At the completion of radiotherapy no palpable masses could be demonstrated. However, his general condition continued to deteriorate, and he died 12 September 1968.

Case 10 (67098): This 69 year-old Latin American man underwent an orchiectomy in June 1967 following a 12-month history of progressive enlargement and pain in the left testis. The initial pathologic diagnosis was seminoma, and he was referred to Anderson Hospital. A review of the tissue obtained at the time of orchiectomy demonstrated diffuse histiocytic lymphoma. The physical exam was within normal limits, but a chest X-ray revealed a mediastinal mass. However, he did not complete his evaluation and was subsequently lost to follow-up.

Case 11 (69206): This 57 year-old Caucasian man had an orchiectomy in November 1967 after a three-month history of swelling of the right testis. A diagnosis of diffuse histiocytic lymphoma was established and he was referred to Anderson Hospital on 27 November 1967 where the diagnosis of diffuse histiocytic lymphoma was confirmed. Physical examination, as well as an excretory urogram and bone marrow aspiration, were interpreted as within normal limits. A chest X-ray revealed a mediastinal mass and a bilateral pedal lymphangiogram demonstrated extensive involvement of the pelvic and periaortic lymph nodes. He was given a single injection of cyclophosphamide and Vincristine intravenously and two weeks later treatment with radiotherapy was started. He received 3,000 rads total tumor dose to the pelvis and six weeks later radiotherapy to the retroperitoneal lymph nodes was started. However, therapy was discontinued after he had received less than 2,000 rads tumor dose due to a decrease in his platelet count. His condition continued to deteriorate and he is presumed to have died in the spring of 1968.

Case 12 (75156): This 74 year-old Caucasian man consulted his physician for a recurrent right inguinal hernia of three months duration. He was found to have a large scrotal mass and in March 1969 underwent a right orchiectomy. A diagnosis of diffuse histiocytic lymphoma was established and he was referred to Anderson Hospital. At the time of his initial investigation on 21 March 1969, the only positive finding on physical examination was an enlarged left testis. He underwent a left orchiectomy on 3 April 1969 for diffuse histiocytic lymphoma of the left testis. He subsequently received 3,000 rads tumor dose to the anterior pelvis over a three-week period. He did well with no other evidence of generalized disease until November 1969, at which time a subcutaneous lesion was noted on the inner aspect of the left arm. The lesion was excised and the diagnosis of diffuse histiocytic lymphoma in the skin and dermis was established. He subsequently received periodic courses of chemotherapy consisting of cyclophosphamide, Vincristine, and Prednisone, but his condition deteriorated and he expired on 10 May 1970.

Case 13 (77840): This 38 year-old Negro male underwent an orchiectomy in August 1969 after a four-month history of progressive enlargement of the left testis. The initial pathologic diagnosis was embryonal cell carcinoma and he was referred to Anderson Hospital. He was seen initially on 13 October 1969 and the physical examination, as well as an excretory urogram, chest X-ray, liver scan, bilateral pedal lymphangiogram, and bone marrow aspiration were within normal limits. The material from the left testis was reviewed and interpreted as diffuse histiocytic lymphoma. He was treated with prophylactic irradiation and received 4,000 rads total tumor dose to the periaortic lymph nodes and left scrotum. One week after completion of radiotherapy, a left supraclavicular lymph node was palpated but histologic examination after its removal revealed only reactive hyperplasia with no evidence of tumor. He was last seen in January 1975 at which time chest and abdominal X-rays were considered normal.

Case 14 (88579): This 77 year-old Caucasian male underwent a left orchiectomy in November 1971 after an eight-month history of progressive enlargement. Initial pathologic diagnosis was diffuse histiocytic lymphoma and he was referred to Anderson Hospital. He was seen initially on 29 November 1971 and physical examination, as well as chest X-ray, metastatic bone survey, films of the nasopharynx, bilateral pedal lymphangiogram and an excretory urogram failed to reveal evidence of metastatic disease. Bone marrow aspiration was normal. He was treated with prophylactic irradiation and received 3,500 rads tumor dose to the para-aortic and left iliac nodes, as well as to the left scrotum. He did well until February 1973 when he developed cutaneous lesions over his left wrist which were biopsied and proven to be diffuse histiocytic lymphoma. At that time he was placed on combination chemotherapy and received intravenous Cytoxan, Vincristine and Prednisone. In June 1973 he was given additional immunotherapy with BCG. The patient remained in partial remission on therapy, but in October 1973 due to persistence of the lesions involving the left wrist, it was elected to treat that area with radiation therapy for which he subsequently received 4,500 rads given dose with electron beam and 3,000 rads tumor dose with the use of the 7 MEV machine to the left wrist. In December 1973, because of continued cutaneous infiltrations of the left forearm, he received an additional 3,000 rads tumor dose to the left arm. He also received radiation therapy to cutaneous lesions involving the right posterior leg. He continued to develop cutaneous metastases in spite of chemotherapy and his course was one of progressive deterioration and he expired on 24 May 1974.

Case 15 (88978): This 70 year-old Latin American male underwent a right orchiectomy on 16 November 1971 with a four-week history of painless enlargement of the testicle. Initial histiological diagnosis was diffuse histiocytic lymphoma and he was referred to Anderson Hospital. Initial evaluation here on 7 December 1971 including physical examination, as well as chest X-ray, complete skeletal survey, excretory urograms, bilateral pedal lymphangiograms and films of the nasopharynx failed to reveal evidence of metastatic disease. Bone marrow aspiration was likewise normal. The patient subsequently received prophylactic irradiation of 3,500 rads tumor dose to the peri-aortic nodes and right iliac chain. He remained in remission without further evidence of metastatic disease. He expired at home, however, on 21 September 1972 and necropsy was not obtained.

Case 16 (97605): This 64 year-old Caucasian male underwent a right orchiectomy for scrotal swelling of two weeks' duration. Initial histologic examination revealed diffuse histiocytic lymphoma and he was referred to Anderson Hospital. He was initially seen on 4 June 1973 and physical examination revealed a large lower abdominal tumor mass in excess of 10 centimeters in diameter with a protuberant abdomen and increased collateral circulation extending up over the chest. An X-ray was negative, as well as a complete skeletal survey. An excretory urogram revealed non-functioning of the right kidney and an inferior venacavogram revealed complete obstruction of the inferior vena cava at its bifurcation. A barium enema further delineated a large mass in the mid-abdomen causing lateral displacement of the small bowel and colon. An upper gastrointestinal series revealed a narrow area in the antral region of the stomach and the possibility of an ulcerated mass at this level was considered. A liver scan was interpreted as normal. A lymphangiogram was not obtained because of the patient's chronic pulmonary problems. He was placed on Cytoxan, Vincristine and Prednisone, with an initial temporary response and has subsequently been lost to follow-up.

Case 17 (99834): This 67 year-old Caucasian male underwent a left orchiectomy in September 1973 for a four-month history of gradual testicular enlargement. Histologic examination revealed diffuse histiocytic lymphoma and he was referred to Anderson Hospital. He was seen initially on 5 October 1973 and physical examination, as well as chest X-ray, complete skeletal survey and an excretory urogram were normal. A bilateral pedal lymphangiogram revealed metastatic disease present in the left iliac and peri-aortic chains. Bone marrow aspiration was negative. He was begun on a combination of Cytoxan, Vincristine and Prednisone with progressive decrease in the size of the involved retroperitoneal lymph nodes. The patient subsequently received 3,000 rads tumor dose to the abdomen. He did well until August 1974, when he developed metastatic disease to the liver and left rib cage. He rapidly deteriorated and expired on 15 September 1974.

Case 18 (105088): This 66 year-old Caucasian male consulted his local physician because of lower abdominal discomfort in July 1974 and during evaluation was noted to have a left testicular mass. He was referred to Anderson Hospital where the initial examination on 26 July 1974 revealed generalized adenopathy present in the left supraclavicular region, bilateral axillary areas and left inguinal region. Examination of the genitalia revealed a markedly enlarged right testicle, which was hard. After preliminary studies including chest X-ray and an excretory urogram were obtained and found to be normal,he was admitted to the hospital and underwent a right inguinal orchiectomy on 29 July 1974. Histologic examination revealed diffuse histiocytic lymphoma of the testis. A bilateral pedal lymphangiogram revealed large bilateral pelvic and right peri-aortic nodes consistent with the diagnosis of metastatic histiocytic lymphoma. A bone marrow aspiration was normal, as well as a liver scan. Excision of the lymph node from the left supraclavicular region likewise showed diffuse histiocytic lymphoma. He was begun on Adriamycin, Vincristine and Prednisone with progressive decrease in the size of the pelvic and peri-aortic nodes. He is currently being maintained on that treatment program without evidence of further metastatic disease.

Case 19 (104179): This 70 year-old Negro male underwent a right orchiectomy in May 1974 after a 3-month history of gradual enlargement of the right testicle. Histologic examination of the removed specimen demonstrated diffuse histiocytic lymphoma and he was referred to this institution. At the time of his initial visit on 10 June 1974 physical examination, chest X-ray, complete skeletal survey, excretory urogram and a bilateral pedal lymphangiogram failed to reveal evidence of metastatic disease. During the course of his evaluation, he developed bilateral cervical lymphadenopathy and re-examination of the lower pharynx revealed tonsillar areas that contained large tumors with necrotic surfaces. These masses were biopsied revealing diffuse histiocytic lymphoma. He was subsequently treated with 4, 600 rads tumor dose to Waldeyer's ring in the upper necks using parallel opposed lateral portals and in addition he received 3, 600 rads given dose to the lower necks using a single anterior portal and 3, 600 rads tumor dose taken at a depth of 3 centimeters to the right inguinal area. Following radiation therapy he developed leukopenia which prevented institution of chemotherapy. In September 1974 he was started on combination Cytoxan, Oncovin and Prednisone, but following each course of chemotherapy, had rather prolonged intervals of myelosuppression. As of 21 January 1975 the patient remained alive and well without further evidence of tumor involvement.

PRIMARY OR SECONDARY?

Malignant lymphoma is the most common metastatic or secondary tumor of the testis, but whether it can arise primarily in an organ normally void of lymphoid tissue remains an enigma to both the pathologist and the clinician. The rare case of a patient with testicular lymphoma living many years after orchiectomy without evidence of generalized disease has been cited as proof of primary testicular origin. In such instances, the reticulum cells are said to be derived from primitive mesoderm present within the gonad which is incited by unknown oncological factors. The usual history of the disease, however, does not favor such a premise. It is likely that all cases presenting initially as testicular tumors represent precocious development of an already disseminated disease which has not yet become clinically manifest. The frequent concomitant findings of bilateral testicular involvement, enlarged lymph nodes, skin and head and neck lesions suggest a generalized disease process. A primary unifocal testicular lesion was excluded initially in seven of our patients when retroperitoneal lymph node involvement was diagnosed by excretory urography or pedal lymphangiography. Mediastinal lymphadenopathy was demonstrated by chest roentgenogram in another patient, and bilateral synchronous testicular involvement was present in one patient without other evidence of disease. The rapid appearance of asynchronous testicular involvement (three patients) as well as lesions involving the skin (four patients), lymph nodes (two patients) and head and neck (three patients) suggests that subclinical generalized disease was present at the time of orchiectomy. Malignant lymphoma of the testis without evidence of extratesticular involvement was present in only two of the 19 patients in this series.

CLINICAL FINDINGS

Age Incidence

Malignant lymphoma occurs occasionally in the younger age group but is predominantly a disease of older men. Waddell (1961), in reviewing the literature, found the youngest patient with a testicular lymphoma to be four years of age. Gowing (1964) has since described the findings in a two year-old boy. The peak incidence in most series has been reported between the ages of 55 and 75 years (Varney 1955; Eckert and Smith 1963; Gowing 1964). In the Anderson Hospital series the patients' ages at diagnosis ranged from 38 to 77 years, with an average age of 64.7 years. The age distribution differs markedly from that of the germinal testicular tumors.

The paucity of cases has prevented definite conclusions to be made regarding the predilection for side of initial involvement. Eckert and Smith (1963) reported equal involvement with regards to side in 32 patients. Gowing (1964) found the initial testicular swelling to involve the right side in 32 patients, the left side in 29 and simultaneous involvement in one. In the Anderson Hospital series the left testis was involved initially in six patients and the right in 11. In two patients the lesions were bilateral at the time of diagnosis. Asynchronous or successive bilateral involvement developed in three patients - seven weeks, two months and five years after initial orchiectomy. A definite tendency for malignant lymphoma to affect both testes has been demonstrated by previous investigators (Hotchkiss and Laury 1950; Abeshouse et al. 1955; Cohen et al. 1955; Gowing 1964).

Clinical Features

As for other types of testicular tumors, there are no pathognomonic signs or symptoms of testicular lymphoma. The usual presenting symp-

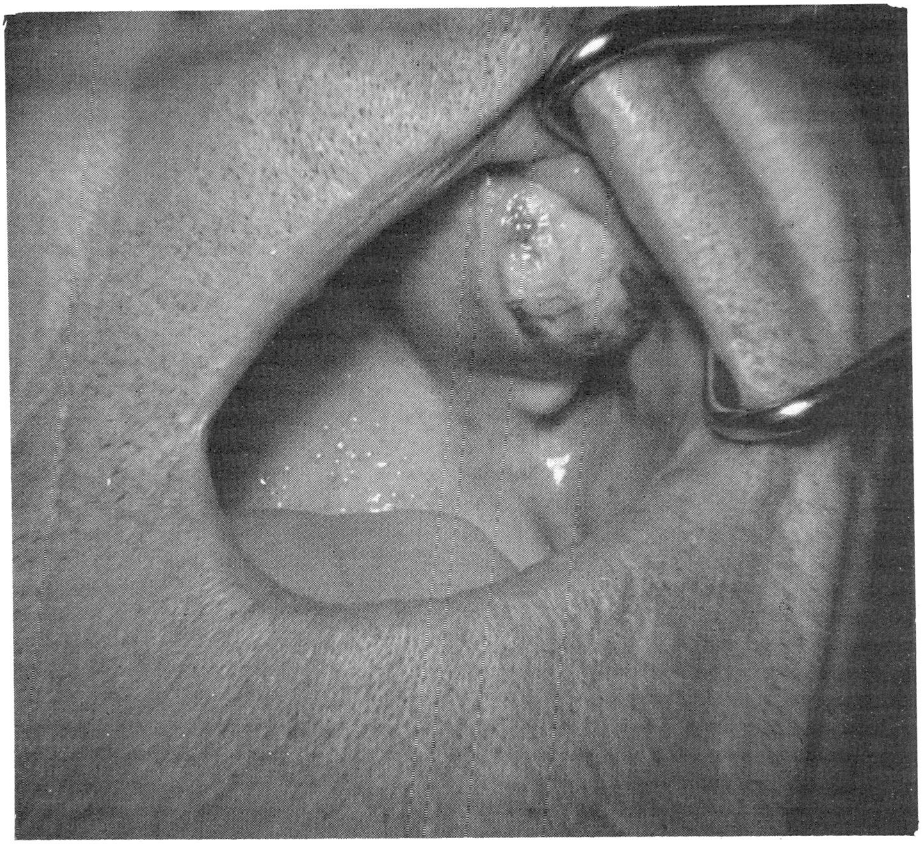

Fig. 12-1. Histiocytic lymphoma involving the hard palate on the left.

tom is one of painless testicular swelling which has been present for a variable period of time and has shown progressive increase in size. The presenting complaint in 16 of our 19 patients was testicular enlargement, which in four instances was associated with pain. The testicular tumor was discovered in one patient at the time of examination for hematuria resulting from a bladder neoplasm, during a routine physical examination in another patient and because of abdominal pain in the remaining patient.

A history of trauma is less frequently obtained than in cases of germinal tumors. Gowing (1964) reported only three of 63 patients in which a history of trauma could be elicited; one many years before, one 20 months before and one shortly before the appearance of the testicular tumor. In addition, no association of malignant lymphoma and cryptorchidism was established. The differential diagnosis is similar to that for other testicular tumors with the lesions being most frequently mistaken for a hydrocele (Cohen et al. 1955; Ellis and o'Conor 1961).

Physical examination, except for the genitalia, is usually unrewarding. Although cutaneous lesions, lymphadenopathy and hepatosplenomegaly were initially absent in all of our patients, the concomitant appearance of both testicular and cutaneous lymphomatous lesions are present not infrequently (Hotchkiss and Laury 1950; Altman and Winkelmann 1960). It has been suggested that the presence of purple-red, nodular or ulcerated cutaneous lesions in association with enlargement of one or both testes is a helpful clinical sign in establishing the diagnosis of malignant lymphoma. Chest roentgenograms taken at the time of diagnosis may reveal evidence of mediastinal adenopathy which was the finding in two of our patients. Excretory urograms are necessary for evaluation of the retroperitoneal lymph node bearing areas. In the eight instances that they were obtained, unsuspected retroperitoneal disease was demonstrated in four patients. Pedal lymphangiograms demonstrated metastatic disease in seven of the 11 patients in whom the procedure was performed. A careful examination of the upper respiratory tract and oral cavity is worthwhile since these sites were involved in two of our patients and have been reported as frequent sites of involvement by others (Varney 1955).

PATHOLOGY

Gross Appearance

The testicle is usually enlarged and hard with a smooth or nodular tunica albuginea appearing intact over the tumor. On sectioning the testis, the cut surface of the tumor has been described as cream-colored, pinkish grey or buff-colored (Gowing 1964). The tumor may be diffuse or may present as one or more discrete nodules. Coagulation necrosis of the tumor is frequently noted. The margins of the tumor are frequently ill-defined and extension into the epididymal and peri-epididymal connective tissue may be present.

Microscopic Appearance

Microscopic sections were examined in all 19 cases of diffuse histiocytic lymphoma presenting as a testicular tumor seen at Anderson Hospital. In six of the cases there were areas of uninvolved testicular tissue which suggested that the testes were at least partially involved in a nodular fashion (Fig. 12-2). In all cases malignant histiocytes were the predominant cell (Fig. 12-3). In two cases there was a significant intermixture of lymphocytes and, to a lesser extent, plasma cells; in five other cases a similar mixture of cell types was present in focal areas. In all cases

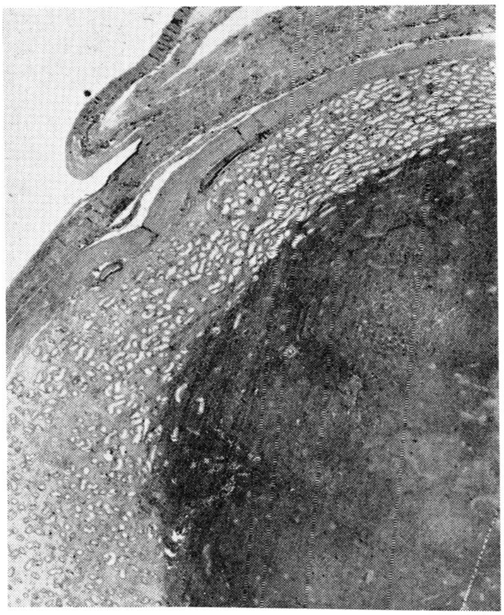

Fig. 12-2. A nodule of lymphoma surrounded by uninvolved testis. H + E x 20.

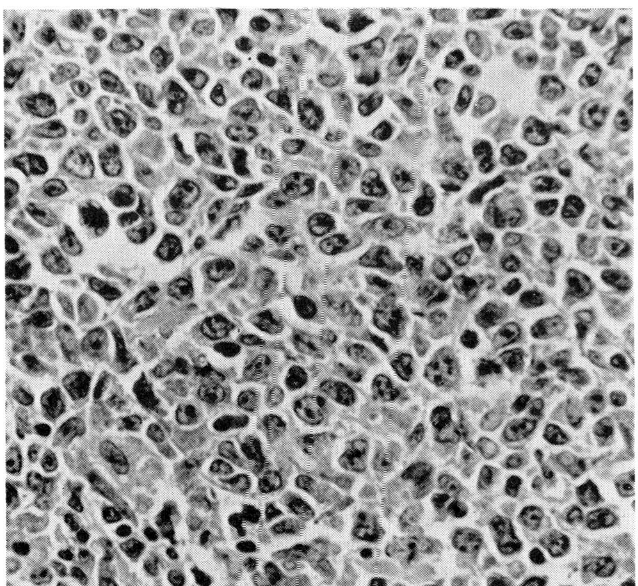

Fig. 12-3. Malignant histiocytes, as illustrated here, predominated in all tumors in this series. H + E x 290.

there was involvement of the walls of some of the seminiferous tubules by the predominant cells, but in every case tubules could be seen in some part of the sea of proliferating cells. The degree of tubular involvement varied from a mild one in which the infiltrated tubules stood out from the dense intertubular cellular infiltrates (Fig. 12-4), to the most severe degree where, in areas, the tubules were difficult to identify (Fig. 12-5). A mixture of cell types tended to be more prominent in those cases showing the most marked degree of tubular involvement. There was involvement of the tunica albuginea in 10 of the 11 cases (Fig. 12-6) and of the epididymis and periepididymal connective tissue in the five cases in which the available histologic sections demonstrated these tissues. Intratubular proliferation of malignant histiocytes, usually admixed with Sertoli cells, was present in the infiltrated tubules of eight cases (Fig. 12-6); there was, however, no intratubular growth of tumor cells in the adjacent normal testicular tissue. Coagulation necrosis of tumor was present in six cases with this microscopic in two and macroscopic in four. Interstitial fibrosis of a significant degree was seen focally in three testes.

In only five of the cases was the original diagnosis lymphoma; in the remaining eight cases the diagnosis was seminoma or embryonal carcinoma. The diagnosis on review of the histologic material at this hospital was lymphoma in nine cases, seminoma in one, and granulomatous orchitis in three. In the latter three cases, all seen in 1964 or before, a question of lymphoma was raised in the report and a lymph node biopsy was suggested. In one of these patients, an excised right inguinal lymph node biopsy exhibited reactive hyperplasia.

DIFFERENTIAL DIAGNOSIS

A correct interpretation of the histologic findings at the time of orchiectomy can be difficult. The incorrect histologic diagnosis of granulomatous orchitis in three of our cases resulted from the use of incorrect histologic criteria. Prior to the publication of the British study of testicular tumors in 1964 (Gowing 1964), lymphomas of the testis were stated to represent a proliferation of one cell type with separation but preservation of the tubules (Dixon and Moore 1952; Melicow 1955). In contrast, granulomatous orchitis was stated to represent a mixture of cell types with prominent involvement of tubules (Spjut and Thorpe 1956). As it happened, the first two of these three cases had the largest number of lymphocytes and plasma cells intermixed with the abnormal histiocytes; in retrospect this appears to be related to the severe degree of tubular involvement present in these two cases. When these three patients developed evidence of diffuse histiocytic lymphoma within a few months of each other, the lack of validity of these criteria was obvious. We now realize that a testicular tumor in which abnormal histiocytes predominate is a lymphoma irrespective of the presence of associated cell types and the presence or absence of involvement of tubules.

The problem of distinguishing diffuse histiocytic lymphoma from seminoma still remains, however. The histologic features of the former which usually help to distinguish it from seminoma are: 1) the histiocytic cells are smaller and have less cytoplasm, 2) special stains fail to reveal intracytoplasmic glycogen in the histiocytic cells as they do in all seminomas except the rare spermatocytic types, 3) invasion of the tunica albuginea is very common in lymphoma but is rare in seminoma, and (4) invasion of the wall of tubules by tumor cells is seen in lymphoma but not in seminoma.

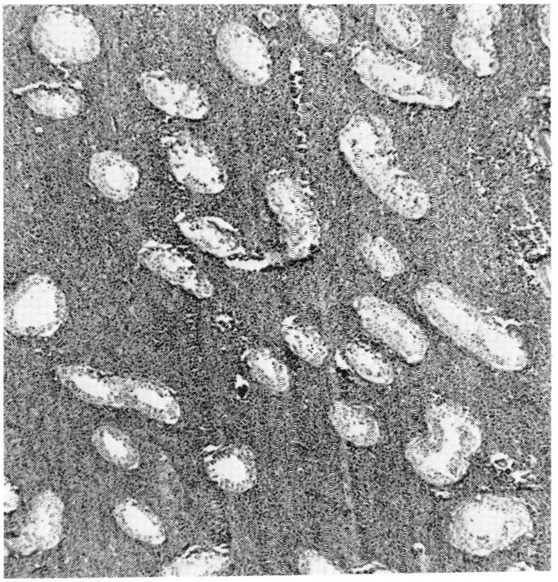

Fig. 12-4. Lymphoma cells surround but do not involve the seminiferous tubules; as a result the tubules stand out against the background of lymphoma cells. H + E x 50.

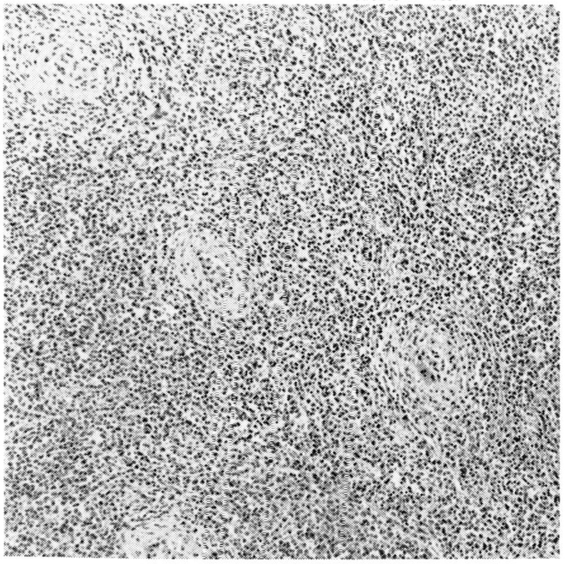

Fig. 12-5. In this tumor involvement of the seminiferous tubules by lymphoma cells makes it difficult to recognize the tubules. H + E x 63.

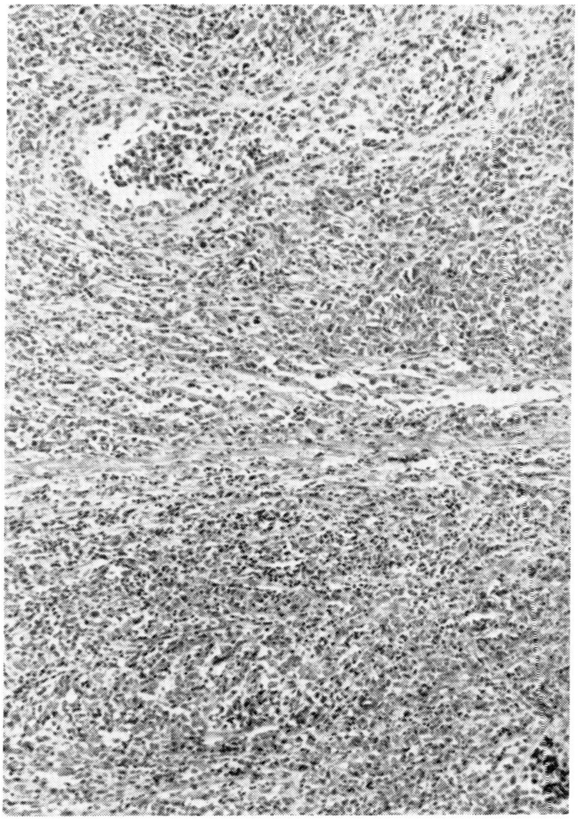

Fig. 12-6. Lymphoma cells are infiltrating the wall of a seminiferous tubule (top) and are present in its lumen; lymphoma cells are also infiltrating the tunica albuginea (lower half). H + E x 75.

TREATMENT

Treatment for malignant lymphoma presenting as a testicular tumor is the same as for other testicular malignant disease, namely radical orchiectomy with high ligation of the spermatic cord at the internal inguinal ring. Thereafter, careful and thorough evaluation of the patient is necessary to exclude the presence of other foci of disease. In addition to the routine clinical and laboratory evaluation, a chest X-ray, excretory urogram, lymphangiogram and skeletal survey films should be obtained.

In the Anderson Hospital series, all patients underwent an orchiectomy as initial therapy. In eight instances, an erroneous initial histologic diagnosis was made, but a review of the excised tissue resulted in establishing the correct diagnosis in four of the cases prior to further therapy. In the remaining four patients, lymphoma was diagnosed only after disease developed in other areas and prompted a review of the previous testicular lesion. Therefore, no consistent mode of therapy was established for this group of patients.

Radiotherapy alone was given to four patients. One died after six months, one was lost to follow-up, one is alive without recurrent disease after 64 months, and one died ten months later without known disease. Combination therapy using the antineoplastic drugs, cyclophosphamide, Vinblastine and Vincristine with radiotherapy was tried in nine patients. All died 6 to 30 months after initial orchiectomy. Chemotherapy was given to four patients; two died at seven months, one was lost to follow-up, and the other is dead after eight years. Two patients received no treatment; one died within three months and the other was lost to follow-up before therapy could be instituted. The median survival for the 15 patients known to have died is 10 months.

The survival rates for our patients is not unlike those from other series. Eckert and Smith (1963) reported a 57 per cent mortality rate within 18 months and only 4 of 35 patients (11.4 per cent) survived for five years. Of 55 patients who were followed for one year or more, Gowing (1964) found 38 (69 per cent) dead with disseminated disease within two years. It is therefore recommended that in the occasional patient without evidence of generalized disease, prophylactic radiotherapy to the retroperitoneal periaortic lymph nodes be given according to the method described by Cohen et al. (1955). Although retroperitoneal lymphadenectomy has been suggested (Gandin and Konwaler 1951), the procedure is not justified for this disease. Patients should be followed at frequent intervals with careful attention directed to the remaining testicle, lymph nodes, skin, liver, spleen and upper respiratory passages so that chemotherapy may be instituted at the first evidence of generalized disease.

CHAPTER 13

SECONDARY NEOPLASMS OF THE TESTIS

by

Douglas E. Johnson and Alberto G. Ayala

Secondary or metastatic tumors of the testis are rare. In a study of 5,000 autopsies, Klinger (1951) found 142 with secondary tumors in the genitourinary tract of which only three involved the testis. However, the majority of the lesions have been found incidentally at necropsy of patients who have died of widespread malignant disease. Less frequently, precocious development of the secondary tumor may precede clinical recognition of the primary disease or may be discovered without knowledge of the previous tumor. Under such conditions, the secondary testicular lesion may be confused both clinically and histologically with a primary testicular neoplasm.

INCIDENCE

Malignant Lymphoma

Malignant lymphoma is the most common metastatic or secondary tumor of the testis and accounts for one to seven per cent of all malignant testicular tumors (see Chapter 12). Sugarbaker and Craver (1940) in reviewing 196 cases of lymphosarcoma found the testis to be the apparent extranodal primary origin of disease in three cases, as well as, the site of later secondary involvement in an additional 1.5 per cent of their cases. The rarity of lymphomatous involvement of the testis was confirmed by Watson et al. (1949) who studied the urological complications in 1,073 cases of lymphoblastoma and found the testis involved in two cases of lymphoma and one case of leukemia.

Multiple Myeloma

Extramedullary plasmacytoma is a relatively rare tumor and only a few cases of testicular involvement have been reported. In 1947, Kirshbaum reviewed the literature and found three cases of metastatic plasma cell myeloma of the testis and reported an additional case. Hayes et al. (1952) observed one case of testicular involvement in 38 cases of multiple myeloma in which necropsies were performed. Their table listing the incidence of extramedullary lesions compiled from a review of the literature from 1892 to 1950 shows that the testis had been involved on five occasions. Melicow and Cahill (1954) reported four additional cases. In two, testicular enlargement was a prominent feature and was the only evidence at the time of metastatic spread from the primary focus in the bone marrow. Osman and Morrow (1966) described a tenth case. In 1969 Weitzner reported a case occurring in an 81 year-old man and reviewed 14 other cases reported in the literature. Levin and Mostofi (1970) reported only 7 cases of surgically resected plasmacytoma out of approximately 6,000 testicular and peri-testicular primary and secondary tumors on file in the American Testicular Tumor Registry.

Plasmacytoma of the testis tends to occur in men in their sixth and seventh decades but cases have been reported as early as 26 years (Levin and Mostofi 1970) and as late as 81 years (Weitzner 1969). Eleven patients have been subjected to orchiectomy with the duration of illness ranging from 2 months to 45 months. Although tumor-free intervals have followed orchiectomy, the prognosis is poor. The duration of time from orchiectomy to death has ranged from 1 month (Ulrich 1939) to 28 months (Gowing 1964). It is doubtful that the lesion is ever primary in the testis, but rather represents a local or initial manifestation of a systemic disorder of plasma cells or plasma cell precursors (Levin and Mostofi 1970).

Other Sarcomas

Other instances of sarcomatous involvement of the testes are very rare. They usually develop as the result of hematogenous spread from a primary sarcoma elsewhere (Dew 1928) or from direct extension of malignant disease arising in the testicular tunics, epididymis or peritesticular tissue (Hinman and Gibson 1924).

Carcinoma

Secondary testicular involvement from metastatic carcinoma is rare; less than 200 cases have been reported (Johnson et al. 1971; Meares and Ho 1973). Price and Mostofi (1957) found less than 60 cases reported prior to 1956 and described an additional 38 cases collected from over 1,600 cases of testicular tumors on file at the Armed Forces Institute of Pathology, Washington, D. C. Collins and Pugh (1964) found six secondary tumors of the testis, exclusive of lymphoma, in 995 testicular tumors referred to the British Testicular Tumor Panel and Registry. At M. D. Anderson Hospital 25 cases of histologically proven secondary carcinoma of the testis have been evaluated. The relative frequency in distribution of the primary lesions in 73 cases collected from the literature, including our own, is summarized in Table XXXI.

The most frequently reported site for a primary carcinoma with metastases to the testis has been the prostate. The first case of prostatic cancer metastasizing to the testicle was described by Semans in 1938. By 1960, a total of 31 cases had been reported (Marble 1960). Additional case reports have subsequently appeared in the literature (Ichikawa et al. 1962; Roque and Goldberg 1967; Wolf and Madsen 1968; Hanash et al. 1969; Malek and Madsen 1969; Jepson et al. 1972; Weitzner 1973). Bronchogenic carcinoma from the lung has been the second most frequently reported tumor to metastasize to the testis (Price and Mostofi 1957; Meares and Ho 1973). Secondary involvement of the testis by malignant melanoma has been recorded only on a few occasions (Coley and Hogue 1961; Weller 1922; Gupta and Grabstald 1965; Lowell and Lewis 1966; Hanash et al. 1969), but was the most frequent metastatic lesion in the Anderson Hospital series. This result reflects the large number of patients with malignant melanoma treated at Anderson Hospital. During the period in which our tumors were collected, 2,275 patients with malignant melanoma were evaluated and autopsies were performed on 223 patients dying with this disease. Other less commonly reported sites have included: kidney (Creevey 1935; Bandler and Roen 1946; Twidwell and Garske 1955); Pienkos and Jablokow 1972), intestine (Belsky and Konwaler 1954; Bodon and Dressler 1967) and stomach (London and Grossman 1949; Murray 1963; and Ford and Tandan 1969).

ANDERSON HOSPITAL SERIES

Metastatic disease involving the testicular parenchyma from a known primary tumor has been demonstrated in at least 64 patients treated at M. D. Anderson Hospital and Tumor Institute, Houston, Texas since 1954. Thirty-nine patients were found to have lesions other than secondary carcinoma with identification of the tumor showing sarcoma in four instances (Figs. 13-1 and 13-2), lymphoma in 19 instances and leukemia infiltration in 16 cases. Leukemic involvement of the testis was diagnosed at necropsy in each instance without prior clinical recognition of the lesion. The pertinent clinical and morphological features are summarized in Table XXXII. In the 25 cases of secondary carcinoma of the testis, the primary tumor arose in the lung in five cases (Figs. 13-3 and 13-4), in the kidney in three cases, in the prostate in two cases (Fig. 13-5), in the adrenal in two cases (Fig. 13-6), in the penis in two cases, and in the bladder and nasopharynx in one case each. There were nine cases of malignant melanoma. The morphological features of these tumors are given in Table XXXIII.

The age at which diagnosis of secondary testicular carcinomatous involvement was made ranged from 3 to 73 years, with the peak incidence in the sixth and seventh decades. The diagnosis was indicated by clinical findings in only eight patients, three of whom were in the pediatric age group. Bilateral testicular involvement was present in eight instances (32 per cent). In the remaining 17 cases, the left side was involved in seven patients, the right side in four patients and the location was not specified in six patients.

ROUTES OF METASTASIS

Metastasis to the testicle can occur by one or more of the following routes: 1) retrograde venous extension or embolism, 2) retrograde lymphatic extension, 3) arterial embolism, 4) retrograde ductal extension, and 5) direct invasion from contiguous growth. Excellent studies of the various routes by which malignant cells reach the testes have been reported (Howard et al. 1957; Hanash et al. 1969). It is difficult, therefore, to explain the apparent rarity of this lesion. Neglect of physicians to carefully record the multiple sites of metastases in patients with disseminated disease, as well as the failure of pathologists to carefully examine the testis during routine autopsies may account for some cases being overlooked. It is unlikely, however, that the paucity of cases results solely from oversight. Instead, it may be that the testicular temperature gradient is sufficient to inhibit neoplastic growth in many potential instances of secondary metastases (Ludwig 1963).

CLINICAL SIGNIFICANCE

Although secondary neoplasms of the testis are rare, precocious development of a secondary tumor occasionally precedes clinical recognition of the primary disease and becomes large enough to simulate a primary testicular tumor (Creevey 1935; Bandler and Roen 1946; London and Grossman 1949; Price and Mostofi 1957). This fact was emphasized in one of our cases. A 66 year-old Caucasian male had an inguinal orchiectomy performed by his local physician for a suspected primary testicular tumor. Initial pathologic examination suggested an embryonal carcinoma and he was referred to Anderson Hospital for further therapy. A secondary testicular lesion was believed to be more in keeping with

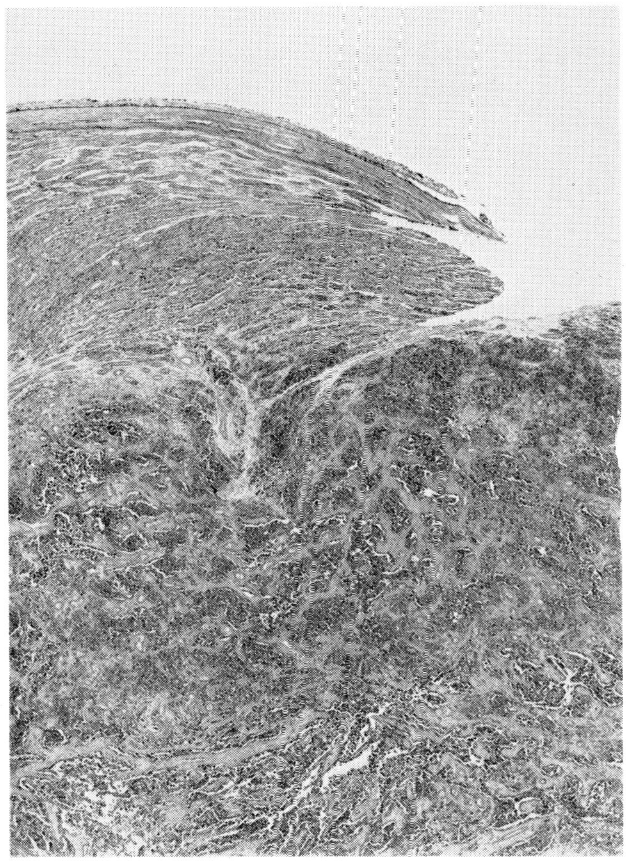

Fig. 13-1. Metastatic alveolar rhabdomyosarcoma from nasopharynx sinus. On the top of the picture there are uninvolved tubules. The lower half exhibits a diffuse infiltrate with characteristic alveolar pattern. 8 X.

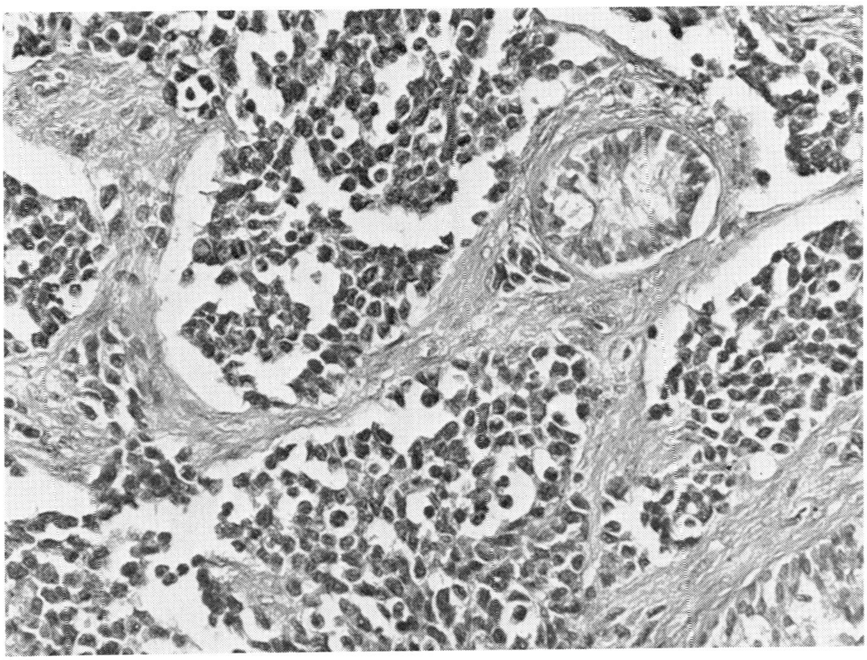

Fig. 13-2. High power picture of metastatic alveolar rhabdomyosarcoma of paranasal sinus. Small hyperchromatic cells infiltrating interstitial tissue. A seminiferous tubule is present in the upper half. 150 X.

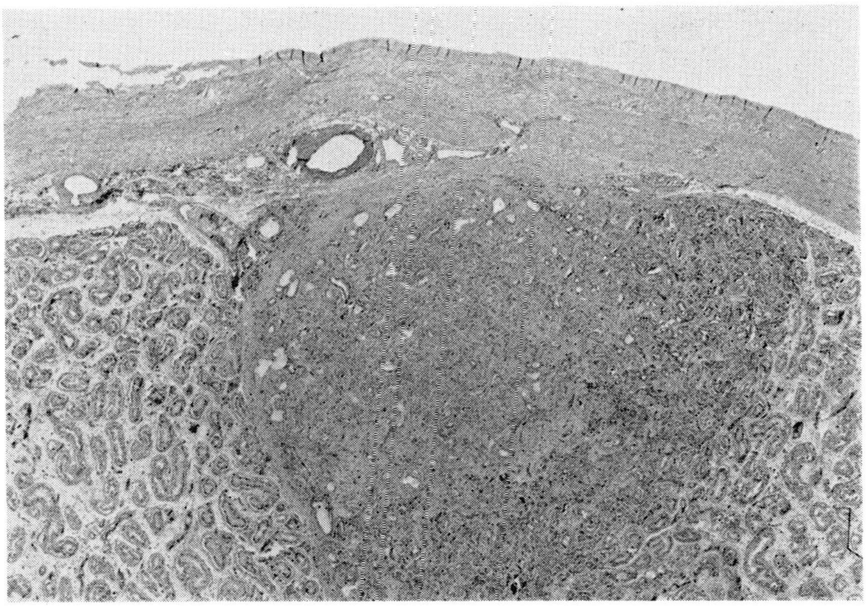

Fig. 13-3. Metastatic adenocarcinoma of lung. Section of testicle demonstrating a nodule composed of metastatic adenocarcinoma.

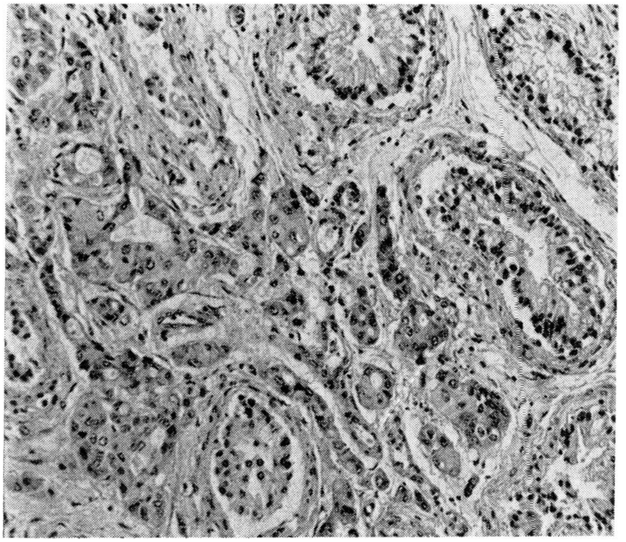

Fig. 13-4. High power view of preceeding picture. Note seminiferous tubules admixed with infiltrating adenocarcinoma. 110 X.

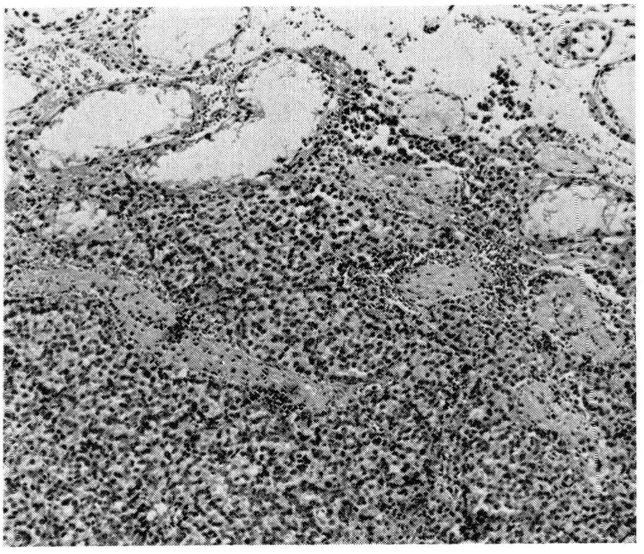

Fig. 13-5. Metastatic adenocarcinoma of prostate. A solid cellular infiltrate with an aborting tendency to form glands or tubules.

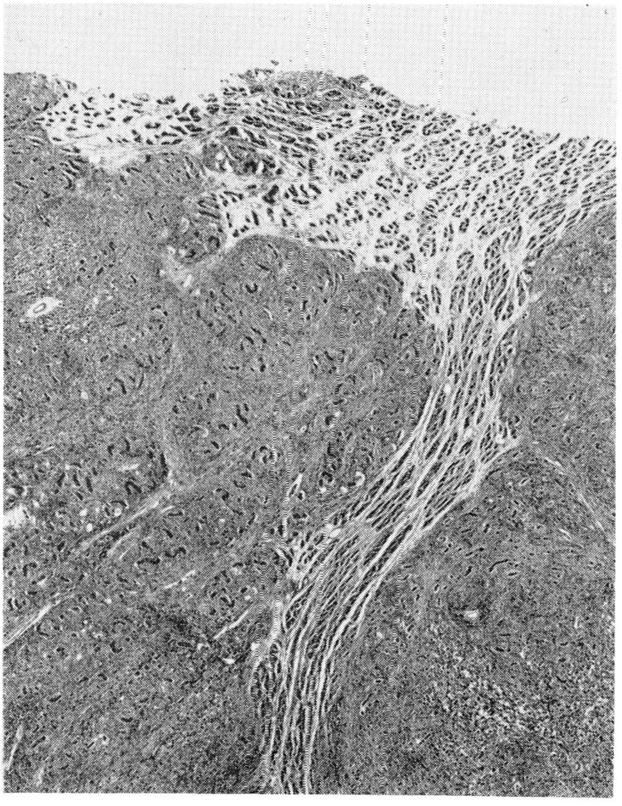

Fig. 13-6. Metastatic neuroblastoma. Low power view demonstrating a diffuse small cell neoplasm which envelops and separates seminiferous tubules. 8 X.

TABLE XXXI

DISTRIBUTION OF
PRIMARY TUMORS*
(87 Cases)

Site of Tumor	No. of Cases
Lung	26
Prostate	17
Skin (melanoma)	12
Kidney	9
Intestine	5
Stomach	3
Adrenal	3
Pancreas	3
Bladder	2
Penis	2
Salivary gland	1
Retina	1
Rectum	1
Nasopharynx	1
Ureter	1

*Based on collected reports from Price and Mostofi 1957 (38 cases), Hanash et al. 1969 (10 cases), M.D. Anderson series (25 cases) and Pienkos and Jablokow 1972 (14 cases).

TABLE XXXII

LEUKEMIC INFILTRATION OF TESTIS*

Age (Years)	Duration of Disease (Months)	Side	Morphologic Type
5	22	Bilateral	Acute Lymphocytic
9	8	N. S. **	Acute Lymphocytic
5	14	N. S.	Acute Lymphocytic
26	3	N. S.	Acute Lymphocytic
23	1	N. S.	Acute Lymphocytic
48	3	Bilateral	Acute Lymphocytic
37	1	N. S.	Acute Granulocytic
27	37	N. S.	Acute Granulocytic
44	2	Left	Acute Granulocytic
23	8	Bilateral	Acute Monocytic
12	6	N. S.	Acute Leukemia (Unclassified)
4	27	N. S.	Acute Leukemia (Unclassified)
54	1	N. S.	Chronic Granulocytic
69	18	N. S.	Chronic Granulocytic
57	19	N. S.	Chronic Granulocytic
2	2	N. S.	Stem cell

*Autopsy Series (16 Cases)
**N. S. - Not Stated

TABLE XXXIII

ORIGIN OF PRIMARY TUMORS

Primary Tumor	Histological Type	No. of Cases
Skin	Malignant melanoma	9
Lung	Bronchogenic	5
Kidney	Wilm's	1
	Hypernephroma	1
	Squamous	1
Prostate	Adenocarcinoma	2
Adrenal	Neuroblastoma	2
Penis	Squamous	2
Bladder	Transitional	1
Nasopharynx	Squamous	1

the patient's age. On physical examination, the prostate was suspicious for malignancy and a prostatic biopsy was positive for adenocarcinoma. A review of the testicular lesion confirmed the diagnosis of adenocarcinoma metastatic from the prostate. Less frequently, a testicular lesion may be discovered without the knowledge of a previous malignancy (Murray 1963). In either case, the secondary lesion may be confused both clinically and histologically with a primary testicular tumor.

A secondary testicular neoplasm should be suspected in any patient over 50 years of age who presents with testicular enlargement since primary testicular tumors occur predominantly in the third and fourth decades. Proper interpretation of the testicular lesion is necessary for early identification of the primary site and implementation of the appropriate therapeutic regime.

CHAPTER 14

EXTRAGONADAL GERM CELL TUMORS

by

Mario A. Luna

Neoplastic disease with morphological characteristics of a primary germ cell tumor developing at an extragonadal site in a patient with normal gonads poses perplexing problems to the clinician, pathologist, and embryologist. It is frequently difficult to determine whether such a tumor is truly extragonadal in origin and arises from primordial germ cells which have failed to undergo normal migration, or represents metastatic disease from an undetected or spontaneously regressed primary gonadal tumor.

Only in the last decade have we come to have a greater appreciation of the spectrum of extragonadal germ cell tumors. We are now in possession of well documented cases of mature teratoma, malignant teratoma, embryonal carcinoma, choriocarcinoma and seminoma, pure or in various mixtures that occur as primary tumors in the anterior mediastinum, retroperitoneum, presacral area and pineal region (Friedman 1951; Oberman and Libcke 1964; Pachter and Cattes 1964; Abell et al. 1965; Conklin and Abell 1967; Simson et al. 1968; Huntington and Bullock 1970; Utz and Buscemi 1971; Schantz et al. 1972; Johnson et al. 1973; Martini et al. 1974; Sickles et al. 1974).

It will be the intent of this presentation to provide a clinically oriented overview of the extragonadal germ cell tumors with emphasis directed to malignant neoplasms occurring in males.

Histogenesis

The histogenesis of malignant germ cell tumors arising in extragonadal sites is still controversial. Numerous theories have been proposed, although none have been universally accepted. Currently the most popular theory considers that these tumors are derived from germinal cells misplaced in their migration during early embryonic development (Witschi 1948; Mintz 1961). Other authorities deny their origin from germ cells and believe that they arise from foci of pluripotential embryonic tissue which have escaped from the influence of the primary organizer during fetal life (Willis 1962).

It was demonstrated by Witschi in 1948 and confirmed in 1957 by Mintz and Russell, that germ cells originate in the yolk sac endoderm and migrate widely throughout the embryo before localizing in the gonadal ridges. These observations provide positive evidence in support of the misplaced germ cell hypothesis first suggested by Askanazy (1907) more than 60 years ago.

No explanation has been offered to clarify the striking preference of the malignant germinal tumors for the male, while the incidence of the benign counterpart is approximately the same in both sexes. Similar contrasting ratios of malignant and benign teratomatous tumors in the two sexes are seen also in the gonadal tumors. It has been suggested that the environment in the female gonads predisposes germ cell neoplasms to differentiation, whereas in the male the environment fosters undifferentiated growth. This hypothesis could be extended to extragonadal germ cell tumors. It is conceivable that in the female the same genetic material has greater potential to differentiation, possibly because of a more suitable endocrine environment.

Pathogenesis

The rarity of these tumors has caused some skepticism regarding primary extragonadal origin. This attitude has prevailed since Prym in 1927, found a small fibrotic nodule in the right testis of a patient with a disseminated choriocarcinoma. He concluded that this nodule represented the complete regression of the primary tumor which eventually had been replaced by a scar but not until after metastases had occurred. Subsequently, and in support of this thesis, there have been several publications in patients with testicular germinal neoplasms in which different degrees of regression and maturation have been demonstrated in the primary tumor contrasting with the rapid growth of the metastases (Rather 1954; Azzopardi et al. 1961; Azzopardi and Hoffbrand 1965; Meares and Briggs 1972).

These studies have led to the current skepticism regarding the extragonadal origin of germinal tumors and prompted many investigators to deny their existence until after careful clinical and microscopic examination of the testes have failed to reveal any abnormality. This attitude is justified with germinal tumors localized in the inferior retroperitoneum but should not apply to tumors diagnosed within the anterior mediastinum or pineal gland. It is extremely rare for germinal testicular neoplasms to metastasize solely to these sites (Lynch and Blewett 1953; Luna and Johnson 1975).

Abell and associates (1965) stated that a seminoma may be considered primary in the retroperineum if there is no detectable tumor in the testis at the time of operation or on subsequent examinations and if one of the following criteria is met: (1) the presence of non-neoplastic gonadal tissue in the capsule of or immediately adjacent to the neoplasm or (2) an encapsulated neoplasm with adjacent lymph node involvement but without neoplasm in the lower aortic, iliac, or pelvic lymph nodes. We would agree with these stipulations in principle. However, from a practical viewpoint, any retroperitoneal or mediastinal mass occurring in a patient without a detectable or subsequent appearance of a tumor in either testis and in whom the absence of metastatic disease in the lower aortic, iliac or pelvic lymph nodes has been demonstrated should be considered as a primary extragonadal tumor if it meets the histologic criteria for such a malignancy.

In our series a distinct and well-defined fibrous scar was demonstrated in only 2 of our 21 patients from whom testicular tissue was available for review. In no instance was an occult tumor or a microscopic focus of malignant disease present. Our results, as well as reports in the literature, strongly suggest, therefore, that these tumors more often arise primarily at extragonadal sites (Oberman and Libcke 1964; Abell 1965; Simson et al. 1968; Houston 1971; Utz and Buscemi 1971; Martini et al. 1974; Sickles et al. 1974).

Pathology

Grossly, the tumors are mainly solid although most have areas of cystic degenerative changes. The malignant neoplasms lack encapsulation and usually invade or surround contiguous structures. The most frequent sites of metastases are the regional lymph nodes, lungs, liver and bones. The high frequency of bone metastases deserves emphasis since it is uncommon for testicular germinal tumors to spread to bone (Oberman and Libcke 1964; Martini et al. 1974). In those patients in whom distant metastases had occurred, the lesions were morphologically similar to the primary neoplasm.

The histology of these tumors is identical to that of the germinal tumors of the testis (Chapter 1); pathologists are familiar with their morphology. However, two points should be emphasized: the first and probably the most important is the consideration of the diagnostic possibility; the second is the absolute necessity of examining numerous histologic sections since tumors apparently monophasic are frequently found to be mixed in additional sections.

Before a lesion is labelled a seminoma, either primary or metastatic, it must meet strict histological criteria. It should not be a diagnosis of exclusion and it should not be made on the basis of poorly preserved or poorly fixed tissue (Schantz et al. 1972). Practically all seminomas evoke a peculiar fibrous and granulomatous reaction, often with giant cells of Langhan's type, that in itself is quite characteristic. Areas of coagulation necrosis may be a prominent feature. The use of periodic acid-Schiff stain, with and without prior diastase digestion for glycogen is helpful in distinguishing seminoma from lymphoma since glycogen is absent in lymphomas.

Clinical Presentation

The overwhelming majority of the patients affected by primary malignant extragonadal germinal tumors are males and the diagnosis is often established during the third decade of life. The symptoms and signs depend on the location of the tumor and of the anatomical structures involved by the disease. With mediastinal tumors, the most frequent complaints are chest pain, cough or dyspnea, although the tumor is often discovered by routine chest roentgenogram. The clinical manifestations of a neoplasm in the retroperitoneum are generally not severe. Abdominal pain is the most common symptom since these neoplasms grow slowly and produce few symptoms until they reach a large size and are easily palpable on physical examination.

The majority of teratomatous neoplasms in the sacrococcygeal region are visible at birth or make their appearance in infancy. Previous studies have emphasized the greater occurrence of sacrococcygeal teratomas in females (Hickey and Martin 1964; Conklin and Abell 1967; Chretiene et al. 1970; Silva-Duarte et al. 1973). Lesions present at birth are nearly always benign whereas those that appear later in infancy are usually malignant and in adult life there is about an equal chance of the lesions being malignant or benign. There is some evidence to suggest that the tendency for malignant change increases rapidly from birth and this has prompted the admonition that excision should follow diagnosis as soon as possible, preferably before the patient is four months old (Hickey and Martin 1964).

In the pineal body the majority of the neoplasms occur in children and young adults; males and females are equally affected. These tumors produce characteristic signs and symptoms including increased intracranial pressure, Parinaud's sign, diplopia and hearing impairment. When diabetes insipidus, visual field defects, hypopituitarism and hypothalamic signs are superimposed upon this clinical constellation, the presence of neoplasm in the suprasellar region is extremely likely (Nishiyama et al. 1966; Simson et al. 1968).

Clinical Behavior

The behavior of the various types of germ cell tumors in extragonadal sites depends upon their location and extension within the body, the sex and age of the host and the histologic type. The mature and immature teratoma usually behave in a benign fashion provided the material is not disseminated by rupture at the time of surgical exploration. Embryonal carcinoma is a very aggressive tumor when it arises in children and young adults and frequently causes death but it is not always fatal in infant boys (Conklin and Abell 1967). Teratocarcinoma, choriocarcinoma and mixed germ cell tumors are poorly controlled and patients with these lesions have a poor prognosis. Local recurrence and local invasion of major contiguous anatomical structures with early distant metastases are the features of these tumors.

The prognosis for patients with pure seminoma is relatively good with long survivals having been documented by several authors (Abell et al. 1965; Simson et al. 1968; Schantz et al. 1972). In this tumor, local control of the disease is good with surgery and radiation therapy, but distant spread usually to lymph nodes and bones is always fatal (Utz and Buscemi 1971; Johnson et al. 1973; Martini et al. 1974).

Diagnosis and Treatment

Our experience suggests that neither routine castration with serial sectioning of the testes nor random testicular biopsies are warranted in these patients in order to establish an extragonadal origin for the malignant disease. We do recommend, however, gonadal exploration in those patients in whom examination suggests the presence of a testicular abnormality (Johnson et al. 1973). After the spermatic cord has been isolated and a noncrushing clamp has been applied to prevent escape of malignant cells during manipulation, the testis is palpated carefully. When necessary, a small incision is made in the tunica albuginea and intratesticular digital examination is performed. All suspicious thickenings, scars and irregularities are biopsied and frozen histologic sections are obtained. In the absence of malignant disease the tunica is closed with interrupted sutures and the testis returned to its scrotal compartment. Postoperative swelling or subsequent atrophy has not been a problem.

The diagnosis and treatment for extragonadal germ cell tumors should parallel that which is currently in use for similar histologic lesions arising within the testis. A careful and thorough evaluation of the patient is necessary to exclude the presence of other foci or disease. In addition to the routine clinical and laboratory evaluation, a chorionic gonadotropin titer, alpha-fetoprotein determination, chest X-ray film, IVP, lymphangiogram and skeletal survey films should be obtained. In cases of pure seminoma, regional radiotherapy (Bagshaw et al. 1969) followed by cyclic systemic chemotherapy is indicated (Martini et al. 1974). In cases of nonseminomatous disease, surgical excision followed by systemic chemotherapy is recommended. Although the prognosis is generally poor, an occasional patient may be expected to survive free of disease for many years (Utz and Buscemi 1971; Schantz et al. 1972; Johnson et al. 1973; Martini et al. 1974).

Anderson Hospital Series

Thirty-two patients with extragonadal germ cell tumors were registered at the University of Texas System Cancer Center, M. D. Anderson

Hospital and Tumor Institute from March 1944 to December 1973. There were 27 males and only 5 female patients. Two tumors were benign. Of the 32 tumors, 13 arose in the anterior mediastinum, 12 in the retroperitoneum, 4 in the sacrococcygeal area, 2 in the pineal region; and in 1 case an accurate assignment of the origin was not detectable because metastases were so generalized.

The tumors which arose in the anterior mediastinum consisted of 6 mixed germinal tumors, seminoma in 3 cases, malignant teratoma in 2 cases, choriocarcinoma in 1, and benign cystic teratoma in 1 case. The retroperitoneal neoplasms included 4 mixed germinal tumors, 3 seminomas, 2 malignant teratomas, 2 choriocarcinomas, and 1 embryonal carcinoma. The sacrococcygeal tumors were: 2 malignant teratomas, 1 mature teratoma and embryonal carcinoma in 1 case. The pinealomas were malignant teratoma and seminoma. The case with an undetermined origin was choriocarcinoma.

The age at which the diagnosis of malignant disease (30 cases) was established ranged from 2 to 57 years with an average age of 29.4 years. There were no pathognomonic signs or symptoms for the disease. Symptoms were usually of short duration, and reflected local extension of the malignant process. A history of bilateral undescended testes was obtained in 1 case but spontaneous testicular descent occurred in this patient at age 8 years. Unilateral cryptorchidism was present in 1 case of pinealoma. The two benign tumors occurred in females of 2 and 17 years of age, one was found on a routine chest film and the other was present at birth in the sacrococcygeal region.

Urinary gonadotropin levels, measured by pregnancy test, were obtained in 18 patients and were positive in 4 instances; all had choriocarcinoma, pure or mixed with other germinal tumors.

In most cases, the disease was far advanced at the time of diagnosis. Consequently, no consistent mode of therapy was established for this group of patients. Generally, treatment paralleled that which was currently in use for similar morphological lesions arising primarily in the testis.

Twenty patients have died from their disease within 1 to 47 months after diagnosis. The mean survival for these patients was 12.4 months. Ten patients with malignant tumors are alive 8 to 78 months after diagnosis. Only 3 patients have survived more than 4 years, all having had pure seminoma. The two patients with benign cystic teratoma are alive 4 and 10 years after diagnosis.

The testes were carefully step-sectioned in 21 cases and at least 30 representative microscopic slides were available for review from each testis. Only 2 cases showed a well-defined fibrous scar, measuring 2 cm and 1.5 cm in largest dimension. Both patients had retroperitoneal seminomas. The scars consisted of relatively acellular collagenous tissue with occasional, barely visible ghosts of seminiferous tubules. A few histiocytes containing yellow, finely granular pigment surrounded the scar tissue. The pigment probably represented lipofuscin. In 4 other cases there was moderate interstitial cell hyperplasia with thickening of the tubular basement membranes. In no case was malignant disease or other significant pathology noted within the testes. These findings support the premise that in the majority of cases, these tumors arise primarily at extragonadal sites.

BIBLIOGRAPHY

Abelev GI: Alpha-foetoprotein: biological and clinical aspects. Bull. (International Union Against Cancer) 12:1, 1974.

Abelev GI, SD Perova, NI Kramkova, ZA Postnikova and IS Irlin. Production of embryonal alpha 1 globulin by transplantable mouse hepatomas. Transplantation 1:174, 1963.

Abell MR, JV Fayos and I Lampe: Retroperitoneal germinomas (seminomas) without evidence of testicular involvement. Cancer 18:273-290, 1965.

Abell MR and F Holtz: Testicular neoplasms in infants and children. I. Tumors of germ cell origin. Cancer 16:965-981, 1963.

Abeshouse BS, A Tiongson and M Goldfarb: Bilateral tumours of testicles; review of literature and report of case of bilateral simultaneous lymphosarcoma. J Urol 74:522-532, 1955.

Acevedo HF, EA Campbell, EL Saier, JC Frich Jr, LP Merkow, DW Hayeslip, SP Bartok, RC Graver and JL Hamilton: Urinary cholesterol v. its excretion in men with testicular and prostatic neoplasms. Cancer 32:196-205, 1973.

Ackerman LV and JA del Regato: Cancer of the male genital organs. In Cancer, the C. V. Mosby Co., St. Louis, Missouri, 1954.

Agarwal S, SS Chouhan and VK Pratap: Orchioblastoma (adenocarcinoma) of the infant testis. Indian J Cancer 4:247-253, 1967.

Ahrens Jr EH: Personal communication, 1971.

Akisada M, A Tasaka and R Mikami: Lymphography in sarcoidosis: comparison with roentgen findings in the chest. Report of 15 cases. Radiology 93:1273-1280, 1969.

Allaire F, E Thieme and D Krost: Cancer chemotherapy with 5-fluorouracil. Cancer Chemother Rep 14:59-75, 1961.

Allen Jr B and L Skaist: Testicular tumors in infants and children: a case report. J Urol 86:795-797, 1961.

Allibone EC, CK Anderson and MW Authurton: Macrogenitosomia Praecox due to an interstitial cell tumour of the testis. Arch Dis Child 44:84-87, 1969.

Al-Sarraf M, K Kithier and VK Poulik Vaitkevicuis: The effect of cytotoxic drugs on alpha one feto-protein in cancer patients. Clin Res 20:3, 1972.

Altman BL and M Malament: Carcinoma of the testis following orchiopexy. J Urol 97:498-504, 1967.

Altman J and RK Winkelmann: Lymphosarcoma of skin and testis. AMA Arch Dermatol 82:943-947, 1960.

Anderson RE and C Huston: Tumors of the testicle in childhood. Amer J Surg 95:445-450, 1958.

Ansfield FJ, BC Korbitz, HL Davis Jr and G Ramirez: Triple drug therapy in testicular tumors. Cancer 24:442-446, 1969.

Anson BJ and EH Daseler: Common variations in renal anatomic affecting blood supply, form and topography. Surg Gynec & Obstet 112:439-449, 1961.

Arcadi JA: Testicular neoplasms in father and son. J Urol 110:306, 1973.

Arduino LJ and MA Glucksman: Interstitial-cell tumor of the testis associated with Klinefelter's syndrome: a case report. J Urol 89:246-248, 1963.

Arean VM and JA Kreager: Paratesticular rhabdomyosarcoma. Amer J Clin Path 43:418-427, 1965.

Arvay N and JD Picard: La Lymphographie. Paris. Masson & Cie, 1964.

Arvola I and HG Lilius: Malignant testicular tumours presenting with severe acute pain. Ann Chir Gynaec Fenn 61:30-32, 1972.

Askanazy M: Die teratome nach ihrem bau, ihrem Verlauf, ihrer Genese und in Vergleich zum experimentellen Teratoid. Verh Deutsch Ges Path 1:39-82, 1907.

Azzopardi JG, FK Mostofi and EA Theiss: Lesions of testes observed in certain patients with widespread choriocarcinoma and related tumors. Am J Path 38:207-225, 1961.
Azzopardi JG and AV Hoffbrand: Retrogression in testicular seminoma with viable metastases. J Clin Path 18:135-141, 1965.
Bader LV and NSF Proctor: Interstitial cell tumor in a cryptorchid testis. AMA Arch Path 78:260-266, 1964.
Bagg HJ: Experimental production of teratoma testis in fowl. Amer J Cancer 26:69-84, 1936.
Bagshaw MA, WT McLaughlin and JD Earle: Definitive radiotherapy of primary mediastinal seminoma. Amer J Roentgen 105:86-94, 1969.
Bailey H: Physical signs. In Clinical Surgery. John Write & Sons Ltd., Bristol, 1960.
Bailey TB, SM Pinsky, BT Mittemeyer, AA Borski and M Johnson: A new adjuvant in testis tumor staging: gallium - 67 citrate. J Urol 110:307-310, 1973.
Bandler CG and PR Roen: Solitary testicular metastasis simulating primary tumor and antedating clinical hypernephroma of the kidney: report of a case. J Urol 55:663-669, 1946.
Barranco SC and RM Humphrey: The effects of Bleomycin on survival and cell progression in Chinese hamster cells in vitro. Cancer Res 31:1218-1223, 1971.
Batsakis JG: Tumors of testis in infancy and childhood. Arch Path 72:27-35, 1961.
Baum S, KM Bron, L Wesler and HL Abrams: Lymphangiography, cavography, and urography, comparative accuracy in the diagnosis of pelvic and abdominal metastases. Radiology 81:207-218, 1963.
Beard JH and WH Cooner: Teratoma of the testis in an infant. Southern Med J 59:627-628, 1966.
Belan A, P Malek and J Kolc: Cine demonstrations of lymphaticovenous anastomoses in dogs. Fortschr Roentgenstr 992:168, 1963.
Bellman S and B Oden: Regeneration of surgically divided lymph vessels. Acta Chir Scand 116:99, 1956.
Belsky JB and BE Konwaler: Testicular metastasis from carcinoma of the colon. J Urol 72:712-715, 1954.
Bergstrand CG and B Czar: Demonstration of new protein in serum from the human fetus. Scan J Clin Lab Invest 8:174, 1956.
Betts JW: Teratoma of testis. Brit J Urol 26:168-171, 1954.
Bhargava MK and DG Reddy: Tumors of the testis. II. Tumors of the testis in childhood. Cancer 19:1655-1665, 1966.
Bishop PMF, DP Van Meurs, DRC Willcox and D Arnold: Interstitial cell tumor of the testis in a child; report of a case and a review of the literature. Brit Med J 1:238-242, 1960.
Bismuth V, JP Deprez-Curely, R Bourdon and A Lambling: Chylous nontumoral ascites - the value of lymphography. Ann Radiol (Paris) 6:817, 1963.
Blalock A, CS Robinson, RS Cunningham and ME Gray: Experimental studies on lymphatic blockage. Arch Surg 34:1049, 1937.
Blandey JP, HF Hope-Stone and AD Dayan: Tumors of the testicle, Grune and Stratton, Inc., New York, N. Y., 1970.
Blodkhin N, L Larionov, L Perenodchikova, L Chebotareva and N Merkulova: Clinical experiences with sarcolysin in neoplastic diseases. Ann NY Acad Sci 68:1128-1132, 1958.
Blum RH, SK Carter and K Agre: A clinical review of Bleomycin: a new antineoplastic agent. Cancer 31:903-914, 1973.

Blundon KE, S Russi and CR Bunts: Interstitial-cell hyperplasia or adenoma. J Urol 70:759-767, 1953.

Boatman DL, DA Culp and VB Wilson: Testicular neoplasms in children. J Urol 109:315-317, 1973.

Boctor ZN, SS Kurohara, AO Badib and GP Murphy: Current results from therapy of testicular tumours. Cancer 24:870-875, 1969.

Bodon GR and JAW Dressler: Metastatic carcinoma of the right testicle from primary carcinoma of the appendix. J Urol 97:885-887, 1967.

Boehme EJ, RO Bagley and AF Pumphrey: Malignant teratoma of the testicle in an infant four months of age. Calif Med 74:397-398, 1951.

Bormel P and HB Mays: Testicular tumors in infancy and childhood: report of two cases. J Urol 86:119-124, 1961.

Borski AA and JC Kimbrough: Cystic adult teratoma of the testis associated with failure of the urogenital union. US Armed Forces Med J 5:266-267, 1954.

Bourgeaux C, F Martin, F Cabanne, M Bordes, H Bastien and P Sizaret: Alpha-fetoproteine et tumeurs testiculaires. Path Biol 22:313-318, 1974.

Bourquin J: Anatomical pathology of the lymph nodes following lymphography. Radiol Clin (Basel) 38:383-401, 1969.

Bowles WT: Inguinal node metastases from testicular tumor developing after variocelectomy. J Urol 88:266-267, 1962.

Bracken RB, DE Johnson and ML Samuels: Alpha-fetoprotein determinations in germ cell tumors of testis. (In press)

Brady EA, W Jarrett and KD Backwinkel: Bilateral testicular tumors: spindle cell sarcoma and seminoma: case report. J Urol 90:215-219, 1963

Brizzi E, R De Dominicis and G Nori Bufalini: Lymphography in the cadaver. (With observations on the lymphatic drainage of the testis). Bull Soc Ital Biol Sper 41:136-138, 1965.

Brown NJ: Miscellaneous tumours of mainly epithelial type. Brit J Urol 36: supp. 70-77, 1964.

Bruun S and A Engeset: Lymphadenography: a new method for the visualization of enlarged lymph nodes and lymphatic vessels (Preliminary report). Acta Radiol 45:389-395, 1956.

Bunge RG and JT Bradbury: An early human seminoma. J Amer Med Ass 193: 960-962, 1965.

Busche FM and ES Sayegh: Roentgenographic visualization of human testicular lymphatics: a preliminary report. J Urol 89:106-110, 1963.

Busche FM, ES Sayegh and OW Shenault Jr: Some uses of lymphangiography in the management of testicular tumors. J Urol 93:490-495, 1965.

Butler JJ: Histopathology of malignant lymphomas and Hodgkin's disease. In Leukemia-Lymphoma. A collection of papers presented at the 14th Annual Clinical Conference on Cancer, 1969, at the University of Texas M. D. Anderson Hospital and Tumor Institute at Houston. Year Book Medical Publishers, Inc., Chicago, Illinois, 1970, pp. 123-142.

Cairns HWB: Neoplasms of the testicle. Lancet 1:845-850, 1926.

Caldwell WL: Why retroperitoneal lymphadenectomy for testicular tumors? South Med J 62:1232-1236, 1969.

Caldwell WL: Lymphadenectomy for testicular tumors. JAMA 218:98, 1971.

Camin AJ, RI Dorfman, JH McDonald and IM Rosenthal: Interstitial-cell tumor of the testis in a seven year-old child. AMA J Dis Child 100:389-399, 1960.

Campbell DC: Testicular tumors. Med Bull European Command 7:653-656, 1950.

Campbell HE: Incidence of malignant growth of the undescended testicle. Arch Surg 44:353-369, 1942.

Campbell HE: The incidence of malignant growth of the undescended testicle: a reply and re-evaluation. J Urol 81:663-668, 1959.

Carleton RL, NB Friedman and EJ Bomge: Experimental teratomas of the testis. Cancer 6:464-473, 1953.

Castro JR: Lymphadenectomy and radiation therapy in malignant tumors of the testicle other than pure seminoma. Cancer 24:87-91, 1969.

Castro JR: Tumors of the testis. In Fletcher GH: Textbook of Radiotherapy, 2nd Ed., Lea & Febiger, Philadelphia, 1973, pp. 737-751.

Castro JR and M Gonzalez: Results in treatment of pure seminoma of the testis. Amer J Roentgen 111:355-359, 1971.

Celis A, J Kuthy and E del Castillo: Importance of the thoracic duct in the spread of malignant disease. Acta Radiol 45:169, 1956.

Champlin HW: Similar tumors of testis occurring in identical twins. JAMA 95: 96-97, 1930.

Charbit A, EP Mailaise and M Tubiana: Relation between the pathologic nature and growth of human tumors. Europ J Cancer 7:307-315, 1971.

Chiappa S, C Uslenghi, G Bonadonna, P Marano and G Ravasi: Combined testicular and foot lymphangiography in testicular carcinoma. Surg Gynec & Obstet 123:10-14, 1966.

Chiappa A, C Uslenghi, G Galli, G Ravasi and G Bonadonna: Lymphangiography and endolymphatic radiotherapy in testicular tumors. Brit J Radiol 39:498-512, 1966.

Chitty EC: Case of abdominal testis complicated by tumor formation and acute torsion of cord. Malayan Med J 8:203, 1933.

Chitwood Jr EM: Chorioepithelioma of testis with bilateral choroidal metastasis. AMA Arch Ophthal 50:363-367, 1953.

Chretiene PB, JD Milan, FW Foote and TR Miller: Embryonal adenocarcinoma of the sacrococcygeal region. Cancer 26:522-533, 1970.

Chute R, JA Baron Jr and CA Olsson: The transverse upper abdominal "Chevron" incision in urological surgery. Trans Amer Ass Genitourin Surg 29: 14-17, 1967.

Clemmesen J: A doubling in mortality from testis carcinoma in Copenhagen 1943-1962. Acta Path Microbiol Scand 72:348-349, 1968.

Clinical Screening Co-operative Group of the European Organization for Research on the Treatment of Cancer: Study of clinical efficiency of Bleomycin. Brit Med J 2:643-645, 1970.

Cohen BB, G Kaplan, AF Liber and B Roswit: Reticulum-cell sarcoma with primary manifestation in testis: report of 4 cases. Cancer 8:136-142, 1955.

Cohen AE and GC Tomskey: A survey of testicular tumors. J Urol 85:613-616, 1961.

Coleman PN and KC McKeown: A case of bilateral testicular tumours: seminoma of one testis with teratoma in the other. Brit J Surg 42:219-221, 1954.

Coley WB and JP Hogue: Melanotic cancer: a report of 91 cases. Ann Surg 64: 206-214, 1961.

Collins DH and KM Cameron: Interstitial cell tumour. Brit J Urol 36:62-69, (suppl), 1964.

Collins DH and RCB Pugh: Classification and frequency of testicular tumours. Brit J Urol 36:1-11 (suppl), 1964.

Collins DH and T Symington: Sertoli cell tumour. Brit J Urol 36:52-61 (suppl), 1964.

Condit PT: Personal communication, 1971.

Conklin J and MR Abell: Germ cell neoplasms of sacrococcygeal region. Cancer 20:2105-2117, 1967.

Cook FE, DD Lawrence, JR Smith and EJ Gritti: Testicular carcinoma and lymphangiography. Radiology 84:420-427, 1965.

Cooper JF, WF Leadbetter and R Chute: The thoracoabdominal apprcach for retroperitoneal gland dissection: its application to testis tumors. Surg Gynec & Obstet 90:486-496, 1950.

Copeman M: Chorionepithelioma teratoma of testis. Breast hypertrophy preceding palpable testicular tumor. Brit J Surg 47:328-329, 1959.

Correa O and EYB Tallman: Tumores del testiculo en Chile. XIIIe Congres Soc Internat d'Urol 2:96-97, 1965.

Cox R: Radiotherapy in malignant diseases of testicle and penis. Brit J Urol 26:350-363, 1954.

Creeny CD: Confusing clinical manifestations of malignant renal neoplasms. Arch Int Med 55:895-916, 1935.

Crowe GG: Hemoperitoneum due to rupture of a seminoma in an abdominal testis. Brit J Surg 39:188-189, 1951.

Culp DA: Testicular neoplasms: an analysis of 113 cases. J Urol 70:282-295, 1953.

Culp DA, RG Frazier and JJ Butler: Sertoli-cell tumor in an infant. J Urol 76: 162-167, 1956.

Cunningham JH: New growths developing in undescended testicles. J Urol 5: 471-477, 1921.

Dalgaard JB and F Hesselberg: Interstitial cell tumours of the testis. Two cases and survey. Acta Path Microbiol Scand 41:219-234, 1957.

Darbari BS and BP Saxena: Adenocarcinoma of the infant's testis. Indian J Pediat 27:400-403, 1960.

Davidson JW: Lymphography in malignant disease. Radiological aspects. Canad Med Ass J 97:1283-1289, 1967.

Davies JNP, S Elmes, MSR Hutt, LAR Mtimavalye, R Owor and L Shaper: Cancer in an African community 1897-1956. Brit Med J 1:259-264, 1964.

Davis Jr AE: Rhabdomyosarcoma of the testicle. J Urol 87:148-154, 1962.

Dean AL: The diagnosis and treatment of testis tumors. New York J Med 51: 485-492, 1951.

Dean AL: Early diagnosis of tumors of the genito-urinary organs. Connecticut Med J 15:959, 1951.

De La Balze FA, RA Mancini, F Arriloge, IA Andrado, P Vilar, AJ Guitman and OW Davidson: Puberal maturation of the normal human testis: a histologic study. J Clin Endocrinol 20:266-297, 1960.

De Roo T: Lymphografie. Netherland, Van Corcum & Co., 1964.

Deshmukh SS, DS Pardanani, AB Bhattacharya and KN Chitnis: Orchioblastoma - A case report. J Postgrad Med 13:123-124, 1967.

DeVita VT, AA Serpick and PP Carbone: Combination chemotherapy in the treatment of advanced Hodgkin's disease. Ann Intern Med 73:881-895, 1970.

Dew H: Sarcomatous tumors of the testicle. Surg Gynec & Obstet 46:447-458, 1928.

Dixon FJ and RA Moore: Tumors of the male sex organs. Armed Forces Inst Path FASC 32:48-103, Washington, D. C., 1952.

Dixon FJ and RA Moore: Clinicopathologic study. Cancer 6:427-454, 1953.

Dockerty MB and JT Priestley: Lymphosarcoma of the testis: Report of 4 new cases. J Urol 48:514-523, 1942.

Dodd GD, AD Patrick, AJ Ballantyne, ML Ibanez and P Chau: The dissemination of tumors of the head and neck via the cranial nerves. Radiol Clin N Amer 8:445-471, 1970.

Dodd GD, FN Rutledge and S Wallace: Postoperative lymphocysts. Amer J Roentgen 108:312-323, 1970.

Dodson AI and JW Hooper Jr: Bilateral concomitant seminoma. J Urol 72:424-427, 1954.

Dolan PA and EB Moore: Improved technique of lymphangiography. Amer J Roentgen 88:110, 1962.

Door DR, AE Nordholt and TE Heerde: Testis-tumoren bij broers bijna gelijktijdig tot maligne groei gek omen. Ned T Geneesk 115:1046-1049, 1971.

dos Santos R: Phleborgraphie d'une veine cane inferieure sutures. J d'urol 39: 586-587, 1935.

Dow JA and FK Mostofi: Testicular tumours following orchiopexy. Southern Med J 60:193-195, 1967.

Doyle GB: Embryonal carcinoma of the testis in an infant. Brit J Urol 27:287-291, 1955.

Dunlap DJ and JA Ochsner: Bilateral successive embryonal carcinoma of the testis. J Urol 97:738-740, 1967.

Dutta LP and J Mahanta: Orchioblastoma. J Indian Med Ass 51:354-355, 1968.

Dykhuizen RF, FW George, S Kurohara, M Rotner, CR Sargent and JK Varney: The use of cobalt 60 telecurietherapy of X-ray therapy with and without lymphadenectomy in the treatment of testis germinal tumors: a 20-year comparative study. J Urol 100:321-328, 1968.

Earle JD, MA Bagshaw and HS Kaplan: Supervoltage radiation therapy of the testicular tumors. Am J Roentgenology, Radium Therapy and Nucl Med 117:653, 1973.

Eckert H and JP Smith: Malignant lymphoma of the testis. Brit Med J 2:891-894, 1963.

Editorial. An epidemic of testicular cancer? Lancet 2:164-165, 1968.

Ekman H, A Fritjofsson and J Johansson: Treatment of testicular tumours. Urol Internat 20:129-142, 1965.

Ekman H, G Giertz, G Johnson and G Notter: Tumors of the testicle: a report from Sweden on combined surgico-radiotherapeutic treatment. XIII Congres Soc Internat d'Urol 2:26-62, 1965.

Ellis WJ and VJ O'Conor Jr: Primary reticulum cell sarcoma of the testis. Quart Bull Northwest Univ Med Sch 35:87-88, 1961.

Ellner HJ, I LeCompte and AM Putra: Bilateral primary testicular tumours. Northwest Med 65:314-316, 1966.

Elwi AM and H El-Katib: An attempt to produce experimental testicular tumor in the albino rat by zinc sulphate with methyl cholanthrene. J Egypt Med Ass 43:853-860, 1960.

Emery JL: Chorionepithelioma in new-born male child with hyperplasia of interstitial cells of testis. J Path and Bact 64:735-739, 1952.

Engeset A: An experimental study of the lymph node barrier. Extrait de Acta Union Internat. Contre Le Cancer 15:3-4, 1959.

Engeset A: Irradiation of lymph nodes and vessels. Acta Radiol 1:1-125 (suppl. 229), 1964.

Evans W: Developmental stages of embryo-like bodies in teratoma testis. J Clin Path 10:31-39, 1957.

Evans CC and HD Kaufman: Unusual presentation of seminoma of the testis. Brit J Surg 58:703-704, 1971.

Falin LI: Experimental teratoma testis in the fowl. Amer J Cancer 38:199-211, 1940.

Falin LI and WW Anissimona: Zur Pathogenese der experimentellen teratoiden Geschwulste der Geschlechtsdrusen. Ztsch f Krebsf 50:339-351, 1940.

Ferber B, VH Handy, PR Gerhard and M Solomon: Cancer in New York State, Exclusive of New York City, 1941-1960. New York State Department of Health, Bureau of Cancer Control (1962).

Fergusson JD: Tumours of the testis. Brit J Urol 34:407-421, 1962.
Fergusson JD: Some clinical statistics of testicular tumour. XIIIe Congres Soc Internat d'Urol 2:72-75, 1965.
Field TE: Malignancy and the ectopic testicle in Army patients. J Royal Army Med Corps 108:189-192, 1962.
Field TE: The role of trauma in the actiology of testicular neoplasms. J Royal Army Med Corps 109:1-4, 1963.
Field TE: Common error occurring in the diagnosis of testicular neoplasms and the effect of these errors on prognosis. J Royal Army Med Corps 110: 152-155, 1964.
Flynn PT and AO Severance: Bilateral interstitial-cell tumors of testis. Cancer 4:817-822, 1951.
Foldi M: Personal communication, 1971.
Fons SD, R Otis and RT Ogden: Germinal testicular tumors. Amer J Roentgen 92:152-159, 1964.
Ford ML and B Tandan: Metastatic tumor of the spermatic cord and testis from carcinoma of the stomach. Southern Med J 62:352-354, 1969.
Fraimow W, S Wallace, RR Greening and R Cathart: Changes in pulmonary function due to lymphangiography. Radiology 85:231-241, 1964.
Fraley EE and AS Ketcham: Teratoma of testis in an infant. J Urol 100:659-660, 1968.
Friedman NB and RA Moore: Tumors of the testis: a report of 921 cases. Military Surg 99:573-593, 1946.
Friedman M and MC Purkayashtha: Recurrent seminoma of testis: causes and treatment of late metastasis, recurrence or second primary tumor. J Urol 84:360-368, 1960.
Friedman NB: The comparative morphogenesis of extragenital and gonadal teratoid tumors. Cancer 4:265-276, 1951.
Fuchs WA: Lymphographie and tumor diagnostik. Springer-Verlag, Germany, 1965.
Fuglsang F and AS Ohlsen: Androblastoma predominantly feminizing: with report of case. Acta Chir Scand 112:405-410, 1957.
Gandin MM and BE Konwaler: Lymphosarcoma of the testicle. Ann West Med & Surg 5:55-58, 1951.
Gangai MP: The AZ titer as an aid in the treatment of testicular tumors. J Urol 91:589-591, 1965.
Gangai MP: Testicular neoplasms in an infant. Cancer 22:658-662, 1968.
Ganina KP: Effects of trauma under conditions of hormonal disturbance on the formation of tumors of the testicle. Unio Internat Cong Cancer 20:1504-1507, 1964.
Garber HE and GI Kauffer: Torsion of an intra-abdominal testicular seminoma. J Urol 98:684-685, 1968.
Garvey FK and TB Daniel: Bilateral interstitial cell tumor of testicles. J Urol 66:713-719, 1951.
Garvin CH: Malignant tumors of testes. J Nat Med Assoc 54:225-233, 1962.
Gehring GG, FR Rodriquez and DM Woodhead: Malignant degeneration of cryptorchid testes following orchiopexy. Transactions of the 52nd Annual Meeting of the South Central Section of the American Urological Association, Inc., 30-40, 1973.
Gerster A: Sarcoma of retained testicle, with twisted pedicle. Ann Surg 27: 649, 1898.
Gerwig WH, LK Countryman, I Harrison and RG Gottschalk: Interstitial-cell tumor of the testis. Amer J Surg 107:760-763, 1964.
Ghormley KO and JL Jacek: Testicular tumors. Wisconsin Med J 53:241-243, 1954.

Giarola A: Protection of reproductive capacity as a factor in therapy for undescended testicle. Fertil & Steril 18:375-380, 1967.
Giersten JC: Malignant testicular tumor following mumps orchitis. Acta Path Microbiol Scand 42:7-14, 1958.
Gilbert JB and JB Hamilton: Studies in malignant testis tumors. III. Incidence and nature of tumors in ectopic testes. Surg Gynec & Obstet 71:731-743, 1940.
Gilbert JB: Tumors of the testis following mumps orchitis: case report and review of 24 cases. J Urol 51:296-300, 1944.
Glassburn JR, S Prasasvinichia, RC Nuss, MN Croll and LW Brady: Correlation of ^{198}au abdominal lymph scans with lymphangiograms and lymph node biopsies. Radiology 105:93-96, 1972.
Gold WM, J Youker, S Anderson and JA Nadel: Pulmonary-function abnormalities after lymphangiography. New Eng J Med 273:519-525, 1965.
Gonder MJ and EJ Fadell: Gonadal stromal tumor in an infant. J Urol 84:357-359, 1960.
Gonick P and JM Lancaster: Bilateral consecutive testicular neoplasms. US Armed Forces Med J 10:232-234, 1959.
Gordon-Taylor G and NR Wyndham: On malignant tumours of the testicle. Brit J Surg 35:6-7, 1947.
Gowing NFC: Malignant lymphoma of the testis. Brit J Urol 36:85-94 (suppl), 1964.
Gowing NFC and AD Morgan: Paratesticular tumours of connective tissue and muscle. Brit J Urol 36:78-84 (suppl), 1964.
Grabstald H, AP Rhamy and CB Dryden Jr: Tumors of the testis: a study of 115 cases. Southern Med J 50:1347-1353, 1957.
Gray CP, JR McDonald and GJ Thompson: Chorioepitheliomatous elements occurring in teratoma. Amer J Surg 79:653-659, 1950.
Gray CP, GJ Thompson and JR McDonald: The clinical findings in 127 cases of teratoma of the testis. J Urol 64:690-696, 1950.
Griffith DP and CE Carlton: Lymphocyst: unusual cause of ureteral obstruction. J Urol 103:43-45, 1970.
Griswold MH, CS Wilder, SJ Cutler and ES Pollack: Cancer in Connecticut 1935-1951. Connecticut State Department of Health, 1955.
Gross RE: Surgery of infancy and childhood, W. B. Saunders Co., Philadelphia, Pa., 1953.
Grove JS: The cryptorchid problem. J Urol 71:735-741, 1954.
Grumet RF and B MacMahon: Trends in mortality from neoplasms of the testis. Cancer 11:790-797, 1958.
Gupta TD and H Grabstald: Melanoma of the genitourinary tract. J Urol 93:607-614, 1965.
Guthrie J: Histological effects of intra-testicular injections of cadmium chloride in domestic fowl. Brit J Cancer 18:255-260, 1964.
Guthrie J: Observations of the zinc induced testicular teratomas of fowls. Brit J Cancer 18:130-142, 1964.
Haidle CW: Fragmentation of Deoxyribonucleic acid by Bleomycin. Molecular Pharm 7:645-652, 1971.
Haines JS and H Grabstald: Tumor formation in atrophic testes. Arch Surg 60:857-860, 1950.
Halley JBW: Pathology and survival in testicular neoplasia. Cancer 16:1269-1280, 1963.
Hamburger C: On the nature of gonadotrophins in cases of malignant tumors of the testis. Acta Path Microbiol Scand 18:457-484, 1941.
Hamburger C, F Bang and J Nielsen: Studies on gonadotropic hormones in cases of testicular tumours. Acta Path Microbiol Scand 13:75-102, 1936.

Hamburger C: Testosterone treatment and 17-ketosteroid excretion. V. Administration of testosterone per rectum. Acta Endocr Kbh 28(4):529-536, 1958.

Hamburger C and SG Johnson: Studies on urinary gonadotropins. III. Qualitative differences between young males and of postmenopausal women. Acta endocr Kbh 26(1):1-29, 1958.

Hamilton JB and JB Gilbert: Studies in malignant tumors of testes. IV. Bilateral testicular cancer. Cancer Res 2:125-129, 1942.

Hamlin JA, AR Kagan and NB Friedman: Lymphomas of the testicle. Cancer 29:1352-1356, 1972.

Hanash KA, JA Carney and PP Kelalis: Metastatic tumors to testicles: routes of metastasis. J Urol 102:465-468, 1969.

Hansen JL: Tumour of undescended testicle in an infant. J Amer Med Ass 199: 944-945, 1967.

Harper JGM, SB Dewing and G Nagamatsu: Bilateral carcinoma of the testis: a report of three cases. J Urol 71:634-637, 1954.

Harvald B and M Hauge: Heredity of cancer elucidated by a study of unselected twins. JAMA 186:749-753, 1963.

Hausfeld KF and D Schrandt: Malignancy of testis following atrophy: report of three cases. J Urol 94:69-72, 1965.

Hayes DW, WA Bennett and FJ Heck: Extramedullary lesions in multiple myeloma. Arch Path 53:262-272, 1952.

Hendrix RC: Neoplasms in children: a review of necropsy in 244 cases. Univ. Michigan Med Bull 22:524-529, 1956.

Herman P, D Beninghoff and J Schwart: A physiologic approach to lymph flow in lymphography. Amer J Roentgen 91:1207, 1964.

Herr HW, I Silber and DC Martin: Management of inguinal lymph nodes in patients with testicular tumors following orchiopexy, inguinal or scrotal operations. J Urol 110:223-224, 1973.

Herrmann WL, F Buckner and A Baskin: Interstitial-cell tumor of the testis with gynecomastia. J Clin Endocr 18:834-842, 1958.

Heuson JC: Addison's disease secondary to occult metastatic seminoma. Cancer 19:1754-1759, 1966.

Hickey RC and RG Martin: Sacrococcygeal teratomas. Ann NY Acad Sci 114: 951-957, 1964.

Hickinbotham PFJ: Malignant tumours of the testicle. Brit J Urol 22:87-102, 1950.

Higgins CC and FW Arber: Malignant tumours of the testicle. Canad Med Ass J 69:124-131, 1953.

Higginson J and AG Oettle: Cancer incidence in the Bantu and races of South Africa: report of a cancer survey in Transvaal (1953-1955). J Nat Cancer Inst 24:589, 1960.

Hinman F: The operative treatment of tumors of the testicle. JAMA 63:2009-2014, 1914.

Hinman F: The radical operation for teratoma testis. Surg Gynec & Obstet 37: 495-508, 1919.

Hinman F, TE Gibson and AA Kutzmann: The radical operation for teratoma testis. Surg Gynec & Obstet 37:429-451, 1923.

Hinman F: The prognosis and treatment of tumors of the testis. J Urol 34:72-84, 1935.

Hinman Jr F: The implications of testicular cytology in the treatment of cryptorchidism. Amer J Surg 90:381-386, 1955.

Hinman Jr F: Optimum time for orchiopexy in cryptorchidism. Fertil & Steril 6:206-214, 1955.

Hinman F and FH Benteen: The relationship of cryptorchidism to tumor of the testis. J Urol 35:378-381, 1936.

Hinman F and TE Gibson: Tumors of the epididymis, spermatic cord and testicular tunics. Arch Surg 8:100-137, 1924.

Hinman Jr F and GI Smith: Leydig cell neoplasia in experimental testicular atrophy. J Urol 83:706-712, 1960.

Hira NR: Rare presentation of testicular neoplasm. Brit J Clin Pract 19:533-534, 1965.

Hobson BM: The excretion of chorionic gonadotrophin by men with testicular tumours. Acta Endocrinol 49:337-348, 1965.

Hope-Stone HF, JP Blandy and AD Dayan: Treatment of tumours of the testis. Brit Med J 1:984-989, 1963.

Hopkins GB and DH Parry: Metastasizing Sertoli-cell tumor (androblastoma). Cancer 23:463-467, 1969.

Hopkins GB: Interstitial cell tumor of the testis: case report and review of the literature. J Urol 103:449-451, 1970.

Horn Jr RC and HT Enterline: Rhabdomyosarcoma: a clinicopathological study and classification of 39 cases. Cancer 11:181-199, 1958.

Hosney SH: Seminoma of the testis presenting as traumatic epididymitis. J Irish Med Ass 54:120-121, 1965.

Host H and T Stokke: The treatment of malignant testicular tumors at the Norwegian Radium Hospital. Cancer 12:323-329, 1959.

Hotchkiss RS and RB Laury: Concomitant bilateral malignant testicular tumors. J Urol 63:1086-1092, 1950.

Houser R, RJ Izant Jr and L Persky: Testicular tumors in children. Amer J Surg 110:876-892, 1965.

Houston RR: Primary retroperitoneal seminoma without gonadal involvement. J Urol 106:841-844, 1971.

Howard DE, WK Hicks and EW Scheldrup: Carcinoma of the prostate with simultaneous bilateral testicular metastases: case report with special study of routes of metastases. J Urol 78:58-64, 1957.

Howden PF: Carcinoma of the testicle. New Zeal Med J 67:215-217, 1968.

Hreschyshyn MM and RR Sheehan: Lymphangiography in patients with pelvic cancer and lymphomas. Proc Amer Ass Cancer Res 3:121, 1960.

Hreschyshyn MM and RR Sheehan: The use of lymphography as a diagnostic method. Radiology 76:47-53, 1961.

Hudack S and PD McMasters: Normal and pathological permeability of lymphatic capillaries in human skin. Proc Soc Exper Biol & Med 29:944-945, 1932.

Huffman LF: Interstitial cell tumor of testicle: report of case. J Urol 45:692-698, 1941.

Hull EW, CG Moertel and PP Carbone: Serum a-fetoprotein (a-FP) in cancer patients. Clin Res 17:403, 1969.

Hunt LD, BM Harvard and JH Glenn: Experimental testicular tumorigenesis. J Urol 87:438-443, 1962.

Huntington RW and WK Bullock: Extragonadal endodermal sinus. Cancer 25:1368-1376, 1970.

Hurley JV: Testicular tumours with special reference to their association with urinary gonadotrophins. Aust New Zeal J Surg 31:180-188, 1962.

Hutter AM, JJ Lynch and BL Shnider: Malignant testicular tumors in brothers: a case report. JAMA 199:1009-1010, 1967.

Hyman GA, JE Uhmana and DV Hebef: Factors to be considered in the clinical evaluation of a new chemotherapeutic agent. Cancer Chemother Rep 16:397-400, 1962.

Ichikawa T, Y Kummamoto and M Asano: A case of prostatic carcinoma with metastases to the skin and both testes. J Urol 87:941-950, 1962.

Jackson JR and D Magner: Spermatocytic seminoma - a variant of seminoma with specific microscopical and clinical characteristics. Cancer 18:751-755, 1965.

Jackson L, S wallace, B Schaffer, S Dramer and A Weiss: The diagnostic value of lymphangiography. Ann Intern Med 54:870-871, 1961.

Jacobs EM: Combination chemotherapy of metastatic testicular germinal cell tumors and soft part sarcomas. Cancer 25:324-332, 1970.

Jacobs EM, FD Johnson and DA Wood: Stage III metastatic malignant testicular tumors: treatment with intermittent and combined chemotherapy. Cancer 19:1697-1704, 1966.

James DC and RD Shupe: Interstitial cell tumor of testicle with report of case. J Urol 63:718-723, 1950.

Jamieson JK and JF Dobson: The lymphatics of the testicle. Lancet 1:493, 1910.

Jemine EE: Hyperplasia and neoplasia of interstitial cells of testicle. Arch Surg 35:967-998, 1937.

Jensen Jr OJ: Testicular tumors. JAMA 149:1-12, 1952.

Jepson PM, HG Labitzke and AJ Bischoff: Solitary testicular metastasis from carcinoma of the prostate. Brit J Urol 44:594-599, 1972.

Jing BS and C Gianturco: Notes on lymphangiography technique. Amer J Roentgen 109:190-196, 1970.

Job TT: Lymphatico-venous communications in common rats and their significance. Amer J Anat 24:467, 1918.

Johnson DE, CR Kuhn and GA Guinn: Testicular tumors in children. J Urol 104:940-943, 1970.

Johnson DE, DR Pohl and H Rivera-Correa: Varicocele: an innocuous condition? Southern Med J 63:34-36, 1970.

Johnson DE, DM Woodhead, DR Pohl and JR Robison: Cryptorchism and testicular tumorigenesis. Surgery 63:919-922, 1968.

Johnson GC: Testicular tumors: a review and report of 93 cases. Stanford Med Bull 15:248-258, 1957.

Johnson DE, JJ Butler and JK Luce: Histiocytic reticulum cell sarcoma presenting as a testicular tumor. J Urol 107:425-428, 1972.

Johnson DE, DE Fuerst and HS Gallager: Mesothelioma of the tunica vaginalis. South Med J 66:1295-1297, 1973.

Johnson DE, L Jackson and AG Ayala: Secondary carcinoma of the testis. South Med J 64:1128-1130, 1971.

Johnson DE, JP Laneri, CF Mountain and MA Luna: Extragonadal germ cell tumors. Surgery 73:85-90, 1973.

Johnson DE and J Morneau: Bilateral sequential germ cell tumors of the testis. Urology 4:567-570, 1974.

Johnstone G: Prepubertal gynecomastia in association with an interstitial cell tumour of the testis. Brit J Urol 39:211-220, 1967.

Jolly H: Sexual precocity: American lectures in endocrinology. Charles C Thomas, Springfield, Ill., 1955, p. 224.

Jones A: Testicular tumours: a clinico-pathological survey. Ulster Med J 24:27-36, 1955.

Jones TC and NB Friedman: Pathologic and clinical features of canine testicular tumours. Bull Int AM Mus 31:36-53, 1950.

Julien R: Etude des tumeurs du testicule chez l'enfant. Paris. Jouve et Cie., 1925.

Jungck EC, AM Thrash, AP Ohlmacher, AM Knight and LY Dyrenforth: Sexual precocity due to interstitial-cell tumor of the testis: report of 2 cases. J Clin Endocr 17:291-295, 1957.

Kaplan G, BB Cohen and B Roswit: Malignant testicular tumors. Amer J Roentgen 66:405-419, 1951.

Kaplan G and B Roswit: Clinical notes, suggestions and new instruments. JAMA 144:1557-1560, 1950.

Katsuyuki T, Y Sagawa and I Arakawa: Therapeutic effect of Bleomycin for skin tumors. Gann 61:207-218, 1970.
Kaufman JJ: The diagnosis of testicular tumors. Cancer 12:2-6, 1967.
Kaufman JJ: Treatment of testicular tumors. Cancer 17:54-59, 1967.
Kaufman JJ and DE Burke: Abdominal venography. Amer J Roentgen 76:807-812, 1956.
Kaufman JJ, DE Burke and WE Goodwin: Abdominal venography in urological diagnosis. J Urol 75:160-168, 1956.
Keller AZ: Testicular cancers in blacks and whites by cell types, laterality, survivorship and age. J Nat Med Assoc 66:49-52, 1974.
Kiely JM, BD Massey Jr, EG Harrison Jr and DC Utz: Lymphoma of the testis. Cancer 26:847-852, 1970.
Kithier K, J Lusher, J Brought and MD Poulik: Effect of therapy on the serum level of alpha-1 fetoprotein in embryonal cell carcinoma. J Pediatrics 81: 71-75, 1972.
Kimbrough JC and FF Cook: Carcinoma of the testis. JAMA 153:1436-1438, 1953.
Kimbrough JC and JC Denslow: Malignant disease of the testicle. J Urol 65: 611-614, 1951.
Kinmouth JB: Lymphangiography in man. Method of outlining lymphatic trunks at operation. Clin Sc 11:13-20, 1952.
Kinmouth JB: Lymphangiography in clinical surgery and particularly in the treatment of lymphoedema. Ann Roy Coll Surg 15:30, 1954.
Kirshbaum JD: Metastatic plasma cell myeloma of the testicles. Urol Cutan Rev 51:456-459, 1947.
Kittridge RD, R Burger, N Finby and J Draper: An illustration of an approach to the diagnosis of pelvic disease. J Urol 89:607-610, 1963.
Kittridge RD, S Hashim, HB Robott, TB Van Itallie and N Finby: Demonstration of lymphatic abnormalities in the patient with chyluria. Amer J Roentgen 90:159, 1963.
Kleinsmith LJ and GB Pierce: Multipotentiality of single embryonal carcinoma cells. Cancer Res 24:1544-1552, 1964.
Klinger ME: Secondary tumors of genito-urinary tract. J Urol 65:144-153, 1951.
Klugo RC, JH Fisher and AB Retik: Endodermal sinus tumors of the testis in infants and children. J Urol 108:359-361, 1972.
Koehler PR: Typical fatal reactions after lymphangiogram. Cancer Chemother Rep 52:113-118, 1968.
Koehler PR, WA Meyers, JF Skelley and B Schaffer: Body distribution of ethiodol following lymphangiography. Radiology 82:866-871, 1964.
Koehler PR, JL Fabrikant and RJ Dickson: Observations on the behaviour of testicular tumors with comments on racial incidence. J Urol 87:577-579, 1962.
Kohler FP and JJ Murphy: Rhabdomyosarcoma of the male genital tract. J Urol 82:500-503, 1959.
Koppikar DD and MV Sirsat: A malignant sertoli cell tumour of the testis. Brit J Urol 45:213-217, 1973.
Krain LS: Testicular cancer in California from 1942 to 1969: the California tumor registry experience. Oncology 27:45-51, 1973.
Krantz S, JA Ward, J Mendeloff and E Haltiwanger: Germinal cell tumors of the testis: a report of 102 cases. Amer J Roentgen 93:138-144, 1965.
Kranz WC: Seminoma metastatic to the maxilla. Oral Surg 21:196-200, 1966.
Kulvin MM: Chorionepithelioma of choroid metastatic from tumor in testicle. Amer J Ophthal 34:217-225, 1951.
Kurohara SS, AO Badib, JH Webster, LSJ Martin and MW Woodruff: Prognostic factors in the common testis tumors. Amer J Roentgen 103:827-836, 1968.

Kurohara SS, FW George III, RF Dykhuisen and KL Leary: Testicular tumors: analysis of 196 cases treated at the U. S. Naval Hospital, San Diego. Cancer 20:1089-1098, 1967.

Lafferty JO and EP Pendergrass: Carcinoma of the testicle with metastasis to bone. Amer J Roentgen 63:95-101, 1950.

Lameer C: Diagnostic information versus risks in lymphography. Radiol Clin (Basel) 38:329-334, 1969.

Larson DL, AE Rodin, DK Roberts, WK O'Steen, AS Rapperport and SR Lewis: Perineural lymphatics, myth or fact. Amer J Surg 112:488-491, 1966.

Laskowski J: Feminizing tumours of testis: general review with case report of granulosa cell tumour of testis. Endokr Pol 3:337-343, 1942.

Leadbetter WF: Diagnosis and treatment of tumors of the testis. Amer J Surg 95:341-352, 1958.

Le Comete (1851) Quoted by JS Grove: The cryptorchid problem. J Urol 71: 735-741, 1954.

Leducq J, B Debaud and J Gest: Apport de la lymphographie dans l'appreciation des metastases ganlionnaries des tumeur du testicle. Bull du Cancer 55: 301-305, 1966.

Leiter E and H Brendler: Loss of ejaculation following bilateral retroperitoneal lymphadenectomy. J Urol 98:375-378, 1967.

Lenzi M and G Bassani: Effect of radiation of lymph and lymph vessels. Radiology 80:814-817, 1963.

Lesson CR: An electron microscope study of cryptorchid and scrotal human testes, with special reference to pubertal maturation. Invest Urol 3:498-511, 1966.

Levin HS and FK Mostofi: Symptomatic plasmacytoma of the testis. Cancer 25: 1193-1203, 1970.

Lewis L, Quoted by Haines JS and H Grabstald: Tumor formation in atrophic testes. Arch Surg 60:857-860, 1950.

Lewis EL, RE Johnston, RR Rowe and JC Kimbrough: Retroperitoneal lymph node resection: the intercostoinguinal approach. J Urol 67:338-341, 1952.

Lewis LH and CG Stockard: Feminizing testis tumors. J Urol 64:518-523, 1950.

Li MC, WF Whitmore Jr, R Golbey and H Grabstald: Effects of combined drug therapy on metastatic cancer of the testis. JAMA 174:1291-1299, 1960.

Li FP and JF Fraumeni: Testicular cancers in children: epidemiologic characteristics. J Nat Cancer Inst 48:1575-1581, 1972.

Li MC, R Hertz and DM Bergenstal: Therapy of choriocarcinoma and related trophoblastic tumors with folic acid and purine antagonists. New Eng J Med 259:66-74, 1958.

Lipworth L and A Dayan: Rural preponderance of seminoma of the testis. Cancer 23:1119-1121, 1969.

Livesay JE, HE Branch and WL Eaton: Interstitial cell carcinoma of the testis. Am J Roentgen 115:728-731, 1972.

Livingstone J: A case of cancer of both testicles, which terminated favourably by the supervention of scurvy. Edinburgh Med & Surg J 1:163-165, 1805.

Ljvraga P: Sui cosidetti teratomi sperimentali del testicolo da zinco. Pathoologica 26:726-735, 1934.

Lockhart J, AG Armas and HJ Pollero: Cavography in cases of testis tumors. J Urol 83:438-444, 1960.

London MZ and SN Grossman: Secondary testicular tumor resembling Krukenberg tumor, a case report. Western Sect Amer Urol Assn Trans 16 28-31, 1949.

Lopis S, TH Bothwell and MB Swerdlaw: Insulin-resistant diabetes: report of a case with an associated interstitial-cell tumour of the testis. South African Med J 26:681-684, 1952.

Lowell DM and EL Lewis: Melanospermia: a hitherto undescribed entity. J Urol 95:407-411, 1966.
Lownes JB and P Leberman: Tumors of the testis in brothers. Urol Cuntan Rev 43:205-206, 1939.
Ludwig J: Experimentelle and statistische untersuchungen uber metastatische Hodengeschwulste. Schweiz Med Wschr 93:1740-1743, 1963.
Luedtke WE: Lymphoblastoma of the testis. Report of a case of reticulum cell sarcoma. J Kansas Med Soc 65:450, 1964.
Luna MA and DE Johnson: Postmortem findings in testicular tumors. To be published, 1975.
Lynch MJG and GL Blewett: Choriocarcinoma arising in male mediastinum. Thorax 8:157-161, 1953.
MacDonald AE: Choroidal chorioepithelioma secondary to teratoma of the testicle. Arch Ophthal 16:672-676, 1936.
MacDonald JS: Lymphography in renal tumors. Brit J Radiol 88:110, 1962.
Mackay B, JL Bennington and RW Skoglund: The adenomatoid tumor: fine structural evidence for a mesothelial origin. Cancer 27:109-115, 1971.
MacKay EN and AH Sellers: A statistical review of malignant testicular tumours based on the experience of the Ontario Cancer Foundation Clinics 1938-1961. Canad Med Ass J 94:889-899, 1966.
MacKenzie AR: Chemotherapy of metastatic testis cancer: results in 154 patients. Cancer 19:1369-1376, 1966.
Macnicol MF, G Rebello, JR Kirkpatrick and IF MacLaren: Reticulum cell sarcoma of the testis. J Roy Coll Surg Edinb 19:116-120, 1974.
Maddison FE: Lymphatic cannulation without dye. Radiology 88:362-363, 1967.
Magner D and AJS Bryant: Adenocarcinoma of the testis occurring in infants. Arch Pathol 51:82-89, 1951.
Magner D, JS Campbell and FW Wiglesworth: Testicular adenocarcinoma with clear cells occurring in infancy. A distinctive tumour. Canad Med Ass J 86:485-488, 1962.
Mahaffy RG: A comparison of the diagnostic accuracy of lymphography, cavography and pelvic venography. Brit J Radiol 37:422-429, 1964.
Mahon FB Jr, F Gosset, RG Trinity and PO Madsen: Malignant interstitial cell testicular tumor. Cancer 31:1208-1212, 1973.
Maier JG, KE Buskirk, MH Van Sulak, RH Perry and DT Schamber: An evaluation of lymphadenectomy in the treatment of malignant testicular germ cell neoplasms. J Urol 101:356-359, 1969.
Maier JG, MH Sulak and BT Mittemeyer: Seminoma of the testis: analysis of treatment success and failure. Amer J Roentgen 102:596-602, 1968.
Maier JG and DT Schamber: The role of lymphangiography in the diagnosis and treatment of malignant testicular tumors. Am J Roentgenology, Radium Therapy and Nucl Med 114:482-491, 1972.
Maier JG and KE Van Buskirk: Treatment of testicular germ cell malignancies. JAMA 213:97-98, 1970.
Malassez M: Lymphadenome du testicule. Bull Soc Anat Paris 52:1176, 1877.
Malek GH and PO Madsen: Carcinoma of the prostate with unusual metastases. Cancer 24:194-197, 1969.
Malek P: Some questions of the pathophysiology of the lymphatic system. Rev Czech Med 5:153, 1959.
Mann AS: Bilateral exophthalmos in seminoma. J Clin Endocr 27:1500-1502, 1967.
Marble EJ: Testicular metastasis from carcinoma of the prostate: review of literature and report of a case. J Urol 84:369-375, 1960.
Marin-Padilla M: Histopathology of the embryonal carcinoma of the testis. Arch Pathol 85:614-622, 1968.

Markland C: Testicular tumors. In Current Problems in Surgery. Year Book Medical Publishers, Inc., Chicago, Illinois, 1968.

Martin MM, JJ Canary and PA Balsamo: Virilizing tumor of the testis in one twin. J Clin Endocr 22:345-351, 1962.

Martini N, RB Golbey, SI Hajdu, WF Whitmore and EJ Beatie: Primary mediastinal germ cell tumors. Cancer 33:763-769, 1974.

Masson P: Deux cancers leydigiens de l'homme. Rev Canad Biol 2:168-243, 1943.

Matsumoto K, K Nakauchi and K Fujita: Radiation therapy for the embryonal carcinoma of testis in childhood. J Urol 104:778-780, 1970.

Mawas C, D Buffe, O Schweisguth and P Burtin: Alpha-1-foeto-protein and children's cancer. Rev Europ Etud Clin Biol 16:430-435, 1971.

Mayers MM: Interstitial cell tumors of testicle: report of three cases. J Urol 68:834-843, 1952.

McCullough DL, CE Carlton and HM Seybold: Testicular tumors in infants and children: report of 5 cases and evaluation of different modes of therapy. J Urol 105:140-148, 1971.

McLean PA and H Browne: Bilateral simultaneous seminoma of the testicles: a case report. J Irish Med Assoc 66:514-515, 1973.

Meares EM and Tzu Leung Ho: Metastatic carcinomas involving the testis: a review. J Urol 109:653-655, 1973.

Meares EM Jr and EM Briggs: Occult seminoma of the testis masquerading as a primary extragonadal germinal neoplasm. Cancer 30:300-306, 1972.

Melicow MM: Embryoma of the testis. Report of a case and a classification of neoplasms of the testis. J Urol 44:333-334, 1940.

Melicow MM: Classification of tumors of testis: clinical and pathological study based on 105 primary and 13 secondary cases in adults, and 3 primary and 4 secondary cases in children. J Urol 73:547-574, 1955.

Melicow MM: Classification of tumors of testis. J Int Coll Surg 25:187-201, 1956.

Melicow MM: New British classification of testicular tumors: a correlation, analysis and critique. J Urol 94:64-68, 1965.

Melicow MM and GF Cahill. Plasmacytoma. J Urol 71:103-113, 1954.

Mendelson D and A Serpick: Combined chemotherapy of testicular tumors. J Urol 103:619-623, 1970.

Merren DD, SA Vest and CH Lupton Jr: Treatment of malignant tumors of the testis. J Urol 65:128-135, 1951.

Merrin C, E Sarcione, M Bohne and DJ Albert: Alphafetoprotein in testicular tumors. J Sur Research 15:309-312, 1973.

Michalowsky I: Eine experimentelle Erzeugung teratioder Geschwulste der Hoden beim Hahn. Zweite Mitteilung. Virchows Arch (Path Anat) 267:27-62, 1928.

Milner WA and JB Gilbert: Painful malignant tumor of testis with and without hemorrhage. J Urol 64:697-704, 1950.

Mintz B: Formation and early development of germ cells. Symposium on the germ cells and earliest stages of development. Milan, Fondazione A. Baselli, Instituto Lombardo, 1961.

Moore RA: Tumors of the testis. J Kansas Med Soc 51:70A-75A (suppl), 1950.

Moore RA: Teratoid tumors of testis. J Urol 65:693-708, 1951.

Most J: Ueber die lymphgefasse and lymphdrusen des hodens. Arch Anat (Anat Abt) 113:123, 1899.

Mostofi FK: Infantile testicular tumors. Bull NY Acad Med 28:684-687, 1952.

Mostofi FK, EA Theiss and DJ Ashley: Tumors of specialized gonadal stroma in human male patients. Cancer 12:944-957, 1959.

Murry LM: Metastasis of gastric carcinomal to the spermatic cord and testis. J Christ Med Ass India 38:511-512, 1963.
Murugasu JJ: A case of seminoma with unusual metastasis. Singapore Med J 2:38-41, 1961.
Myers Jr GH and BR MacPherson: Histologically similar testicular neoplasms occurring in brothers. J Urol 108:757-759, 1972.
Nagamatsu GR: New extraperitoneal approach for bilateral retroperitoneal lymph node dissection in testis tumor. J Urol 90:588-590, 1963.
Naranjo CA, SJ Kandzari and DF Milam: Reticulum cell sarcoma with primary manifestation in the testicle. South Med J 67:346-348, 1974.
Nation EF, HA Edmundson and RA Mammack: Interstitial cell tumors of testis: report of 3 new cases. Arch Surg 48:415-422, 1944.
Navarro RB and HM Martinez: XIIIe Congres de la Societe Internat d'Urol 2: 96, 1965.
Nelson JW and EH Ruffolo: Testicular seminoma as a cause of paraplegia: a case report. J Urol 95:70-73, 1966.
Newns GH: Precocious sexual development due to an interstitial-cell tumour of the testis. Brit J Surg 39:379-381, 1952.
Nielsen J: Classification, interpretation and diagnosis of testicular tumors. Acta un Int Contra 9:877-882, 1953.
Nielsen H, M Nielsen and NE Skakkebaek: The fine structure of a possible carcinoma - in-situ for the seminiferous tubules in the testis of four infertile men. Acta Path Microbiol Scand 82:235-248, 1974.
Nishimura R, I Knodo, T Oyamatsu, H Kondo, T Morita and M Hirokawa: Contribution to the diagnosis and treatment of testicular tumors. Yokohama Med Bull 15:231-241, 1964.
Norris JM and RE Scully: Endocrine Pathology of the Ovary. The C. V. Mosby Co. , St. Louis, Missouri, 1958.
Notter G and NE Ranudd: Treatment of malignant testicular tumours - a report of 355 patients. Acta Radiol NS 2:273-301, 1964.
Nusbaum M, S Baum, RC Hedges and WS Blakemore: Roentgenographic and direct visualization of the thoracic duct. Arch Surg 88:105, 1964.
Oberman HA and JH Libcke: Malignant germinal neoplasms of the mediastinum. Cancer 17:498-507, 1964.
O'Connell HV and CF Geschickter: Tumors of the testes: five-year follow-up study. US Armed Forces Med J 1:719-732, 1950.
Oettle AG: Tumours of the testis in South Africa. Leech 34:142-148, 1964.
Osman R and JW Morrow: Myeloma of testicle. J Urol 96:352-355, 1969.
Osman R and JW Morrow: Reticulum cell sarcoma with primary manifestation in the testicle: three case reports. J Urol 102:230-232, 1968.
Ostergaard E: Feminizing tumor of testis: presumably aberrant adrenocortical tumor. J Clin Endocr 7:438-445, 1947.
Ottaviani G: Osservazioni anatomobiologiche sue vasi linfatici. Monitore Zoologico Italiano 9:54-58 (suppl), 1947.
Pachter MR and R Cattes: "Germinal" tumors of the mediastinum: a clinicopathologic study of adult teratomas, teratocarcinoma, choriocarcinomas and seminomas. Dis of Chest 45:301, 1964.
Pack GT and RG LeFevre: The age and sex distribution and incidence of neoplastic diseases at the Memorial Hospital, City of New York. J Cancer Res 14:167, 1930.
Packham DM: Torsion of an intra-abdominal seminoma of the testis. Brit J Surg 52:25-27, 1965.
Parker RG: Treatment of apparent solitary pulmonary metastases. J Thorac Surg 36:81-87, 1958.

Parker RG and JB Holyoke: Tumors of the testis. Amer J Roentgen 83:43-65, 1960.

Passanante BM, GR Guerra and H Alarcon: Acute abdomen in a case of torsion of an intra-abdominal seminoma of the testicle. Missouri Med 65:362-364, 1968.

Pastan I and RM Friedman: Actinomycin-D: inhibition of phospholipid synthesis in chick embryo cells. Science 160:316-317, 1968.

Patton JF, CB Hewitt and N Mallis: Diagnosis and treatment of tumors of the testis. JAMA 171:2194-2198, 1959.

Patton JF and N Mallis: Tumors of the testis. J Urol 81:457-461, 1959.

Patton JF, DN Sietzman and RA Zone: Diagnosis and treatment of testicular tumors. Amer J Surg 99:525-532, 1960.

Patton JF, DM Seitzman and CB Hewitt: Tumors of the testis: diagnosis and treatment. Postgrad Med 33:440-445, 1963.

Patriquin HB: The lymph nodes - normal neoplastic: radiologic-pathologic correlation. J Canad Ass Radiol 18:452, 1969.

Paul M: Malignant testicular tumour in a child aged sixteen months. Ceylon Med J 2:178, 1952.

Perch GA and H Kirshman: A testicular tumor of specialized gonadal stroma. J Urol 97:880-884, 1967.

Persky T: Testicular tumors in children. Paper given at Third Annual Radiotherapy Symposium, Miami, Florida, January 24, 1969.

Perttala Y: Prognosis of cancer of the testis. Follow-up study of 69 cases. Ann Chir Gynaec Fenn 53:349-356, 1964.

Pessin SB: The lower urinary tract and male genitalia. In Pathology (ed) WAD Anderson, The C. V. Mosby Co., St. Louis, Missouri, 1957.

Phelan JT, LB Woolner and AB Hayles: Testicular tumors in infants and children. Surg Gynec & Obstet 105:569-576, 1957.

Philip PP: Feminizing tumours of the testis. Postgrad Med J 36:190-196, 1960.

Picard JD: Lymphography in the course of chyluria (Apropos of 30 cases). J Urol Nephrol (Paris) 73:761-780, 1967.

Pienkos EJ and VR Jablokow: Secondary testicular tumors. Cancer 30:481-485, 1972.

Pierce GB: Teratocarcinomas. A problem in developmental biology. Canad Cancer Conf 4:119-137, 1961.

Pierce GB: Ultrastructure of human testicular tumors. Cancer 19:1963-1983, 1966.

Pierce GB, WK Bullock and RW Huntington Jr: Yolk sac tumors of the testis. Cancer 25:644-658, 1970.

Pierce GB and FJ Dixon Jr: Testicular teratomas. I. Demonstration of teratogenesis by metamorphosis of multipotential cells. Cancer 12:573-583, 1959.

Pierce GB, FJ Dixon and EL Verney: Teratocarcinogenic and tissue-forming potentials of the cell types comprising neoplastic embryoid bodies. Lab Invest 9:583-602, 1960.

Pierce Jr GB and AR Midgley Jr: The origin and function of human syncytiotrophoblastic giant cells. Amer J Pathol 43:153-173, 1963.

Pitts N: Clinical data accumulated by Pfizer for NDA for Mithramycin in: Proc of Chemother Conf on Mithramycin. Carter SA and M Friedman (eds), Bethesda, Maryland. National Cancer Institute of the National Institute of Health, 1970, pp. 33-34.

Podis AD: Malignant testis tumors of infancy. Southern Med J 59:1415-1419, 1966.

Pohl DR, DE Johnson and JR Robison: Bilateral testicular rupture: report of a case. J Urol 99:772-773, 1968.

Pomer FA, RE Stiles and JH Graham: Interstitial cell tumors of the testis in children. New Eng J Med 250:233-237, 1954.
Pomerantz M: Lymphiography. Surg Clin N Amer 49:1415-1423, 1969.
Pomerantz M and WS Kise: Lymphangiography: its use in the diagnosis and treatment of urologic disorders. J Urol 91:190-195, 1964.
Price Jr EB and FK Mostofi: Secondary carcinoma of the testis. Cancer 10: 592-595, 1957.
Price Jr EB: Papillary cystadenoma of the epididymis: A clinicopathologic analysis of 20 cases. Arch Path 91:456-470, 1971.
Prosser TM: Tumours of the testis. J Roy Coll Surg Edinburgh 9:85-106, 1964.
Prym P: Spontanheilung lines bosartigen, wahrscheinlich chorionephiteliomatosen gewachs imhoden. Virchows Arch 265:239-258, 1927.
Pugh RC: Tumours of the testis - some pathological considerations. Brit J Urol 34:393-406, 1962.
Pugh RCB and JP Smith: Teratoma. Brit J Urol 36:28-44 (suppl), 1964.
Raines SL and TG Hurdle: Tumors of the testis. J Urol 73:363-372, 1955.
Ram MD and JJ Burn: Solitary malignant lymphoma of the testis. Brit J Surg 56:80-82, 1969.
Ramkissoon RA, NO Chamberlain, EL Baker and ER Jennings: Diagnostic significance of urinary lactic acid dehydrogenase. J Urol 91:603-605, 1964.
Rappaport H: Tumors of the hematopoietic system. Armed Forces Inst of Pathol, Washington, D. C., 1966, p. 99.
Rasmussen KE: Retinal and cerebral fat emboli following lymphography with oily contrast media. Acta Radiol 10:199, 1970.
Rather LV, WR Gardiner and JB Frerichs: Regression and maturation of primary testicular tumors with progressive growth of metastases: a report of 6 new cases and a review of the literature. Stanford Med Bull 12:12-24, 1954.
Raven RW: Tumours of the testis in two brothers. Lancet 2:870-871, 1934.
Ravich L, PH Lerman, JW Drabkin and J Noya: Embryonal carcinoma of testicle in childhood; review of literature and presentation of two cases. J Urol 96:501-507, 1966.
Ray B, AG Huvos and WF Whitmore Jr: Unusual malignant tumors of the scrotum: review of 5 cases. J Urol 108:760-766, 1972.
Reddy DB and I Ranganayakamma: Review of 56 cases of testicular tumours. Indian J Cancer 3:255-271, 1966.
Rees GM and WP Cleland: Surgical treatment of pulmonary metastases from testicular tumours. Brit Med J 3:467-470, 1971.
Reichert FL: The regeneration of the lymphatics. Arch Surg 13:871, 1926.
Reinhard RE and ARW Climie: Testicular tumors - the Harper Hospital experience, 1947-1959. Harper's Hospital Bull., Detroit, Michigan, 18: 302-304, 1960.
Remzi D: Tumors of the tunica vaginalis. South Med J 66:841-842, 1973.
Resnick MI, DJ Walvoord and GJ Bulkley: Testicular tumor presenting as inferior vena caval thrombosis. J Urol 109:656-658, 1973.
Rezek P and HC Hardin Jr: Bilateral interstitial-cell tumor of the testicle: report of one case observed fourteen years. J Urol 74:628-635, 1955.
Richards G and AM Neville: Steroid metabolism in vitro by an interstitial cell tumour and the attached prepubertal testis. J Endocr 59:637-649, 1973.
Roberts JB: Excision of the lumbar lymphatic nodes and spermatic vein in malignant disease of the testicle. Ann Surg 36:539-549, 1902.
Robson CJ, AW Bruce and J Charbonneau: Testicular tumors: a collective review from the Canadian Academy of Urological Surgeons. J Urol 94:440-444, 1965.

Roque MP and HW Goldberg: Metastatic carcinoma of the prostate. Unusual sites. Chicago Med Sch Quart 27:42-45, 1967.

Rosas-Uribe A, MA Luna and GA Guinn: Paratesticular rhabdomyosarcoma. Am J Surg 120:787-791, 1970.

Rose TF: Unusual early symptomatology of primary malignant testicular neoplasms. Med J Austral 1:164-166, 1960.

Ross MM and JW Morrow: Yolk sac carcinoma of the testis. J Urol 108:109-111, 1972.

Rosvoll RV and JR Woodart: Malignant Sertoli-cell tumor of the testis. Cancer 22:8-13, 1968.

Roswit B, J Sorrentino and R Yalow: The use of radio-active phosphorus (p^{32}) in the diagnosis of testicular tumors: a preliminary report. J Urol 63:724-728, 1950.

Rouviere H: Anatomy of the Human Lymphatic System. (Translated by MJ Tobias), Edwards Bros., Ann Arbor, Mich., 1938.

Rusche C: Clinical data on 131 cases. J Urol 68:340-353, 1952.

Rusche C: Twelve cases of testicular tumors occurring during infancy and childhood. J Pediatr 40:192-199, 1952.

Rusznìak I, M Foldi and G Szabo: Lymphatics and Lymph Circulation. Pergamon Press, Inc., Long Island City, N. Y., 1960.

Rutledge F, GD Dodd Jr and FB Kasilag Jr: Lymphocysts: a complication of radical pelvic surgery. Amer J Obstet & Gynec 77:1165-1175, 1959.

Ruttiman A (ed): Progress in Lymphology - Proceedings of the International Symposium on Lymphology, Zurich, July 19-23, 1966. Georg-Thieme, Verlag, Stuttgart, Germany, 1967.

Ruttiman A and MD Del Buono: Schenz de Lymphographie. Georg-Thieme, Stuttgart, Germany, 1964.

Sacchi E: Di un caso di giantismo infantile (psdomacrosomia) con tumore del testicolo. Riv sper di freniat 21:149-161, 1895.

Saint Donat, Quoted by Melicow MM: Classification of tumors of testis. J Int Coll Surg 25:187-201, 1956.

Salm R and SR Adlington: Seminoma in identical twins. Brit Med J 2:962-965, 1962.

Samuels ML and CD Howe: Vinblastine in the management of testicular cancer. Cancer 25:1009-1017, 1970.

Sandeman TF: Testicular tumours. J Coll Radiol Aust 8:134-151, 1964.

Santos RT: Testicular tumors. Phillipine J Surg & Surg Spec 18:101-105, 1963.

Sayegh E, T Brooks, E Sacher and F Busch: Lymphangiography of the retroperitoneal lymph nodes through the inguinal route. J Urol 95:102-107, 1966.

Schaffer B, R Burton, J Gould et al.: Urologic applications of lymphangiography. J Urol 87:91-96, 1962.

Schaffer B, PR Koehler, CR Daniel et al.: A critical evaluation of lymphangiography. Radiology 80:917-930, 1963.

Schantz A, W Sewall and B Castleman: Mediastinal germinoma. Cancer 30: 1189-1194, 1972.

Schiff BL: Tumors of testis with cutaneous metastases to scalp. Arch Derm 71:465-467, 1955.

Schmidt JD: Significance of total urinary lactic dehydrogenase activity in urinary tract diseases. J Urol 96:950-970, 1966.

Schmitz WH: Diagnosis and management of intrascrotal masses. J Omaha Mid-West Clin Soc 14:71-77, 1953.

Schoonees R and CB Stell: A case of interstitial-cell tumour of the testis presenting with acute epididymo-orchitis. South African Med J 42:53-54, 1968.

Schrek R: Racial distribution of cancer; tumors of kidney, bladder, and male genital organs. Ann Surg 120:809-812, 1944.

Schwartz JW and N Mallis: Teratoma testis: report of 100 consecutive cases. J Urol 72:404-410, 1954.
Schwartz JW and JF Reed Jr: The pathology of cryptorchidism. J Urol 76:429-435, 1956.
Scully RE: Spermatocytic seminoma of testis. Cancer 14:788-794, 1961.
Scully RE: Gonadoblastoma: a review of 74 cases. Cancer 25:1340-1356, 1970.
Scully RE and AR Parham: Testicular tumors: Interstitial cell and miscellaneous neoplasms. Arch Pathol 46:229-242, 1948.
Seddon JA: Acute epididymo-orchitis and teratoma of testis. Brit Med J 1: 1885-1886, 1962.
Selvaggi FP, RT Young, R Brown and AL Dick: Interstitial cell tumor of the testis in adults: two case reports. J Urol 109:436-439, 1973.
Semans JH: Carcinoma of prostate with metastasis in testis. J Urol 40:524-529, 1938.
Servelle M: Pathology of the thoracic duct. J Cardiac Surg 4:704, 1963.
Servelle M and M Deysson: Reflex of the intestinal chyle in the lymphatics of the leg. Ann Surg 133:234, 1951.
Shambron E and N Zheutlin: Radiographic studies of the lymphatic system. Arch Int Med 104:589-593, 1959.
Sharma KC, JF Gaeta, ID Bross, RH Moore and GP Murphy: Testicular tumors. NY State J Med 72:2421-2425, 1972.
Shepherd RTH: Germ cell tumours of the testis. Clin Radiol 17:280-288, 1966.
Shivde AV and RV Junnarkar: Primary lymphosarcoma of testis. Report of a case. J Urol 103:762, 1970.
Shively JA: Assay of gonadotropins in the diagnosis of neoplasms. U. S. Armed Forces Med J 1:505-513, 1950.
Short M and JI Coe: Malignant interstitial-cell tumor of the testis: a case report. J Urol 89:851-855, 1963.
Sickles EA, RE Belliveau and PH Wiernik: Primary mediastinal choriocarcinoma in the male. Cancer 33:1196-1203, 1974.
Silber SJ, S Cittan and G Friedlander: Testicular neoplasm in father and son. J Urol 108:889, 1972.
Silverberg SG, JW Thompson, G Higashi and AM Baskin: Malignant interstitial-cell tumor of the testis. Case report and review. J Urol 96:356-363, 1966.
Silva-Duarte CA, ML Cristina and J Roza de Oliveira: Extragonadal embryonal carcinomas. Path Europ 8:187-191, 1973.
Silvert D: Embryonal carcinoma of testis in infants and children. Report of two cases. J Urol 78:269, 1957.
Simson LR, I Lampe and MR Abell: Suprasellar germinomas. Cancer 22:533-544, 1968.
Skakkebaek NE: Possible carcinoma-in-situ of the testis. Lancet 2:516-517, 1972.
Skinner DG and WF Leadbetter: The surgical management of testis tumor. J Urol 106:84-93, 1971.
Smart WR and RF Escamilla: Simultaneous bilateral testicular seminomas: report of a case after a 10-year follow-up period with discussion of substitution androgen therapy. J Urol 86:614-619, 1961.
Smith AM and KT Riese: Infarction of the testis in the newborn: report of two cases and review of the literature with regard to differential from testicular tumor. Conn State Med J 22:180-183, 1958.
Smith JB: Alpha-fetoprotein: occurrence in certain malignant diseases and review of clinical applications. Med Clin N Am 54:797-803, 1970.
Smith JB and RT O'Neill: Alpha-fetoprotein - occurrence in germinal cell and liver malignancies. Am J Med 51:767-771, 1971.

Smithers DW and ENK Wallace: Radiotherapy in the treatment of patients with seminomas and teratomas of the testicle. Brit J Urol 34:422-435, 1962.
Smithers D: The treatment of patients with seminomas and teratomas of the testis. J Roy Coll Surg, Edinburgh 17:133-147, 1972.
Sohval AR: Histopathology of cryptorchidism. Am J Med 16:346-362, 1954.
Sohval AR: Testicular dysgenesis in relation to neoplasm of the testicle. J Urol 75:285-291, 1956.
Sohval AR: Testicular dysgenesis as an etiologic factor in cryptorchidism. J Urol 72:693-702, 1954.
Spark RP: Leiomyoma of epididymis. Arch Path 93:18-21, 1972.
Spjut HJ and JD Thorpe: Granulomatous orchitis. Amer J Clin Pathol 26:136-145, 1956.
Spratt JS and PF Yuen: Retroperitoneal lymph node dissection and resection of pulmonary metastases for testicular cancers. Case reports. Missouri Med 63:981-985, 1966.
Staubitz WJ, TC Jewett Jr, IV Magoss, GS Worthington and S Phalakornkule: Management of testicular tumors in children. J Urol 94:683-686, 1965.
Staubitz WJ, IV Magoss, JT Grace and WG Schenk III: Surgical management of testis tumors. J Urol 101:350-355, 1969.
Staubitz WJ, IV Magoss, OJ Oberkircher, MH Lent, FD Mitchell and WT Murphy: Management of testicular tumor. JAMA 166:751-758, 1958.
Staubitz WJ, OJ Oberkircher and MS Brick: Precocious puberty in case of bilateral interstitial cell tumor. J Urol 69:562-570, 1953.
Stephens RA: Clinical presentation of testicular tumours. Brit J Urol 34:448-453, 1962.
Sterns DB and SK Gordon: Visualization of testicular lymphatics in the dog: clinical application: preliminary study. J Urol 84:347-356, 1960.
Stevens LC: Embryology of testicular teratomas in strain 129 mice. J Nat Cancer Inst 23:1249-1295, 1959.
Stevens LC: Origin of testicular teratomas from primordial germ cells in mice. J Nat Cancer Inst 38:549-552, 1967.
Stevens LC: Experimental production of testicular teratomas in mice. Proc Natl Acad Sci US 52:654-661, 1964.
Stevens LC: The biology of teratomas including evidence indicating their origin from primordial germ cells. Annee Biol 1:585-610, 1962.
Stewart JR and MA Bagshaw: Malignant testicular tumors appearing simultaneously in identical twins. Cancer 18:895-898, 1965.
Sugarbaker ED and LF Craver: Lymphosarcoma: a study of 196 cases with biopsy. JAMA 115:17-23, 1940.
Sulak MH: Classification of different pathologic types. JAMA 213:91-93, 1970.
Sum PW, B Roswit and SM Unger: Skeletal metastases from malignant testicular tumors. Amer J Roentgen 83:704-708, 1960.
Sumner WA: Malignant tumor of testis occurring 29 years after orchiopexy: case report and review of the literature. J Urol 81:150-152, 1959.
Suzuki H, K Nagia, H Yamaki, N Tanaka and H Umezawa: On the mechanism of action of Bleomycin: scission of DNA in vitro and in vivo. J Antib Tokyo Ser A 22:446-448, 1969.
Swanson GE: Lymphangiography in chyluria. Radiology 81:473, 1963.
Symington T and N Wallace: Hormone investigations in cases of testicular tumour. Brit J Urol 36:103-106 (suppl) 1964.
Szymanowski (1868), Quoted by Johnson DE, DM Woodhead, DR Pohl and JR Robison: Cryptorchism and testicular tumorigenesis. Surgery 63:919-922, 1968.
Talerman A: Malignant sertoli cell tumor of the testis. Cancer 28:446-455, 1971.

Talerman A and WG Haije: Alpha-fetoprotein and germ cell tumors: a possible role of yolk sac tumor in production of alpha-fetoprotein. Cancer 34:1722-1726, 1974.

Talerman A, JGAH Kaalen and W Fokkens: Rural preponderance of testicular neoplasms. Brit J Cancer 29:176-178, 1974.

Tananbaum B, RS Sanford, A Elquezabal and ME Klinger: Testicular tumor: presenting sign of lymphoma. Cancer 29:1223-1229, 1972.

Tarvares A: Puberdade precoce e ginecomastia por tumor de celulos intersticiais do testiculo. Acta Gynaec et Obstet hips lusit 2:321, 1952.

Tatarinov YS: Content of embryo specific alpha one protein in fetal and neonatal sera and sera from adult humans with primary carcinoma of the liver. Fed Proc Trans (suppl) pt 2(25):T344, 1966.

Teilum G: Classification of testicular and ovarian androblastoma and Sertoli-cell tumors; a survey of comparative studies with consideration of histogenesis, endocrinology and embryological theories. Cancer 11:769-782, 1958.

Teilum G: Endodermal sinus tumors of ovary and testis: comparative morphogenesis of so-called mesonephroma ovarie (Schiller) and extraembryonic structure of rat placenta. Cancer 12:1092-1105, 1959.

Templeton AC: Testicular neoplasms in Ugandan Africans. Afr J Med Sci 3: 157-161, 1972.

Teoh TB, JK Stewart and RA Willis: The distinctive adenocarcinoma of the infant's testis; an account of 15 cases. J Path Bact 80:147-156, 1960.

Teter J: An unusual gonadal tumour (gonadoblastoma) in a male pseudohermaphrodite with testicular dysgenesis. J Obstet Gynaec Brit Comm 97:238-242, 1960.

Tetoni E, A Bologna and VN Calavita: Diagnostica linfografica. Minerva Chir 22:785-796, 1967.

Thackray AC: Seminoma. Brit J Urol 36:12-27 (suppl), 1964.

Thomas GJ and AJ Bischoff: Tumors of the testis: analysis of 80 cases. J Urol 72:411-423, 1954.

Thomas TV: Surgical implications of retroaortic left renal vein. Arch Surg 100: 738-740, 1970.

Thomford NR, LB Wolner and OT Clagett: The surgical treatment of metastatic tumors in the lungs. J Thorac & Cardiovasc Surg 49:357-363, 1965.

Thompson HT: The clinical prognosis in testicular tumors: an analysis of 48 cases. J Urol 69:299-306, 1953.

Thompson IM: Lymphadenectomy for testicular tumor. Arch Surg 83:746-748, 1961.

Thompson IM, J Wear Jr, C Almond, FJ Schewe and J Sala: An analytical survey of one-hundred and seventy-eight testicular tumors. J Urol 85:173-179, 1961.

Thompson JR: Infantile teratoma testis - report of one case and review of the literature. Brit J Surg 42:437-439, 1955.

Thompson HT and AM Goldstein: Resection in the treatment of pulmonary metastases from testicular tumours and its influence on the overall survival rate. Brit J Surg 56:349-351, 1969.

Threefoot SA, WT Kent and BF Hatchett: Lymphatico-venous and lymphatico-lymphatic communications demonstrated by plastic corrosion models of rats and by post-mortem lymphangiography in man. J Lab Med 61:9-22, 1963.

Thurzo R and J Pinter: Cryptorchism and malignancy in men and animals. Urol Int 11:216-231, 1961.

Tobin CE: The renal fascia and its relation to the transversalis fascia. Anat Rec 89:295-311, 1944.

Tong EC: Improved technique of lymphatic cannulation for lymphography. Experience with 300 cases. Amer J Roentgen 107:877-880, 1969.

Treves N: Gynecomastia. Cancer 11:1083-1102, 1958.

Tsuji I, F Nakajima, T Nishida, Y Nakanoya and K Inoue: Testicular tumors in children. J Urol 110:127-129, 1973.

Tulinius H, N Day and CS Muir: Rarity of testis cancer in negroes. Lancet 1: 35-36, 1973.

Twidwell JE and GL Garske: Testicular tumor: metastatic from hypernephroma. Proc N Cent Sect Amer Urol Ass 164:173, 1955.

Ujiki GT, WN Brandand PH O'Brein: Effect of lymphangiography on metastasis. Radiology 91:877-880, 1968.

Ulm AH and JW Draper: Bilateral primary tumors of testis: a report of four cases. J Urol 86:421-427.

Ulrich H: Multiple myeloma. Arch Intern Med 64:994-1016, 1939.

Umezawa H, Y Suhara, T Takita and K Maeda: Purification of Bleomycins. J Antib Ser A 19:210-215, 1966.

Umezawa H, K Maeda, T Takeuechi and Y Okami: New antibiotics, Bleomycin A&B. J Antibiotics Ser A 19:200-209, 1966.

Umezawa H: Natural and artificial Bleomycins: chemistry and antitumor activities. Pure and Appl Chem 28:665-680, 1971.

Umezawa H, T Takeuechi, S Hori, T Sawa and M Ishizuki: Studies on the mechanism of antitumor effect of Bleomycin on squamous cell carcinoma. J Antib 25:409-420, 1972.

Umiker WO: Interstitial cell hyperplasia in association with testicular tumors: a study of its relationship to urinary gonadotropins, testicular atrophy and histological type of tumor. J Urol 72:895-903, 1954.

Utz DC and MK Buscemi: Extragonadal testicular tumors. J Urol 105:271-274, 1971.

Valeyeva ZT: Some reflexes in the lymphatic system. Sechenov Physiol J USSR 47 No. 3, 1961.

Vallega L and F Magrassi: Su di un caso di seminoma bilaterale del testicolo in criptorchide. Contributo clinico. Osped Ital chir 15:135-142, 1966.

Van Welkenhuyzen P and J Henry: Etude de 175 cas de cancer du testicule traites au centre des tumeurs de Bruxelles de 1925 a 1963. XIIIe Congres Societe Internat d'Urol 2:44-51, 1965.

Varney DC: Lymphosarcoma of testis. J Urol 73:1081-1088, 1955.

Vechinski TO, WH Jaeschke and H Vermund: Testicular tumors. An analysis of 112 consecutive cases. Amer J Roentgen 95:494-514, 1965.

Viamonte M, D Altman, R Parks, E Blum, M Bevilacqua and L Recher: Radiographic-pathologic correlation in the interpretation of lymphangioadenograms. Radiology 80:903-916, 1963.

Villani U: Concordant tumors of the testicles in monozygotic twins. Urol Int 22: 353-365, 1967.

Waddell RW: Testicular lymphoblastomas in children: report of a case and review of the literature. J Urol 85:956-959, 1961.

Wahlqvist L, L Hulten and M Rosencrantz: Normal lymphatic drainage of the testis studied by funicular lymphography. Acta Chir Scand 132:454-465, 1966.

Wakeley C: A case of benign teratoma of the testicle in an infant. Brit J Surg 26:443-444, 1938.

Wallace S: Dynamics of normal and abnormal lymphatic systems as studied with contrast media. Cancer Chemother Rep 52:31-58, 1968.

Wallace S: Lymphatico-venous anastomoses: clinical significance. Progress in Lymphology II, Georg-Thieme Verlag, Stuttgart, 1970, pp. 87-91.

Wallace S: The paralymphatic system. Progress in Lymphology II. Georg-Thieme Verlag, Stuttgart, 1970, p. 42.

Wallace S and L Jackson: Diagnostic criteria for lymphangiographic interpretation of malignant neoplasia. Cancer Chemother Rep 52:125-145, 1968.

Wallace S, L Jackson, G Schaffer, J Gould, RR Greening, A Weiss and S Kramer: Lymphangiograms: their diagnostic and therapeutic potential. Radiology 76:179-199, 1961.

Wallace S and BS Jing: Lymphangiography: diagnosis of nodal metastases from testicular malignancies. JAMA 213:94-96, 1970.

Walter DC, G Bras and SEH Brooks: The incidence of malignant neoplasms in Jamaica, West Indies. Acta Un Int Cancer 20:595-598, 1964.

Walton AJ: Testicular tumours. Med Illus 8:322-325, 1954.

Ward JA, S Krantz, J Mendeloff and E Haltiwanger: Interstitial-cell tumor of the testis: report of two cases. J Clin Endocr 20:1622-1632, 1960.

Warren S and KW Olshausen: Interstitial cell growths of testicle. Amer J Pathol 19:307-331, 1943.

Watson EM, HR Sauer and MG Sadugor: Manifestations of the lymphoblastomas in the genito-urinary tract. J Urol 61:626-641, 1949.

Weitzner S: Adenocarcinoma of infantile testis. Amer J Dis Child 108:662-666, 1964.

Weitzner S: Metastatic plasma cell myeloma in testis. Rocky Mountain Med J 66:48-50, 1969.

Weitzner S: Survival of patients with secondary carcinoma of prostate in the testis. Cancer 32:447-449, 1973.

Weller CU: Unusual cardiac and cerebral metastases in melanosarcoma. J Cancer Res 7:313-327, 1922.

Wershub LP: The human testis: a clinical treatise. Charles C Thomas, Springfield, Ill., 1962.

Westcott JW: Reticulum cell sarcoma with primary manifestation in the testis. J Urol 96:243-246, 1966.

Whitmore WF: Some experiences with retroperitoneal lymph node dissection and chemotherapy in the management of testis neoplasms. Brit J Urol 34: 436-447, 1962.

Whittle RJM: Tumours of the testicle. Brit J Radiol 30:7-12, 1957.

Wiljasalo M: Lymphographic differential diagnosis of neoplastic diseases. Acta Radiol 247:11-143 (suppl), 1965.

Wiljasalo M: Lymphographic polymorphism in Hodgkin's disease. Acta Radiol 289:1-89 (suppl), 1969.

Williams Jr DC: Testicular tumors. J Med Ass Georgia 44:177-179, 1955.

Willis RA: An experimental study of possible influence of injury in the genesis of tumours of the gonads. Brit J Exp Path 15:234-236, 1934.

Willis RA: Borderland of embryology and pathology, 2nd ed., Butterworth Inc., Washington, D. C., 1962, 641 pp.

Wilson JM and DM Woodhead: Prognostic and therapeutic implications of urinary gonadotropin levels in the management of testicular neoplasia. J Urol 108:754-756, 1972.

Wilson W: Chemotherapy of human solid tumors with 5-fluorouracil. Cancer 13: 1230-1239, 1960.

Witschi E: Migration of the germ cells of human embryos from the yolk sac to the primitive gonadal folds. Contrib Embryol Carnegie Inst #209:67-80, 1948.

Witus WS, JH Sloss and WL Valk: Inguinal node metastasis from testicular tumours developing after orchiopexy. J Urol 81:669-671, 1959.

Wolf H and PO Madsen: Metastases to the external genitalia from carcinoma of the prostate: a report of two cases. J Urol 99:198-202, 1968.

Wolfel DA: Lymphatico-venous communications. Amer J Roentgen 88:766-768, 1965.

Woodhead DM, DE Johnson, DR Pohl and JR Robison: Aggressive management of advanced testicular malignancy: experience with 147 patients. Milt Med 136:634-638, 1971.

Wright DG: Gynecomastia caused by testicular tumors. Proc Roy Soc Med 60: 479, 1967.

Wyatt J and L McAninch: A chemotherapeutic approach to advanced testicular cancer. Canad J Surg 10:421-426, 1967.

Yoffey JM and FC Courtice: Lymphatics, lymph and the lymphomyeloid complex. Academic Press, Inc., London, 1970.

Young JA and AW Bohne: Seminoma in non-twin brothers. J Urol 107:1000-1001, 1972.

Young PG, BM Mount, FW Foote Jr and WF Whitmore Jr: Embryonal adenocarcinoma in the prepubertal testis: a clinicopathologic study of 18 cases. Cancer 26:1065-1075, 1970.

Yuval, EA Eidelman, SI Beer and E Vure: Local excision of a virilising Leydig-cell tumour of the testis. Brit J Urol 46:237-240, 1974.

Zeidman I, BE Copeland and S Warren: Experimental studies on spread of cancer in lymphatic system. Absence of lymphatic supply in carcinoma. Cancer 8:123-127, 1955.

Zondag HA: Enzyme activity in dysgerminoma and seminoma: a study of lactic dehydrogenase isoenzymes in malignant diseases. Rhode Island Med J 47: 273-281, 1964.

Zondek B: Gonadotropic hormone in the diagnosis of chorioepithelioma. JAMA 108:607-611, 1937.

INDEX